Nursing a Radical Imagination

Examining the historical context of healthcare while focusing on building a more just, equitable world, this book proposes a radical imagination for nursing and presents possibilities for speculative futures embracing queer, feminist, posthuman, and abolitionist frames.

Bringing together radical and emancipatory perspectives from an international selection of authors, this book reflects on the realities created by the COVID-19 pandemic, recognizing that our situation is not new but the result of ongoing hegemonies and injustices. The authors attend to the history of nursing and related institutions, examining the assumptions, ideologies, and discourses that shape the discipline and its place within healthcare. They explore the impact of this context on contemporary nursing and look at alternative visions for the future. The final section specifically focuses on ways that we can move forward.

Envisioning new possibilities for nursing, this innovative volume is a vital resource for practitioners, scholars, and students keen to promote social justice within and without nursing. It is an important contribution to nursing theory, philosophy, and history.

Jess Dillard-Wright is an Assistant Professor at the University of Massachusetts Amherst Elaine Marie College of Nursing. She/they is also the 21–22 University of California Irvine Center for Nursing Philosophy Fellow.

Jane Hopkins-Walsh is a primary care pediatric nurse practitioner at Boston Children's Hospital, USA, and a PhD candidate at Boston College Connell School of Nursing.

Brandon Brown is a bedside nurse, teacher, clinical assistant professor, and doctor of education student at the University of Vermont in Burlington, USA.

Routledge Research in Nursing and Midwifery

For more information about this series, please visit: https://www.routledge.com/Routledge-Research-in-Nursing/book-series/RRIN

Nursing a Radical Imagination

Moving from Theory and History to Action and Alternate Futures

©2023

Jess Dillard-Wright,
Jane Hopkins-Walsh, and
Brandon Brown

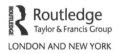

Routledge
Taylor & Francis Group

LONDON AND NEW YORK

First published 2023
by Routledge
4 Park Square, Milton Park, Abingdon, Oxon OX14 4RN

and by Routledge
605 Third Avenue, New York, NY 10158

Routledge is an imprint of the Taylor & Francis Group, an informa business

British Library Cataloguing-in-Publication Data
A catalogue record for this book is available from the British Library

ISBN: 978-1-032-15853-2 (hbk)
ISBN: 978-1-032-37313-3 (pbk)
ISBN: 978-1-003-24595-7 (ebk)

DOI: 10.4324/9781003245957

Typeset in Goudy
by MPS Limited, Dehradun

Contents

Figures

Tables

Boxes

Contributors

Blythe Bell is a PhD candidate at the University of Victoria.

Candace Burton PhD, RN, AFN-BC, FNAP is a qualitative and mixed methodology researcher whose scholarship examines stress, trauma, gender, and health inequities in nursing science and practice. She is an Associate Professor at the University of California Irvine.

Emmanuel Christian Tedjasukmana is a Staff Nurse at the University of Vermont Medical Center.

Ruth De Souza is a Vice-Chancellor's Research Fellow at RMIT University in Melbourne, Australia.

Thomas Foth is an Associate Professor at the University of Ottawa.

Cory Ellen Gatrall is a PhD candidate with the Elaine Marieb College of Nursing at the University of Massachusetts Amherst.

DaJanae Gresham-Ryder is a Clinical Nurse II at the UC Davis Medical Center.

Dave Holmes, RN, PhD, FAAN, FCAN is a Professor and University Research Chair with the School of Nursing at the University of Ottawa(Canada). He conducts critical qualitative research in the fields of forensic nursing and public health.

Danisha Jenkins, PhD, RN is a Nurse Leader and Researcher at the University of California, Irvine, whose scholarship focuses on institutions and biopolitics, particularly at the intersection of nursing and law enforcement.

Venika Marwaha has several years of direct patient care experience as in the acute and community health setting with her most recent being in project management and production scheduling in the biotech industry.

Jon McIntyre is a PhD candidate at the University of California, Irvine School of Nursing with research interests in power, control, and resistance in nursing.

Patrick McMurray is a Nurse Specialistat the University of North Carolina Medical Center, and is a PhD in Nursing Student at Virginia Commonwealth Univesity.

Evy Nazon is an Associate Professor at the Université du Québec en Outaouais.

Amélie Perron is a Full Professor with the School of Nursing at the University of Ottawa.

Em Rabelais is an Interdependent Scholar.

Jamie B. Smith is a Research Associate at the Institute for Clinical Nursing Science, Charité Universitätsmedizin, Berlin.

Claire Valderama-Wallace is an Assistant Professor at California State University East Bay.

Rachel (Rae) Walker is Associate Professor and PhD Program Director with the Elaine Marieb College of Nursing at the University of Massachusetts Amherst.

Eva Willis is a Research Associate at the Institute for Clinical Nursing Science, Charité Universitätsmedizin, Berlin.

Acknowledgments

We have so many folks to thank that it is hard to know where to begin. This is a collective act of love and resistance. We thank all of the authors who risked joining us in this wild adventure: Jamie, Ruth, Eva, Claire, DaJanae, Venika, Candace, Dave, Danisha, Jon, Thomas, Evy, Em, Rae, Patrick, Christian, Cory Ellen, Blythe, and Amélie. As educators and nurses and humans, we have all been shouldering the weight of the COVID-19 pandemic in ways diffracted and differentiated by virtue of our positionalities. We appreciate and acknowledge the commitment, the enormity of which was amplified in these pandemic times. We also wish to embrace those folks who joined us for segments of the adventure but who, for a variety of reasons, had to redirect their efforts: Chloe, Lucinda, Natalie, Odette, and Mick—we love and appreciate you, feeling your presence and solidarity as we bring this thing home.

We would like to thank Grace McInnes and Evie Lonsdale for their support in bringing this vision to life.

We can't let this go by without thanking our families, chosen and blood. We love you. We appreciate you. We couldn't do it without you.

Finally, we send gratitude to the universe of folks we know and we don't know, whose ideas and visions and dreams and joys and sorrows nourish this rhizome as we build toward collaborative liberation.

Introduction

Jess Dillard-Wright, Jane Hopkins-Walsh, and Brandon Brown

Imagination is generative, opening up possibilities for realities that are yet to manifest. In *Freedom Dreams*, historian of social movements Robin D. G. Kelley (2002) wrote "I inherited my mother's belief that the map to a new world is the imagination, in what we see in our third eyes rather than the desolation that surrounds us" (p. 3). Radical imagination, following the collective vision of radical scholar-activists Max Haiven and Alex Khasnebish (2014), is simply "the ability to imagine the world, life, and social institutions not as they are but as they might otherwise be. It is the courage and the intelligence to recognize that the world can and should be changed. The radical imagination is not just about dreaming of different futures. It's about bringing those possibilities back from the future to work on the present, to inspire action and new forms of solidarity today" (2014, p. 4). Learning from the past, imagining the future, building in the present.

Radical imagination is not a new idea, nor do we claim this concept as in any way proprietary. Here we note that, when we use "we" in this introduction, we are speaking of ourselves as editors. In thinking about imagination as generative possibility, we draw inspiration from a wide array of thinkers across space, time, and discipline. Folks like Arundhati Roy and Angela Davis have sparked critical fires in our collective thinking, which was further fueled by abolitionist Mariame Kaba, feminist educator bell hook, sociologist of medicine Ruha Benjamin, critical posthuman feminist Rosi Braidotti, and more. Our kernel of radical imagination seeks to center queer, feminist, Indigenist, abolitionist, dissident, and other otherwise marginal perspectives as we aim to upend white, cishteropatriachal, ableist, anthropocentric, capitalist, pernicious norms. Imaginations that do not not center these things are not and cannot be radical. We envision radical imagination as shared collective mutual relational experiences long existing outside of the academy and unbound from elitist ideas based on power and privilege.

Yet in speaking of the folks that inspire us, we know that for some, articulating dissident perspectives came—and comes—with the threat of incarceration and even death under systems of white supremacy, colonialism, and extractive relentless capitalism. We risk almost nothing. We enter this book project riding the ancestral waves of inherited power and unearned privilege

DOI: 10.4324/9781003245957-1

conferred on us as white nurses and scholars working and living in the United States (US). This privilege is accentuated by the systems of white supremacy that overdetermine the US healthcare (non)system and within the elite spaces of nursing academe around the world. These declarations are not excuses, recognizing the empty indulgence of settlers' move to innocence (Tuck & Yang, 2012). Rather, we recognize that these positionalities constitute the material realities in which we are ensconced. This means we must continually commit to confront, dismantle, and challenge white supremacy, including within ourselves, as we navigate the critically important work of imagining a more just nursing present-future. We have asked authors who contributed to this anthology to position themselves in relation to their scholarship as a starting point toward transparent anti-oppressive scholarship. To this end, in the following text, we position ourselves as editors further in relation to this book project.

Jess Dillard-Wright lives and works in Springfield, MA, the traditional home of the Algonkian people known as the Agawam and is an assistant professor in Elaine Marieb College of Nursing at the University of Massachusetts Amherst. Jess is a white, fat, queer, settler-colonizer, genderqueer, feminist, antiracist, abolitionist, nurse dissident, activist-scholar working to disrupt the violence of hegemonic whiteness, the pernicious influence of capitalism, and the constraints of cisheteropatriarchy in nursing and beyond. She/they relish the connections that spring forth from this collaboration and the learning, unlearning, relearning that has accompanied this rhizome.

Jane Hopkins-Walsh (she/her/hers) is a US-based, cisgender, heterosexual woman, nondisabled, white settler colonizer nurse who resides and works on the stolen land of the Massachusett people. Jane is a nurse-activist-artivist-scholar who strives to unlearn white supremacy while actively working toward an antiracist, anti-oppression, and anticolonial nursing present-future. She embraces art as a vehicle for making marks and meaning, and she embodies daily practices of protest and joy through music, movement, and playing with color and fiber.

Brandon Brown, MSN, RN-BC, CNL (he/him/his), is a bedside nurse, teacher, clinical assistant professor, and doctor of education candidate living on the unceded lands of the Abenaki People. Brandon is gay, cisgender, white, able-bodied, and a settler-colonizer, who benefits from white-male privilege, white supremacy, capitalism, and dispossessed Indigenous lands. He is a nurse-activist scholar, whose vision for nursing education includes creating equitable and just nursing futures for students and communities rooted in liberatory praxis and planetary-geo-centered care.

Our praxis is a work in progress as we collectively and individually strive to live and write and work in ways that actualize our values. While we do not pretend to have answers, resisting the temptation to embrace quick fixes, we commit to stay with trouble (Haraway, 2016). We hold onto a radical imagination for nursing alongside the authors who have come together in this collection. These commitments led us to co-create the anthology you are currently reading.

Anthology as Radical Imagination

It is our honor and privilege to present this collection of essays from an international group of nurses whose work inspires us daily. As editors, together we have nurtured our collective rhizome, establishing our collaborative ideas as nurse-scholar-activists via publications and presentations at numerous national and international conferences within the backdrop of the pandemic. Over the past several years, we embodied a process—a collective and situated praxis—that can be understood as *nursing* a radical imagination, as we nurtured near daily relational social practices via phone, text, and social media. Through this process, our friendship and ideas about critical scholarship unfolded. Together we have become kin, grown the rhizome, and further connected with a transnational and transcontinental network of like-minded scholars and activists who have agreed to be part of this exciting writing and thinking project. In conversation with other nurses across the globe, the editors and authors cultivate a sustained social media presence outside the hegemony of academia where we actively and collaboratively opine, rage, critique, connect, protest, promote, imagine, and advance our ideas for a radical and emancipatory future for nursing while living and dying on a dying planet. We believe that connectivity is foundational to the project of radical imagination in nursing and together we have imagined ways to connect around this book project.

Drawing upon aesthetic ways of knowing, we also envision arts as an integral part of this radical imagination project, understanding that creativity in forms of mark-making, visual arts, fiber arts, poetry, and music are ways to relationally make meaning unconstrained by the rules of the academy. We have created a website that helps to reflect this, Nursing Futurities located at https://nursingfuturities.org/. An ongoing work-in-progress, there we have linked to ongoing projects, work that inspires us, an interactive art project—the Drift Journal—and more. The Drift Journal will travel to the authors in the book for contributions of human and nonhuman mark making (pet, earth, mineral, water, all marks are invited) and to the hands and homes of other people and places yet to be known—we welcome your marks, too. See the website for how to contribute. The QR code in the "Epilogue is Prologue" that concludes our book will take you to additional resources including the webpage.

The Process of Nursing a Radical Imagination

We would like to share a bit about the process of how this project came to be. We began imagining this anthology through our readings, entangled daydreams, and impassioned yearning for that which is not yet manifest. We share a collective passion for nursing, problematic as it is. We approach our discipline with a critical lens that is based in justice and liberation for people and communities, decentering whiteness, ableism, transmisia, and undoing white supremacy. In envisioning this book, we strove to be inclusive and expansive in our invitations to authors to participate but recognize the book's limitations and shortcomings notably missing representative voices from authors from the global south, from developing nations, and missing authors with diverse identities from both inside and outside the academia. The pandemic time period created challenges for several invited authors, as did work restrictions for those involved in labor organizing, and other authors declined to participate for a variety of reasons. Ultimately we had to recognize the imperfection and messiness of what we could accomplish in organizing an anthology during pandemic times. We give thanks to our authors who endured despite challenges, together we all stumbled forward and we are very excited to share the collective works with readers.

The anthology includes chapters from influential nursing scholars whose work emanates from critical, radical, and emancipatory perspectives spanning three continents and five countries, including the US, Canada, Australia, United Kingdom (UK), and Germany. In addition to cultural and geographic range, many of the chapters are written by nurses from disparate backgrounds, people who are part of groups whose voices and bodies are and have been historically oppressed in and by nursing. The essays contained here are concerned with liberation, an intentional choice, as we sought to amplify diverse voices and de-center the voices of white cis-hetero-patriarchy; the dominant group within the nursing profession.

Our efforts are imperfect and partial: we acknowledge the overrepresentation of voices from the global north, countries with histories of colonization and genocide. We also understand that academic publishing in English marginalizes non–English-speaking people from interacting with this project, pushing us to further imagine multilingual collaborative future projects. In rejections of the neoliberal corporate structures around publishing and knowledge generation, we commit to redirecting any and all profits accumulated from the anthology to support open access publishing of this project. Any further funds will be used to support mutual aid endeavors selected by contributors.

Authors retained their unique voice, style, and language in their individual chapters. We chose not to standardize spelling of certain words; thus, the essays reflect the spelling variations in Canada, the UK, Australia, and the US. This was done to center the authors' situated materialities, while decentering languages and geopolitical boundaries.

Radical Imagination in the COVIDicene

The book before you is definitively a product of the pandemic. The seeds for this edited volume book were planted and grown over the past four years, composting and sprouting among the editors and authors as we try to imagine how to safely and effectively live, work, and nurse the people and communities we accompany, amidst COVID-19 inequities. We grapple with how to educate the next generation of nurses during a politically tumultuous time of rising global authoritarianism, persistent Trumpism, climate disaster, abortion rights restrictions, civil rights erosions, voting rights denials in the US, and around the world. In the background, the COVID-19 pandemic continues to kill people around the planet, yet in the US where the editors live and work, we navigate political misinformation around vaccines realizing that this insipid ableism and disinformation media machinery has far-reaching implications, including for nurses.

Nurses named this pandemic era the COVIDicene (Brown et al., 2021), marked by stark inequities, recognizing that these realities are not new but rather the result of ongoing oppression. The crucible of the COVID-19 pandemic amplifies preexisting injustice, exploiting the faults and fissures constructed through hundreds of years of racialized capitalist extraction, connections to past and present-day imperialism and colonialism throughout the globe. Despite the realities forged by the Covidence, we see potentiality in a radically alternate future. Envisioning radical possibility, we pay homage to Arundahati Roy (2020), whose early pandemic essay, *"The Pandemic is a Portal,"* captivated our collective imaginations, planting insistent seeds of hope back to which we continuously circle.

With *Nursing Futurities: Co-creating a Radical Imagination for Healthcare*, we present a collection of works that are relevant for folks working in nursing and healthcare including those we accompany in care, including each other. We hope these essays are thought-provoking for folks outside of the discipline of nursing. Care practices are embedded and embodied. We understand the givers of care and the recipients of care to be dynamic collaborators, interactive and relational in the work of care and caring. The need for critical perspectives and building a more just, equitable future for nursing, healthcare, communities, the world is at a fever pitch. At the same time, the global movemnent toward authoritarianism with hidden and insidious systems of technological surveillence is simultaneously making justice work difficult and even dangerous. Our thinking and writing practices are political acts and we see these as important nursing interventions connected to the work of nursing care.

A Roadmap

We divided the book into four sections representing essays with ideas based in history, critical present, radical future, and ending with thoughts about speculative paths forward to alternative futures. Our journey begins with attention to the past and the ways in which history shapes our present reality. In order to imagine other possibilities, we first attend to the history of nursing in *Section One titled Towards a Re/Visioned History for Nursing*. This section has three essays that examine the assumptions, ideologies, and discourses that shape the discipline and its place within healthcare more broadly including critiques of neoliberalism and whiteness, and unpacking disciplinary framings of culture and iconic myths tied to nursing's origin story. The authors in Part I employ a critical lens to understand how the past shapes our present, bringing to the forefront how the structures, institutions, systems, and ideas construct our reality.

In attending to histories—and here, please note the indefinite article and plurality implied by "histories"—of nursing, we find links to the present. Complicating our grasp of the past enables us to understand the present in more nuanced, attuned ways. This is not because the past gives us a roadmap to the present/future, as Mariame Kaba (2021) reminds us, but because critically reckoning with the past can enable us to see the present more clearly, confronting and understanding our histories as multiple, as fragmentary, as complex, as contested can lead us to ask better questions as we seek to understand the present and dream of the future.

From these critical nursing histories, our attention turns to Part II, A *Critical Understanding of the Present*, where authors concern themselves with untangling the snares and snarls of our nursing present, enclosed as it is in the crucible of the COVIDicene and the catastrophe of climate disaster and end-stage capitalism. Part II contains four essays that critically explore issues of nursing identity from the vantage point of self and society using philosophy, critical posthumanism, and analyses of politics, power, control, and planetary responsibility. The final makes the invisible visible by showing the impact of healthcare waste on the planet using mixed media visual art using non-biohazardous healthcare waste.

The viewpoint of the critical present brings us next to the third section in the book, titled A *Radical Imagination for Nursing*. This section contains three essays, one of which is divided into two parts. Each essay in this section critically unpacks issues of equity and justice, confronting white supremacy, embracing an antiracist stance to envision what is possible for nursing education and nursing care. The essays in this section connect to critical ideas around culture and safety in different nursing spaces including the academy, classroom, and healthcare system—spaces that are ever more dependent on technological systems like artificial intelligence and surveillance technology.

With this backdrop secured, in the final Part IV called *Getting There: Speculative Paths for the Present-Future*, authors turn to speculative, democratic, abolitionist, and posthuman visions for the future of nursing. The ideas presented in the four essays of this section represent collective voices speaking up and speaking out in nursing, talking about issues that are too often policed and ignored, even punished, representing a radical departure from the business as usual orientation of much nursing and health sciences scholarship.

Connecting the Tendrils of Ideas and Actions

As editors, we approach our nursing work nourishing the verdant tendrils of rhizomatic connection to critical theoretical and philosophical frameworks that include new materialism, post humanism, Black feminism, critical race theory, queer studies, abolition, anarchism, disability justice, reproductive justice, and anti-/de-/excolonialism to name a few. Threads of these theories and philosophies will be evident in many of the essays included here. We encourage readers to think about theory and philosophy as intertwined, not separate, and we hope that readers will consider using more critical approaches as a way to explain and imagine the important work of nursing. Even though the anthology is divided into four parts, readers will notice that each essay touches both the ones they are organized alongside as well as all the others in the anthology, consolidating ideas of rhizomatic thought, and illustrating how all things touch all things (Haraway, 2016). The result *is* anthology—a woven tapestry of critical thought, generative ideas, and radical imagination embroidering together, around, within and across chapters and sections. We hope you enjoy the journey.

References

Brown, B. B., Dillard-Wright, J., Hopkins-Walsh, J., Littzen, C. O., & Vo, T. (2022). Patterns of knowing and being in the COVIDicene: An epistemological and ontological reckoning for posthumans. *Advances in Nursing Science, 45*(1), 3.

Haraway, D. J. (2016). *Staying with the trouble: Making kin in the chthulucene.* Duke University Press.

Kaba, M. (2021). *We do this till we free us: Abolitionist organizing and transforming justice.* Haymarket Books.

Kelley, R. D. G. (2002). *Freedom dreams: The Black radical imagination.* Beacon Press.

Roy, A. (2020, April 3). *The pandemic is a portal.* https://www.ft.com/content/10d8f5e8-74eb-11ea-95fe-fcd274e920ca

Tuck, E., & Yang, K. W. (2012). Decolonization is not a metaphor. *Decolonization: Indigeneity, Education and Society, 1,* 1–40.

Part I

Towards a Re/Visioned History for Nursing

Taking feminist cyborg Donna Haraway's (2016) mantra "It matters what stories make worlds, what worlds make stories" (p. 12) to heart, this anthology opens with histories for nursing. Histories, plural. This is because history is not a singular narrative, settled, decided, and definitive. Instead, history is multiple, polyvocal, multirhythmic, and improvisational, following historian Elsa Barkley Brown's (1991, 1992) theorization. There is power and possibility in this sentiment, recognizing that history is neither -settled nor certain. History tells us about ourselves, both in the instructive nature of thinking about the "facts" of our past as well as in the metanarratives enforced by upholding disciplinary origin myths. None of the three chapters included here push the Nightingale narrative that all too often serves as shorthand for the entrenched history of professionalized nursing. Instead, they that ensue ask readers to consider what they think they know about nursing's history—as a practice, as a discipline, as an act of care—and interrogate the assumptions that construct this history.

This section on history begins with an essay by Thomas Foth and Evy Nazon entitled "Alleviating the suffering of Others: Nursing and humanitarian reason under Neoliberalism." This provocative paper traces the emergence of humanitarianism as a guiding moral sentiment in nursing. Foth and Nazon link moral sentiments to the fusion of Christan values and Enlightenment reason that crystallized in the 18th century. Moral humanitarian sentiment may be directed at people near or far facing abject conditions—those living unhoused or suffering in wartime, for example. And while the acts of care carried out toward the alleviation of the suffering in others may appear benevolent, it is always deeply political. Foth and Nazon implore nurses to consider their own political position, awakening to the ways in which nursing can be mobilized as cover, shielding more dubious political interventions. This, they argue, reflects the ways in which humanitarianism as a stop-gap for meeting basic needs functions as part of the neoliberal project that reinforces the governing discourses. Thus, Foth and Nazon conclude that nurses, in their humanitarian efforts, must attend to the dominant discourses structuring political interventions.

Chapter 2 is an essay that tangles history of nursing with feminist theory, interrogating the ways in which CASSANDRA Radical Feminist Nurses Network, a late 20th-century nursing collective, both resisted and reinforced the

DOI: 10.4324/9781003245957-2

norms imposed by the Victorian legacy of nursing. Jessica Dillard-Wright excavates the function of mythology, hagiography, and historiography in the development of nursing's disciplinary imagination using CASSANDRA as a starting place in "Finding CASSANDRA: Mythology, Hagiography, Historiography for Nursing." Cassandra, a mythical victim in Greek lore, cast into the wilderness, believed to be mad is the eponym for an essay written by Florence Nightingale in the lull between her nursing training and getting to put that training to work. Published in 1969 by Feminst Press under the title *Cassandra: Florence Nightingale's Angry Outcry Against the Forced Idleness of Victorian Women* during the women's liberation movement, this essay inspired the CASSANDRA the feminist collective. Putting nursing's historical narratives in conversation with more contemporary modes of feminist activism, "Finding CASSANDRA" invites readers to consider the ghosts of nursing's past and the ways these ghosts continue to animate nursing's present in order that we might imagine a different present/future.

In Chapter 3, "Madeleine Knows Best: Race and Culture in Nursing History" nurse historian Cory Ellen Gattrall attends to the construction of culture as a concept in nursing. Tracing how nursing understood racialized social difference, Gattrall puts nursing in conversation with the scientific milieu within which nursing was situated during the middle of the 20th century. She links this to the early 20th century beginnings of American public health nursing, considering the ways in which nursing took up questions of race, paralleling other eugenicist sciences of the day. Gattrall then examines the emergence of Transcultural Nursing, a subfield engineered by white nurse theorist Madeleine Leininger, predicated on her own claim that she single-handedly introduced "culture" as a concept to nursing. Reflecting on the legitimacy of this claim, Gatrall sketches the frameworks of culture used contemporaneously by Black and other nurse of color in the 1970s to center health equity. Ultimately, Gattrall arrives at the conclusion that the culture concept in nursing centered white comfort at the expense of antiracist nursing scholarship and praxis, shoring up white supremacy in nursing while alleging to attend to the cultural needs of diverse others.

In order to imagine other possibilities, we first attend to the history of nursing, examining the assumptions, ideologies, and discourses that shape the discipline and its place within healthcare. Recognizing the multiplicity of history creates possibility and repair (Scott, 2017): thinking about the material harms that have been done in the name of nursing and of nursing history gives rise to the possibility of healing those harms in the present/future. It asks that we disassemble the mythologies that feel good and give cover to reveal the complex, competing, and complicit cacophony that construct the history of the present. The chapters assembled here should not be construed as complete, comprehensive, categorical. Rather, these essays represent ideas that challenge nursing's hegemony in some way or another, asking readers to see things from another point of view, another perspective. This section is not without its limitations: the views presented are partial and fragmented, in their own ways failing to escape normative whiteness even as authors critique this impulse. In the end, we can see these histories as a start, not a map, to paraphrase prison abolitionist, educator, and transformative justice visionary Mariame Kaba (2021) suggests, but as a technique for thinking the present/future in different ways, if we choose.

References

Brown, E. B. (1991). Polyrhythms and improvisation: Lessons for women's history. *History Workshop*, *31*, 85–90.

Brown, E. B. (1992). "What has happened here:" The politics of difference in women's history and feminist politics. *Feminist Studies*, *18*(2), 295–312. 10.2307/3178230

Haraway, D. J. (2016). *Staying with the trouble: Making kin in the Chthulucene*. Duke University Press.

Kaba, M. (2021). *We do this till we free us: Abolitionist organizing and transforming justice*. Haymarket Books.

Scott, D. (2017). Preface: A reparatory history of the present. *Small Axe*, *52*, vii–x. 10.1215/07990537-3843914

1 Alleviating the Suffering of Others: Nursing and Humanitarian Reason under Neoliberalism

Thomas Foth and Evy Nazon

Since the mid-19th century, nurses have often been perceived as "heroes" and "angels of mercy" (Kalisch & Kalisch, 1983, p. 6). These kinds of labels are still used by politicians, the general public, and the mass media to describe the commitment of nurses to providing care and healing, despite often compromising their own personal safety (Stokes-Parish et al., 2020). Moral sentiments have emerged out of the combined effects of values like sensibility and altruism that can be understood as emotions inviting us, for example, to care for the poor and the needy in our societies. These sentiments have become an important part of current political discourses, legitimating political actions, particularly when they are directed at the helpless and the sick, whether they live in our local environment, like the drug user or homeless person, or live far away, like victims of famine, epidemics, or war. Philosopher Richard Rorty stated that scholars writing during the Scottish Enlightenment, particularly David Hume, saw a "fundamental moral capacity" as the foundation of reason (Rorty, 1993, p. 129). According to this perspective, the Enlightenment not only instilled a new sensitivity in suffering but also made us "feel called upon to relieve suffering, to put it to an end," which led to "certain standards of universal concern" (Taylor 1981, p. 394, as cited in, Asad, 2015, p. 390). We are moved not by deeper insights of rationality but by sad and sentimental stories. Moral sentiments become the source for (nursing) actions because one wants to correct the situation that provokes the misfortune of others (Asad, 2015; Fassin, 2010).

The history of nursing both in Canada and elsewhere in Western countries suggests that moral sentiments such as charity and humanitarianism have shaped nursing work into that of solidarity, goodness, and global healing (Lynch, 2004). Most recently, ideas of heroism and humanitarianism have been attributed to nurses in the battle against the COVID-19 pandemic (Mohammed et al., 2021). Despite the assumption that humanitarianism is assumed to be benevolent and good, it closely intersects with the history of Christian missionaries, states, and empires (see also Wynter, 2003). New forms of humanitarianism developed by organizations like Médecins Sans Frontières, as well as harm reduction NGOs that put nurses at the forefront in helping the drug user,

DOI: 10.4324/9781003245957-3

the homeless, or the poor, to name just a few, are used to manage populations considered superfluous that are produced through neoliberal politics.

In this paper, we argue that moral sentiments have become a central stake of current politics that help to legitimate political actions. First, we will summarize what could be called a genealogy of humanitarianism, outlining its roots in charitable activities. Then, we present an analysis of humanitarianism and liberalism, where we argue that: (a) humanitarianism and civil society have become an integral part of the "neoliberal project" and of the governing of our current societies, and (b) nurses in their humanitarian care support the neoliberal and biopolitics rationale. Thus, our goal in this article is to describe how the deployment of moral sentiments and humanitarianism in nursing is often used to serve the needs of political interventions.

Humanitarianism, Welfarism, and Liberalism

According to Asad (2015), the state is not only the guarantor of liberal democracy "but also [is] the basis of a wealthy civilization founded on capitalism in which general concern for human wellbeing can flourish" (Asad, 2015, p. 392). Indeed, what will be called "humanitarian reason" can be described as one of the social imaginaries of our times, occupying center stage in our current moral order and inscribed in our modernity. Historians like Thomas Laqueur and Lynn Hunt have described how the idea of humanity emerged in the late-18th century, a sentiment that linked the human and the humane, a characteristic related to compassion, sympathy, and ethics. Humanity from this perspective is the sensibility that emerges in this process, broadening the processes of inclusion and leading to a feeling of connectedness between humans. This development made humanity as an ethical sentiment possible (Hunt, 2007; Laqueur, 1983, 1989, 2009).

However, the emergence of humanitarianism was the result of a very specific historical constellation – the onset of capitalism and capitalist markets and new ways to write about "the Other" in a newly developing genre of novels and medical reports, particularly autopsy reports. This specific historical constellation was the precondition for humanitarian sentiments like sympathy, pity, or compassion toward a stranger to develop. Thus, the idea of the "human" as in humanitarianism or in human rights is a very recent invention. Compassion or sympathy with the unfortunate is symbolized in the Christian parable of the Good Samaritan, who was the only one who cared for a man left for dead in the street by thieves. It is the paradigm for the current politics of compassion and for Western morals even though it goes far beyond Christian doctrine and is still referenced in the present. Recent examples include the "Good Samaritan Drug Overdose Act" as part of the Canadian government's "comprehensive approach" to address overdoses (Government of Canada/Gouvernment du Canada, 2019) or the "Good Samaritan Order" protecting "frontline" healthcare workers responding to the COVID-19 outbreak in the American state of Arizona (GilBride, 2020).

The politics of compassion and the necessity of the state to provide social protection to the most vulnerable citizens in capitalist societies have been used as justification for liberal democracy (e.g., Brown, 2019). With the onset of the "precautionary state" at the end of the 19th century in France and Germany, social services that were up to then provided mostly by charitable, religious, and philanthropic organizations became the responsibility of the secular state, which systematically organized them in a multitude of institutions. As Ewald (1996) demonstrated in his analysis, with the introduction of insurance such as pension plans or workers compensation, the risk of industrial accidents was shifted from the individual employer and employee to society as a whole through the ccontributions of every citizen into these insurance schemes. The so-called welfare state of the 20th century implemented more and more administrative procedures and management to address the "social" needs of the population, splitting them into different entities that were administered by different sets of experts, like those found in health, education, housing, etc.

With the bourgeois revolutions of the 18th century, liberalism led to what critical theorists Jürgen Habermas and Axel Honneth called the emergence of a modern public sphere that was facilitated by the separation of state and civil society (Habermas, 1986). For Habermas, civil society is a realm of "private individuals" communicating freely in a "public context" with the potential development of critical public spheres capable of generating resistance to forms of power. Contrary to this conceptualization, according to Foucault (2004), the idea of civil society emerged within liberalism; it was in the period of the Scottish Enlightenment that Adam Ferguson conceptualized civil society as the necessary counterpoint to the self-interest of the modern, economic subject, which tries to realize maximum profit without considering the consequences for his or her economic opponent. For Foucault, civil society is neither an ideological construct nor an aboriginal reality, a natural given repelling government or opposing the state. Civil society is a "transactional reality" at the interface of political power and the government of populations (Foucault, 2004). With civil society, a mechanism was "naturally" in place that would balance this self-interest and address the social needs of the community but would leave the market to itself without any intervention of the state (Foucault, 2008; Villadsen, 2016). Be this as it may, the function of civil society and the role of humanitarianism dramatically changed in what we will call the neoliberal project.

Humanitarianism, Nursing, and Neoliberalism

We understand neoliberalism as a specific rationale of governmentality that has taken shape in very different forms depending on historical and national contexts (Mirowski, 2015) but the different varieties share similar goals. All of them target populations who depend on social and health services provided by governments. In the healthcare sector, governments systematically have dismantled services in order to reduce the costs of healthcare systems, with devastating effects on parts of the population by making them vulnerable and on the nurses who care for them. These measures have been justified as a way to break "welfare dependency" by privatizing services and implementing profit-making in healthcare. Some nursing scholars refer to a "neoliberal tide"—which they define as a "symbiotic process implying structures, material, and ideologies that foster the growth of its neoliberal values"—aimed particularly at supporting a market economy based on the dynamics of supply and demand in order to achieve cost-effectiveness (Krol & Lavoie, 2014).

But neoliberalism cannot be understood merely as an ideology and the economization of the social but must rather be analyzed as a specific rationality about how to govern our societies, with far-reaching consequences for populations on a global scale. Neoliberalism is a "constructivist project" organized through laws and the institutionalization of a rationality that directs the economy and protects it through laws and other regulations. As social theorist Thomas Lemke put it, "the market [must] be constituted by dint of political interventions" (Lemke, 2001, p. 193). The state must orient its politics to the needs of markets by adapting its monetary policies, its tax regimes, its organization of social services and healthcare, etc., instituting a new form of legitimation for the state, which is now evaluated by its ability to maintain and strengthen "free" markets.

In a neoliberal society, an individual is conceived as *homo oeconomicus*, one who organizes all areas of life according to this market rationality—every individual becomes an entrepreneur of itself, organizing life according to the model of the firm (Rose, 2005). Individuals are conceptualized in terms of human capital and like any other kind of capital, "are constrained by markets in both inputs and outputs to comport themselves in ways that will outperform the competition and to align themselves with good assessments about where those markets may be going" (Brown, 2015, p. 109). The human understood as human capital is responsible for itself and at the same time, becomes a dispensable asset because the neoliberal state grants no guarantee for the life of the individual. The neoliberal state itself must behave as a market actor and is responsible only for safeguarding the conditions for profitable competition. To this end, "the hegemony of *homo oeconomicus* and the neoliberal 'economization' of the political transform both state and citizen as both are converted, in identity and conduct, from figures of political sovereignty to figures of financialized firms" (Brown, 2015, p. 109). Those who are not able to successfully compete against others are left without any support and will ultimately perish.

It is in this context that humanitarianism and civil society become an integral part of the "neoliberal project" and of governing our current societies. Under neoliberalism, the central function of civil society is to guarantee and manifest individual freedom—the feeling of belonging, participation, and action without the state—but it is also necessary for guaranteeing the operation of the market and competition among citizens. It also favors public services provided by nongovernmental organizations (NGOs) instead of state organizations. The central idea in neoliberalism seems to be that if and when different functions of society cannot be organized in accordance with market principles, and "socio-moral" motives and engagements are needed, then a strong civil society in the form of voluntary, philanthropic, Christian organizations is clearly a better alternative to a strong and interventionist state. Civil society is a ground for problematization and for the development of a set of innovative techniques of government; it is both an object and an end of government. It is here that the idea of humanist care in nursing meets the neoliberal rationale of the lean state and serves the interest of the neoliberal transformation of current societies.

Nursing humanitarian organizations like the Canadian Association of Nurses in HIV/AIDS Care (CANAC), an important player in the propagation of Harm Reduction (HR) approaches, see themselves as part of civil society and as critical of governmental politics. Often understood as a space of criticism and resistance against "big government" and bureaucratic organizations, these organizations play a prominent role in contemporary political discourses. But these nurses and activists, using the idea of humanitarianism as a foundation for advocacy, do not realize that they do not really oppose "governments" but rather are an integral part of how we are governed today. In the same vein, the COVID-19 pandemic crisis is remarkable for the increasing importance of nurses' humanitarian actions and moral sentiments. Nurses are part of the moralizing discourses that invite the population to stay at home or to self-distance. Their work has earned them recognition as heroes and this hero discourse is not a neutral expression of public adulation, appreciation, and sentimentality, but rather is a tool employed to accomplish multiple aims. These aims include the enforcement of nurses as model citizens, the normalization of nurses' exposure to risk, and the preservation of existing power relationships (Mohammed et al., 2021). And these limit the ability of "front-line" nurses to decide the conditions of their work, to identify inadequate governmental support, and to understand their role in neoliberal forms of governance.

Genealogy of Humanitarianism

Apart from current societal developments and the neoliberal rationality, humanitarianism has always been part of a different form of governmentality. In what follows, we problemitize humanitarianism and compassionate care through a genealogical perspective. We will begin by describing the Christian roots of humanitarianism and how these roots influenced nursing history. We will use empirical data from the Canadian francophone province of Quebec—a province that is traditionally close to Catholicism and in which most hospitals have been run by the church.

Humanitarianism and its Charitable Roots

Historically, the concept of compassion has been at the heart of nursing care. Compassion was animated by charity, which was rooted in Christianity, and guided action to relieve the suffering of the poor and sick (Lynch, 2004). Beginning in the Western Middle Ages, sickness had spiritual significance, and the sick poor were perceived as deserving of compassionate and charitable care that was undertaken by private, frequently religious initiatives based on a moral and social obligation (Lynch, 2004). As we have discussed elsewhere in more detail (Nazon et al., 2019), nurses became an integral part of this history in the 17th and 18th century. Early nurses in Quebec and elsewhere were mostly religious sisters or Protestant deaconesses and were seen by the church as "servants of Lord Jesus, servants of the sick for Jesus' sake, and servants among one another" (Foth et al., 2014, p. 30). In one of the Catholic communities in Quebec, the religious sisters of Saint-Joseph had an obligation, according to their regulations, to exercise "boundless charity" toward the sick and the poor. As specified in their first Constitutions, they had to be "people fully consecrated to God to serve Him in the exercise of spiritual life and in the practice of perfect charity, and had to be especially dedicated to the service of Jesus Christ in the person of the poor who are its members" [authors' translation] (Archives des Religieuses Hospitalières de Saint-Joseph de Montréal [ARHSJM], 1643, p. 6). The poor were to be the object of all the attention and works of nursing sisters (Archives des Soeurs Grises [ASG], 1981, p. 31). Scholar Colin Jones (1989) believes there was a "charitable imperative" based on moral obligations, religious and cultural foundations, and specific social practices and expectations, which aimed to provide poor relief. This charitable conception of care was inspired by the philosophy of Christian virtue that encouraged healing, but above all, sanctifing and saving souls (Lefève, 2006). The soul was more important than the body and by caring for the souls of the poor as well as their bodily needs, nursing sisters guaranteed their own salvation. Eternal salvation was the reward for those who assisted the poor (ARHSJM, 1643).

The fascination for suffering is linked to Christian genealogy. Christianity valorizes the passion of Christ, which redeems the original sin of men and women and is re-actualized in the sacrifice of martyrs and the mortification of saints. This dolorous genealogy of modernity introduced a break in the use of suffering both in literature and in politics by inverting passion into compassion—the exaltation of one's own suffering into the suffering of others. However, sociologist Robert Castel (1995) argued that charity was a combination of compassion and discipline. He highlighted that charity provided to the poor in hospitals was a means to control the movement of the homeless population and to force them to conduct themselves according to a religious code. Only those indigent people who were thought to *deserve* charity were selected; the lazy, the needy, and those who had the spiritual poverty of *Pauper Christi* were to be left aside.

It is important to emphasize the continuity of the place that suffering occupies in the moral imagination and even its valorization as an experience of salvation, individually or collectively. Fassin (2010) refers to Augustine, who emphasized the ambiguity of valorization, because the spectacle of the suffering of others provokes horror and pleasure at the same time. One feels sadness in watching the misfortune of others and, at the same time, one cannot detach oneself from this vision, because one loves to feel pity. This emotional duality of empathy is a decisive characteristic of humanitarian reason—as one can easily see in the iconic images of agonized bodies like the father and daughter drowned at the Mexican–US border in 2019 (Ahmed & Semple, 2019)—and it seems as if the exposure of suffering enables the mobilization of moral sentiments and access to the transcendent truth of the victims.

The Importance of Capitalism

Deeply rooted in Christian history, the sacredness of life and the valorization of suffering makes any humanitarian government into a political theology, as it highlights the manifestation of religious order and a renewal of Christian heritage as a part of capitalisms' liberal democracies. Historian Thomas Haskell (1992) in *Capitalism and the Origins of the Humanitarian Sensibility* contended that between 1750 to 1850, an unprecedented wave of humanitarian reform sentiments emerged in Western Europe and North America. The most spectacular movement was the abolition of slavery but countless other movements emerged at the same time, including those concerned with animal welfare, child welfare, temperance, women suffrage, etc. These movements questioned the way the poor were assisted, the criminal was punished, or the insane were treated, and often resulted in the reform of practices. Haskell called it the onset of a "new humanitarianism" (p. 108) that was closely linked to the growth of capitalism and industrialization and not the expression of an unselfish desire to assist the unfortunate.

From its inception, humanitarianism was characterized by a deep ambivalence. Whereas humanitarians claimed that their project was courageous and resulted in reforms that ameliorated the living conditions of those living at the margins of society, humanitarianism was also part of an increasing rationalization of capitalist societies that served the interests of the reformers. For example, Foucault (2013) demonstrated in his work that the new humanitarian sensibilities did not aim to punish less but to punish more effectively and that they inserted the power to punish more deeply into the social body. Thus, humanitarian reforms were the consequence of cognitive structures that developed in the context of market transactions, and to understand the emergence of the humanitarian impulse, one has to analyze the close links between the capitalist market and social and economic changes (Haskell, 1992).

The market is the expression of the laws of supply and demand and it transforms the individual's self-interest into the greater good of the nation—the invisible hand in Adam Smith—and therefore public interest regulates itself. The marketplace injected calculations into all areas of life, meaning that every individual had to perform means-end calculations on the consequences of his/her decisions. For capitalism, it was vital that promises made in a contract could be trusted, that other contractual partners were able to fulfill their obligations. Thus, capitalism came with a new form of moralism. In fact, modifications in the market produced a change in perception and in the cognitive style of citizens and it was due to a change in how to perceive and explain causal connections (Amable, 2010).

Moral and political philosophers of the 17th and 18th centuries tried to define the necessary affective supposition of a responsible citizenry and the moral foundations of political control of sentiments. The relationship between politics and sentiments became defining concerns for the art of governing. Francis Bacon, for example, defined the role of the state as one of curtailing dangerous and explosive passions of ordinary men. This is close to Foucault's notion of governmentality and the art of governing that combines governing of a population with the conduct-of-conduct of an affective self (see also Foucault, 2007). Dangerous passions were to be controlled and transformed so that they could serve the interest of the public good.

The Impact of Biopolitics

The capitalist market is only one aspect in the genealogy of humanitarianism. The other dimension of humanitarianism is what Foucault called "biopolitics," which he used to describe the changing characteristics of power that occurred in the 19th century. From that point on, power was concentrated on humans as living beings—what he called the *"étatisation du biologique"* or state control over the biological (Foucault, 1978, 1997, 2003), a form of power that acts on two levels. On the level of disciplinary power or, what Foucault called, the anatomo-politics of the human body, everything is centered around the difficulty of drilling the body and augmenting the abilities of the individual to integrate the body into the (capitalist) economic control systems. On the second level, a new kind of power emerged that Foucault called biopower. It was no longer disciplinary; it was not directed toward the individual body but towards humans as "living beings" (Foucault, 1997, 2003).

It is in this context that medicine interconnected with governmental political thinking, conceptualizing human beings as something unique that could be studied in forms of positive knowledge (Foucault, 2000, 2014a, 2014b). The medical gaze penetrated the bodies of the sick, and autopsies in particular became the preferred technology to penetrate the body and to discover the hidden secrets of the causes leading to death; it was the beginning of establishing an anatomy of pathologies. Death became the objective, real, and undisputable foundation for the description of diseases. Medical science tried to understand the status of a population and to determine how it could be administered. It combined an axis of statistics that grasped the population in terms of, for example, rates of birth, illness, and death, with an axis of administration that established mechanisms to regulate events in widely dispersed heterogenous locales. Medicine developed into a science and a discipline of social spaces (Foucault, 2000). It was in this context that nursing became an important aspect of medical interventions, because nurses as capillaries of productive power (Foucault, 1995) perfectly incorporated both biopolitical dimensions: they were the ones who would discipline the individual and as public health nurses would intervene into families, communities, and the population at large.

Narrative Style and Humanitarianism

The emergence of biopower and the development of medicine into a social science is related to what Laqueur (1989) identified as another reason for the emergence of humanitarianism. This new humanitarianism was based on a particular narrative style, in the form of realistic novels, autopsy reports, clinical reports, and social inquiries, that emerged in the 18th to early 19th century. This style described the pain and dying of ordinary people by providing reasons for the suffering to which readers could easily relate. These narratives induced compassion in the reader because he or she was immediately affected by the reports of the pain or dying of others (see also Hunt, 2007). Laqueur (1989) emphasized that these humanitarian narratives provided very detailed accounts that were considered evidence of their truthfulness. They were the consequence of the empiricism of the 17th century and the new medical gaze that developed at that time based on minute observations and collections of facts about peoples' lives that had been unnoticeable before.

Even though the body played a decisive role in Christianity as an object of mercy, the body in humanitarian narratives differs from the Christian notion. In humanitarian narratives, the individual body, alive or dead, exists in its own right, whereas in Christianity the soul was more important than the body, which was considered nothing more than a vessel for the soul. But what is even more important for our context is that humanitarian narratives became the trigger for political reform because they established a causal chain between human agency and suffering. If one would undertake ameliorative actions now one would be able to reduce suffering, and thus these actions became a moral imperative. This became the leading rationale for nurses to actively promote public hygiene campaigns and to advocate for the moral regulation of urban spaces considered unhealthy because of the immoral conduct of the people living there.

However, what we find interesting are medical case histories and autopsy reports that basically shared the same techniques used in other humanitarian narratives along with their assumptions about agency. Medical reports provided a detailed history of the body and related this history to the social context, thereby generating a way to imagine the misfortune of the other. Even though medical reports were not written for a public audience, as novels were, these narratives nevertheless became the basis for political reformist arguments and newspaper articles. Medical reports accumulated a large amount of detail and ordered it in such way that the pain and suffering of others became real, justifying the need for specific interventions. Medical case histories made "bodies [into] a common ground of humanitarian sensibility" by describing the histories of these suffering bodies. It is important to note that humanitarian action is ostensibly focused on saving lives, but the genealogy of humanitarianism shows that its main attention is on the dead—humanitarianism is a "guide to the mastery of death" (Laqueur, 1989, p. 181). What Laqueur means by this is that humanitarianism became such an important moral obligation through analyzing death and dying. Thus, humanitarianism is guided by the question of how to prevent unnecessary deaths—it is a profoundly biopolitcal perspective and linked to the medical gaze that appeared in the same context—the analysis of dying and death (Foucault, 1994). These accounts had the specific ability to arouse moral concerns in the late-18th century.

Thus, these case histories demonstrated that medicine held a secular mastery over the body and the suffering described in these narratives was meant to induce sympathy. They provided a language and rationale for humane concern. In the 18th century, doctors claimed for themselves the "party of humanity" (Laqueur, 1989, p. 185), a claim that they no longer had to repeat in the 19th century because it was taken for granted. It was then that nursing became the representation of the humanitarian aspect of biomedicine in the form of care. At the end of the 18th century, humanitarian and political claims merged in medical writings using the narrative style of novelists that was mimicked also in the writings of nurses. The call for sympathy was based on the authority of the clinical practitioner and the social and anatomical details provided in these accounts justified the readers' compassion. Laqueur (1989) calls it "scientific sensationalism," which calls for the readers' sympathy and attention by merging a social narrative with forensic medicine.

What we want to highlight here is that narratives do not provoke a moral response but "merely milk sentiments and defer revolutionary action" (Laqueur, 1989, p. 202) because sympathy and compassion are directed to a fictional and distant suffering while the real suffering is left untouched. However, Laqueur (1989), referring to Hume, goes even a step further when he contends that "humanitarians" also "implicitly claim a proprietary interest in those whom they aid" (p. 182), meaning the relationship between humanitarian and the person in need of assistance is itself a form of capitalist relationship. The humanitarians are the ones who speak in the name of the sufferings of the wronged. But moral concern is not so much about the relationship between human beings; it is more about the "pain of a stranger crying out - as if the pain were one's own or that of someone near" (p. 182).

This discussion enables us to get back to where we began in our article, namely to criticize Richard Rorty's "sentimentalist thesis," according to which narratives of suffering induced in their listeners or readers the feelings that became the origins of humanitarianism and human rights and led to broadening struggles to defend them. According to Rorty, human rights and humanitarian sentiments were not the consequences of inalienable rights and reason or the insight that we all belong to the same species, but the impulse to care for strangers was generated by the feeling that we all know how it feels to be in a situation of suffering. Sympathy, not law and reason, is the foundation of our moral human rights culture, which is a success story of the last 200 years "in which it has become easier for us to be moved by sad and sentimental stories" (Rorty, 1993, p. 134, as quoted in, Laqueur, 2009, p. 32). But Sadiya Hartman makes clear for White abolitionists that empathy with Black suffering is a specific form of violence-induced fungibility of Blackness. This fungibility allows for its appropriation by White psyches as "property of enjoyment."

Hartman criticized a "Northern White man's fantasy that replaces the body of the slaves with the bodies of himself and his family, as the slaves are being beaten." (Wilderson, 2010, p. 88).

> By exporting the vulnerability of the captive body as a vessel for the uses, thoughts, and feelings of others, the humanity extended to the slave inadvertently confirms the expectations and desires definitive of the relations of chattel slavery. In other words, the case of Rankin's empathetic identification is as much due to his good intentions and heartfelt opposition to slavery as to the fungibility of the captive body ... In the fantasy of being beaten ... Rankin becomes a proxy and the other's pain is acknowledged to the degree that is can be imagined, yet by virtue of this substitution the object of identification threatens to disappear.
>
> (Hartman, 1997, p. 19)

However, the last two centuries have witnessed an increase in these kinds of narratives that were a precondition for the emergence of the human as an ethical subject (Hunt, 2007). These narratives developed independently from the evolution of human rights law, which rather followed sentimental stories. History shows that narratives expanded "the circle of we" because they re-commended looking at other people and their conditions (Hunt, 2007; Laqueur, 2009). These narratives addressed both the nearby stranger and the distant "other" and elements of causality became embedded in them, establishing a relation between the character in the narratives and the reader/hearer. These sentimental stories were the basis of what Laqueur (1989) called the "broader cultural story" (p. 53) that made visible the lives and living conditions of people who had not been noticed before.

These cultural stories served as justification for humanitarian expansionism and demonstrated how the religious was secularized by its permanent inscription into the heart of secular democracies. Life as the supreme good is the Christian idea of the sacredness of life. Fassin (2010) calls this idea biolegitimacy, the recognition of life as a supreme value above all other values in our societies, with· life being understood as the bare fact of being alive. This is what Benjamin (1965) called the "simple fact of living" and Arendt (1994) called "naked life." It is this biolegitimacy that makes it impossible to think about or to support public health as a collective or common good. Instead, the focus of humani-tarian organizations is on providing help on an individual basis. Simultaneously, moral economies have been constituted around a new relation to suffering and they have become the central element of public life. Whereas in the past, suffering was part of punishment that was carried out in public spectacles, today images and reports about suffering in painful detail are disseminated in public spaces and used as justification for action. Humanitarian government is the heir of this active protest against the suffering of the world (see also Agamben, 1998). New humanitarianism is united under "a common set of morally framed affective goals and practices around suffering, innocence, benevolence, and compassion" (Ticktin, 2011, p. 180). The aim of this new humanitarianism is to provide compassionate care for morally legitimate individual suffering and nursing became part of this global project.

The question is, according to Laqueur, how the "human" became a new moral urgency. Humanitarianism has been criticized exactly because it does not often lead to care for the humans at hand (e.g., Agamben, 1998), as we can see in our societies where large parts of the population live in unliveable conditions such as indigenous communities that are deprived of the minimal means to live by the settler-colonial states who historically and presently benefit from the material resources extracted from these communities. Thus, it seems to be easier to moralize than to act against injustices and the reasons for suffering. The divide between who is included and who is not is very fragile and narratives can be used to exclude in the name of humanity by describing the excluded as non-human. Thus, sympathy, empathy, and other moral sentiments must be understood politically because narratives of suffering authorize and motivate political actions only under specific circumstances.

Conclusion

For decades, moral sentiments and humanitarianism have shaped the history of Western societies. With roots in charitable endeavours, humanitarianism became an important element in the care of the poor, the powerless, and the sick. As we have argued, instead of the expression of an unselfish desire to assist the unfortunate, the emergence of humanitarianism must be considered the result of specific historical constellations and an integral part of the neoliberal and biopolitics project in the government of populations. In particular, nursing humanitarian organizations in civil society are one of the elements in expanding neoliberalism. From this view, humanitarian nursing organizations are more a product of power than a way to resist governments and neoliberalism, being deeply enmeshed within forms and practices of governmentality. If nurses are to participate in humanitarian action and expand nursing action on issues of social justice and advocacy for patients, it is important to keep a critical lens on political interventions. Developing an awareness of political philosophies will give nurses the ability to critique positively and negatively their implications in the humanitarian project.

References

Agamben, G. (1998). Biopolitics and the rights of man. In W. Hamacher & D. E. Wellbery (Eds.), *Homo sacer: Sovereign power and bare life* (p. 136). Stanford University Press.
Ahmed, A., & Semple, K. (2019). Photo of drowned migrants captures pathos of those who risk it all. *New York Times*. Retrieved October 14, 2021, from https://www.nytimes.com/2019/06/25/us/father-daughter-border-drowning-picture-mexico.html

Amable, B. (2010). Morals and politics in the ideology of neo-liberalism. *Socio-Economic Review*, 9(1), 3–30. 10.1093/ser/mwq015

Archives des Religieuses Hospitalières de Saint-Joseph de Montréal [ARHSJM]. (1643). *Constitution des filles hospitalières de Saint-Joseph.* (ARHSJM – 4A011-12-01-01). Montréal, Canada.

Archives des Sœurs Grises [ASG]. (1981). *Constitutions et statuts de l'institut des sœurs de la charité de Montréal "Sœurs Grises"* (ASG – L036; L102). Montréal, Canada.

Arendt, H. (1994). *The origins of totalitarianism.* Harcourt Brace Jovanovich.

Asad, T. (2015). Reflections on violence, law, and humanitarianism. *Critical Inquiry*, 41(2), 390–427. 10.1086/679081

Benjamin, W. (1965). Zur Kritik der Gewalt. In *Zur Kritik der Gewalt und andere Aufsätze. Mit einem Nachwort von Herbert Marcuse* (pp. 29–65). Suhrkamp.

Brown, W. (2015). *Undoing the demos: Neoliberalism's stealth revolution.* In W. Brown & M. Feher (Eds.), *Zone books near future.* Zone Books.

Brown, W. (2019). *In the ruins of neoliberalism: The rise of antidemocratic politics in the West.* Columbia University Press.

Castel, R. (1995). *Les métamorphoses de la question sociale: Une chronique du salariat.* Fayard, 1995.

Constitutions et Statuts de l'Institut des Sœurs de la Charité de Montréal "Sœurs Grises," 31 (1981).

Ewald, F. (1996). *Histoire de l'état providence.* Livre de poche.

Fassin, D. (2010). *La raison humanitaire.* Gallimard Seuil.

Foth, T., Kuhla, J., & Benedict, S. (2014). Nursing during national socialism. In S. Benedict & L. Shields (Eds.), *Nurses and midwives in Nazi Germany: The "Euthanisia programs"* (pp. 27–47). Routledge.

Foucault, M. (1978). *History of sexuality: volume 1, an introduction.* Random House, Inc.

Foucault, M. (1994). *The birth of the clinic: An archaeology of medical perception.* Vintage Books.

Foucault, M. (1997). *Il faut défendre la société. Cours au College de France. 1976.* Gallimard Seuil.

Foucault, M. (1995). *Discipline & punish: The birth of the prison.* Vintage Books.

Foucault, M. (2000). The birth of social medicine. In J. D. Faubion (Ed.), *Power: Essential works of Foucault 1954–1984. Volume three* (pp. 134–156). Penguin Books.

Foucault, M. (2003). Society must be defended: Lecture at the Collège de France, March 17, 1976. In M. Bertani, A. Fontana, & F. Ewald (Eds.), *Society must be defended: Lectures at the Collège de France 1975–1976* (pp. 239–264). Picador.

Foucault, M. (2004). *Naissance de la biopolitique: Cours au collège de France (1978–1979).* Gallimard: Seuil, c2004.

Foucault, M. (2007). *Security, territory, population: Lectures at the collège de France, 1977–78,* G. Burchell (Trans.). Palgrave Macmillan.

Foucault, M. (2008). *The birth of biopolitics: Lectures at the collège de France, 1978–79.* Palgrave Macmillan.

Foucault, M. (2013). *La Société punitive. Cours au Collège de France, 1971–1973.* Gallimard Seuil.

Foucault, M. (2014a). Bio-history and bio-politics. (Richard A. Lynch, Trans.). *Foucault Studies*, (18), 128–130.

Foucault, M. (2014b). The politics of health in the eighteenth century. (Richard A. Lynch, Trans.). *Foucault Studies*, October(18), 113–127.

GilBride, E. (2020). *The "good samaritan order:" Protecting frontline healthcare workers responding to the COVID-19 outbreak*. https://www.jshfirm.com/covid-19-legislative-updates-good-samaritan-executive-order-state-legislation-federal-coronavirus-relief-bill-cares-act/

Government of Canada/Gouvernment du Canada. (2019, April 23, 2019). *About the Good Samaritan Drug Overdose Act*. Retrieved June 30, from https://www.canada.ca/en/health-canada/services/substance-use/problematic-prescription-drug-use/opioids/about-good-samaritan-drug-overdose-act.html?utm_source=Youtube&utm_medium=Video&utm_campaign=EOACGSLCreative1&utm_term=GoodSamaritanLaw&utm_content=GSL

Habermas, J. (1986). *Strukturwandel der Öffentlichkeit*. Sammlung Luchterhand.

Hartman, S. V. (1997). *Scenes of subjection: Terror, slavery, and self-making in nineteenth-century America*. Oxford University Press.

Haskell, T. L. (1992). Capitalism and the origins of the humanitarian sensibility, Part 1 and 2. In T. Bender (Ed.), *The antislavery debate: Capitalism and abolitionism as a problem in historical interpretation* (pp. 107–160). University of California Press.

Hunt, L. A. (2007). *Inventing human rights: A history* (1st ed.). W.W. Norton & Co.

Jones, C. (1989). *The charitable imperative: Hospitals ans nursing in ancien regime and re-volutionnary France*. Routledge.

Kalisch, B. J., & Kalisch, P. A. (1983). Anatomy of the image of the nurse: Dissonant and ideal models [Research Support, U.S. Gov't, P.H.S.]. *ANA Publ, G-161*(G-161), 3–23. https://www.ncbi.nlm.nih.gov/pubmed/6556020

Krol, P., & Lavoie, M. (2014). Beyond nursing nihilism: A Nietzschean transvaluation of neoliberal values. *Nursing Philosophy, 15*(2), 112–124. 10.1111/nup.12025

Laqueur, T. W. (1983). Bodies, death, and pauper funerals. *Representations*, (1), 109–131. 10.2307/3043762

Laqueur, T. W. (1989). Bodies, details, and the humanitarian narrative. In L. Hunt (Ed.), *The new cultural history* (pp. 176–204). University of Califonia Press.

Laqueur, T. W. (2009). Mourning, pity, and the work of narrative in the making of "humanity". In R. A. Wilson & R. D. Brown (Eds.), *Humanitarianism and suffering: The mobilization of empathy* (pp. 31–57). Cambridge University Press.

Lefève, C. L. (2006). La philosophie du soin. *La Matière et l'Esprit, 4*, 25–34.

Lemke, T. (2001). "The birth of bio-politics": Michel Foucault's lecture at the College de France on neo-liberal governmentality. *Economy and Society, 30*(2), 207.

Lynch, K. A. (2004). Behavioral regulation in the city: Religious associations and the role of poor relief. In *Social control in early modern Europe, 1500–1800* (pp. 200–2019). Ohio State Univeristy Press.

Mirowski, P. (2015). Postface: Defining neoliberalism. In P. Mirowski & D. Plehwe (Eds.), *The road from Mont-Pèlerin: The making of the neoliberal thought collective* (pp. 417–457). Harvard University Press.

Mohammed, S., Peter, E., Killackey, T., & Maciver, J. (2021). The "nurse as hero" discourse in the COVID-19 pandemic: A poststructural discourse analysis. *International Journal of Nursing Studies, 117*, 103887. 10.1016/j.ijnurstu.2021.103887

Nazon, É., Perron, A., & Foth, T. (2019). Rethinking the social role of nursing through the work of Donselot and Foucault. *Witness: The Canadian Journal of Critical Nursing Discourse, 1*(1), 49–58. https://witness.journals.yorku.ca/index.php/default/article/view/23

Rorty, R. (1993). Oxford amnesty lecture. In S. Shute & S. Hurley (Eds.), *On human rights: The Oxford amnesty lectures, 1993* (pp. 111–134). Basic Bokks.

Rose, N. (2005). *Powers of freedom: Reframing political thought.* Cambridge University Press.

Stokes-Parish, J., Elliott, R., Rolls, K., & Massey, D. (2020). Angels and heroes: The unintended consequence of the hero narrative. *Journal of Nursing Scholarship, 52*(5), 462–466. 10.1111/jnu.12591

Ticktin, M. (2011). *Casualties of care: Immigration and the politics of humanitarianism in France.* University of California Press.

Villadsen, K. (2016). Michel Foucault and the forces of civil society. *Theory, Culture & Society, 33*(3), 3–26. 10.1177/0263276415581895

Wilderson III, F. B. (2010). *Red, white & black.* Durham, NC: Duke University Press.

Wynter, S. (2003). Unsettling the coloniality of being/power/truth/freedom: Towards the human, after man, its overrepresentation—An Argument. *The Centennial Review, 3*(3), 257–337.

2 Finding CASSANDRA: Mythology, Hagiography, and Historiography for Nursing

Jess Dillard-Wright

As I have written and revised this essay for this anthology, I have struggled to put words to why I think the theme of mythology, hagiography, and historiography is imperative for nursing. This is not because the topic is not important. Rather, the challenge comes in precisely just how important the ideas rooted in our past are that have shaped and continue to shape the nursing present. I share this reflection to situate myself and to contextualize how I understand history, imagination, and disciplinary identity. I am a nurse and midwife. Before my turn to nursing, I studied science, technology, and culture as well as women's history. These lines of flight shape my understanding of the discipline and disciplinary history of nursing. This is also shaped by my lived experiences as a fat and queer and genderqueer parent and partner with considerable educational as well as unearned class and race priviledge navigating in the white spaces of nursing and higher education. I generally assume a critical feminist and poststructuralist—and more recently anarchist and abolitionist—stance that approaches the history of ideas in nursing as both a historical and a philosophical endeavor. This disciplinary unruliness is instructive and animates my impulse to understand why nurses are the way we are and how we devise other narratives, narratives for nursing that create alternate points of entry, alternate lines of flight.

The shifting narratives of nursing in our pandemic times suggests to me that now is the time to interrogate what it means to be a nurse, who is allowed to be a nurse, and how people understand nursing from within, beyond, and opposing disciplinary boundaries. I contribute to this effort in thinking about the historical entanglements between nursing and feminism. My point of entry for this consideration is located with CASSANDRA Radical Feminist Nurses Network (from here I will use "CASSANDRA"), a radical feminist collective mobilized more than 120 years after Nightingale's arrival on the scene. CASSANDRA also links the ancient Greek myth of Cassandra and Florence Nightingale's visions of Victorian womanhood as penned in an essay known as "Cassandra," which documents Nightingale's manifold laments. In this paper, I examine the historical operation initiated by hanging nursing history on the Nightingale origin story and, using CASSANDRA and mythic Cassandra, tease out points of resistance to and compliance with the Nightingale hegemony (de Certeau,

DOI: 10.4324/9781003245957-4

1988). Here, I openly tangle history with theory and philosophy in order to work on some of the pernicious problems that plague nursing.

In this paper, I concern myself with examining the ideological vestigia that remains in our disciplinary embrace of a particularly tenacious Victorian professional origin myth. Our past shapes our present, just as our present shapes the histories we write (Foucault, 1984). Historian Michel de Certeau (1988) further articulated the generativity of the "historiographical operation," which is "bound to the complex of a specific and collective fabrication more than it is the effect merely of a personal philosophy or the resurgence of a past 'reality.' It is the *product* of a *place* [emphasis original]," (p. 64) both geographic and temporal. What is *mobilized* as nursing's disciplinary history shapes nursing's imagination. These ideas, discourses, and ideologies that circulate are neither stable nor immutable. The events that mark our past, following de Certeau (1988), are not irrelevant to history as nursing knows it; however, the "facts" of history are insufficient to account for the historiographies we embrace. As I weave the threads of Ancient Greek Cassandra with Nightingale's "Cassandra" and CASSANDRA of the 20th century, I hope to attend to some of the ways ideas about gender, sexuality, and race entered into and circulate within nursing. In what follows, I tease out the normative ideals and values that structure nursing's imaginary, including gender, sexuality, and race. Before delving into these themes, I also define some of the theoretical terms that I have used to make sense of nursing's history. But first, I will introduce CASSANDRA.

Meet CASSANDRA

As the Equal Rights Amendment (ERA) was due to expire June 30, 1982, a single vote short of ratification, a small but fierce band of radical feminist nurses converged on Washington, D.C. (Hunter & Times, 1982). As the ERA was laid to rest, the 1982 ANA convention unfolded in the nation's capital. And while outside, D.C. roiled in protest, within the halls of the ANA conference hotel, scarce mention of the ERA could be found (Chinn & Berrey, 2014). While the 1982 ANA House of Delegates passed a resolution in support of the ERA ("Resolution on Equal Rights for Women," J. Hunter, 1984, pp. 20–22), the conference was otherwise eerily silent on the question (Chinn & Berrey, 2014, pp. 50–64). CASSANDRA Radical Nurses Network formed in response to this, mobilized by the ANA's unwillingness to engage in women's liberation, perhaps more deeply emblematic of nursing's disciplinary unwillingness to enter into feminist reckoning.

Determined to bring radical feminist identity, politics, and philosophy as a challenge to the hegemonic patriarchal structures that shaped most nursing organizations, CASSANDRA sought to weave new—and reclaim lost—ways of being as nurses. This effort was led by Peggy Chinn, Charlene Eldridge Wheeler, Sharon Deevey, Denise O'Connor, Gretchen LaGodna, and other activist nurses connected to the wider world of radical feminist thought. Local chapters of CASSANDRA were loosely affiliated, threaded together through three-times yearly newsjournals that documented CASSANDRA's happenings and annual Gatherings, national meetings often organized as an informal auxiliary to larger nursing conferences. Together, the nurses of CASSANDRA were committed to building a national network of feminist nurses with a strong radical voice (LaGodna, 1982, p. 1). CASSANDRANs further committed to the preservation of women's writing, sharing skills, feminist research in nursing and beyond, as well as developing new pedagogical modalities free from the "social censorship and bias" commonplace in nursing education (LaGodna, 1982). CASSANDRA also boasted a separatist ethos, which they described as woman-identified, following the Radicalesbians (1970), that limited membership to women, many of whom were lesbians. CASSANDRA was active until 1991, its last embers cooling as Third Wave feminism ignited. And while these aims may now appear modest, the formation of CASSANDRA constituted an act of resistance, a praxis informed by radical feminist separatism and solidarity but one that was also undermined by the replication of some of the self-same problems that plagued nursing as a disicpline, including its persistent whiteness, compulsory heterosexuality, and rigid femininity bound up in its Victorian framing.

CASSANDRA's Victorian Legacy

CASSANDRA, as I have alluded above, is bound up with both ancient Greek mythology and with nursing's chosen Victorian foremother, Florence Nightingale. Shortly after her return from nurse training at Kaiserswerth, Nightingale wrote an essay that would eventually become CASSANDRA's eponym. Upon her return to the family home, Nightingale fell into a miasma of impotent misery compounded by her sister Parthenope's nervous breakdown. This breakdown, Parthenope alleged, was precipitated by Nightingale's unsisterly devotion to nursing (Showalter, 1981). Though no doubt stressful and difficult for the Nightingale family, Parthenope's breakdown had a silver lining in it for Nightingale: Advised by the family's physician, Nightingale's father emancipated her, supporting her independence with a 500 pound annuity. This, it was thought, would end Parthenope's pathological dependence and liberate Nightingale (Showalter, 1981).

In the midst of this domestic crisis, Nightingale penned her essay, "Cassandra." Drawing from her unusually robust classical education, Nightingale found parallels with the ancient Greek myth of Cassandra and her own experiences of womanhood in her time. In this essay, Nightingale (1979) beseeched women to awaken to their predicament, the velvet cage of Victorian femininity under the Separate Spheres doctrine for the elite (Nightingale, 1979). Nightingale's analyses vacillate between denigrating women's work and perceived idleness, on the one hand, while castigating the rigid social mores that confined her given her class status on the other (Nightingale, 1979). In the course of her complaint, Nightingale (1979) envied the liberation of those women who work outside the home, even by necessity—widows, the impoverished, those with ill husbands—wishing for herself the opportunity to exercise her passion, intellect, and morality. Nightingale went on to indict marriage for the limiting institution she understood it to be, a barrier to the independence necessary to exercise passion and industry. Of course, Nightingale's call for emancipation is limited at the same time as it is complex: Only families of means could afford to support their adult daughters outside the family home to pursue their passions absent a husband. And Nightingale was fortunate to rely on her father's allowance to free her to pursue her calling, though we cannot assume the impoverished and widowed women she envied experienced similar luxury (Nightingale, 1979).

The Eponymous Cassandra

The inspiration for Nightingale's essay is rooted in the ancient Greek myth, another symbol of Nightingale's class privilege. By all accounts, Cassandra was a woman gifted with true sight, prophesy (Shamas, 2011). The origin of this gift is usually attributed to Apollo, though this varies from telling to telling. In some accounts, Cassandra was then cursed after spurning the advances of Apollo, with never being believed (Peggy, 1982). Poor Cassandra went mad, cast out into the wilderness to fend for herself, in spite of (or perhaps because of) the truths she could tell (Shamas, 2011). Cassandra also made appearances in Shakespeare's plays and eventually came to constitute a Second Wave feminist touchstone for radical feminists in nursing.

What's in a Name?

Choosing "Cassandra" for a moniker linked CASSANDRA Radical Feminist Nurses Network to both ancient Greek mythology and to Nightingale, building CASSANDRA's place in the canon of nursing history and constructing space for feminists within that history. But while CASSANDRA worked to undermine patriarchal notions of heteronormativity and femininity, and as part of Second Wave feminism's radical encampment, choosing "Cassandra" for an eponym is complex and conflicted, tapping into a familiar narrative. This connects CASSANDRA with a remarkably conventional narrative of nursing history and a mythology that, at least superficially, reinforces silence and misogyny, on the one hand, and recasts the bourgeois origins of professional nursing as radical, on the other. Linking CASSANDRA to Nightingale opens a fissure of possibility, one in which radical possibility exists without challenging nursing's established imagination.

However, well before the first gasps of CASSANDRA, at the earliest stages of the professionalization of nursing in the late 19th century, nursing as a discipline adopted an unspoken commitment to a politics of neutrality. These politics are linked to the gendered episteme that shaped the birth of the professional discipline as controlled, feminine, and caring. Hints of this can be located Nightingale's *Notes on Nursing*, where she implored would-be carers to eschew the rhetoric of women's rights, urging her nurse-sisters "to keep clear of the current jargons now everywhere" in *Notes on Nursing* (Nightingale, 1968, p. 125). This sentiment reflects Nightingale's personal reluctance to support woman suffrage during feminism's so-called First Wave. Nightingale further professed indifference to any alleged wrongs against her sex, a stance that contributed to an image of modern, professional nursing that angelically rose above the venal concerns of something as base as politics (Cook, 1914, p. 385).[1] Nightingale's legacy is complex: Nightingale created and sustained bold and decisive action in the development of a profession by and for women, which seems decidedly feminist by some measures. However, this possibility is undermined by Nightingale's public denigration of early feminist activists and her refusal to work with women of color, evinced in part by her refusal of Mother Mary Seacole (Seacole, 2019). Ultimately, Nightingale's *strategies* paralleled the of woman suffrage—including the subversion of women of color and exclusion of poor women—and early feminist thought. But the *substance* of her thought was clearly less than feminist. Nightingale eventually came to support woman suffrage. This makes Nightingale's Cassandra a precarious eponym for CASS-ANDRA, a radical feminist group, in particular because of the vestigia of the persistant antifeminist impulse in the enduring popularity of *Notes on Nursing* and in the popular image of nursing which has implications for our present (Anderson, 2016, p. 30).

Mythology, Hagiography, Historiography

Early efforts in women's history, contemporaneous with Second Wave feminism (of which CASSANDRA was a part), was characterized by a tendency to construct "Great Woman" narratives, developing line up of sheroes to counterbalance the heroes of Great Man history. Like women's history more broadly, early trends in nursing history replicated a tendency to build heroes, developing a revisionist, Great Woman approach to nursing history that leaves us with a hollow sort of hagiography (Nelson, 1997). This history of canonical saints flattens a rich, conflicted, and dynamic history into something monolithic and static (D'Antonio, 2006; Nelson, 1997). Professional foremothers like Florence Nightingale sanitized nursing, making it an occupation fit for *ladies* and not the exclusive purview of the Sairy Gamps of the time. They did not *invent* nursing, but rather seized nursing and engaged efforts to sanitize the work of nursing, making it palatable and safe for the daughters of middle-class families (Reverby, 1987). The way we choose to present this aspect of nursing is a historical operation in its own right, one that is still in play some 200 years later. A recent commentary by feminist theorist Cynthia Enloe (2021) demonstrates as much, wherein Nightingale rescued nursing from the clutches of the "untrained, drunk, and slovenly" (Enloe, 2021, p. 7).

This particular operation whitewashed nursing, prioritizing genteel attributes in nursing even while nursing educators scrambled to recruit, educate, and retain nurses in the field, a familiar problem that seems remarkably current, no matter the point in history at which we look. This tendency to heroify—or angelicize, when we think of the gendered and religious expectations with which nursing is imbued—gives rise to an ahistoricity for nursing, a discipline beyond space and time, when nothing could be further from the truths. The mythologies of nursing are built on romantic desires that are perhaps informed by but remote from the discipline's daily realities. This is most apparent in nursing's oft-cited reputation as the "most trusted" profession, an honor that is mitigated by profligate misapprehension of what it is that nurses do, emblematic, perhaps, of the proxy maternal role society envisions broadly for nurses, overdetermined by the expectation of self-sacrificial emotional labor (Foth et al., 2018).

Nursing's Great Woman Narratives

Nursing's Great Woman narrative valorizes women like Florence Nightingale and Clara Barton, angels in the hospital as our first heroines, reinforcing a respectable, feminized, feminine image of nursing at the expense of Women of Color and prior gender diversity in the profession (Threat, 2015). The reductive nature of these idols flattens nursing, eliding complexity in favor of easy-to-love (for some) icons exaggerating our most prized nursing values. Nursing is reduced to emotional labor, saturated with ideas like the "greatest mother." Our status as the most trusted profession, while politically salient and flattering, reinforces a limited, romantic, sometimes ill-fitting image. At the same time, this trajectory for early nursing history parallels other kinds of developmental historiographies that seem to start with a "great person" narratives. Early efforts in women's history, for example, started with what pioneering women's historian Gerda Lerner (1975) called "woman worthies" (p. 5), accounting for notable individuals without attending to the lived experiences of most women.

This kind of history for nursing satisfied and satisfies professional efforts at legitimacy, weaving a specific narrative for the purpose of identity-building, cult personalities that rallied enthusiasm and respect, creating community and building heroes (Anderson, 2016). It is also uncritical and nearly universally panegyric in nature, hagiography rather than history. This kind of paean fixes nursing and flattens those "nurse worthies" into static caricatures: the Lady with the Lamp, as in the case of Nightingale; the World's Greatest Mother, at least in propaganda from World War II; the silent and sacrificing super hero of pandemic times. These renderings anchor nursing's ideas about itself. These imaginings bear the imprint of White heteronormative femininity which linger in and through the histories nursing chooses to write.

Nursing's Past Isn't Dead. It isn't Even Past

In thinking about the dimensions of the nursing history that continue to structure the discipline, it is worth noting that, as nursing has pursued legitimacy as a science and profession, it has also embraced what Suzanne Gordon and Siobhan Nelson (2004) have called a rhetoric of rupture. This rhetoric positions nursing's past as outdated, old-fashioned, and something to be left in the past as nursing embraces a present/future inflected with technoptimism and an affinity toward medical hegemony. Evidence of this rhetoric can be found in a recent editorials imploring nurses to "once and for all to discard these residues of our religious, militaristic and highly gendered history and to take our rightful place as leaders of health service delivery" (Carryer, 2019, p. 288). And while I am sympathetic to the project of thinking more expansively about nursing, we cannot leave behind a past that continues to, whether we attend to it or not, shape the current order of things. To this end, I wish to consider, in the section that follows, some of the discourses that shaped and shape nursing. I will then interrogate the ways in which CASSANDRA both resists and reinforces these ideas.

Gender and Sexuality

The mythologies, imagery, and ideologies nursing embraces to construct the discipline and through which it is understood from the outside are steeped in gendered ideals and expectations. Some of this is rooted in professionalized nursing's Victorian origins, which were themselves rooted in both religious and military order as well as class-based respectability. Other aspects are rooted in the persistent, patriarchal binary that shaped what Jo Ann Ashley called the "hospital family," which has evolved over time (Ashley, 1976). Though much is made of the homosocial quality of nursing, little time or effort has been dedicated to understanding how gender is produced in nursing.

Closely linked to the production of gender in nursing is the enforcement of a compulsory heteronormativity (Rich, 1980). The heteronormative construct of the hospital family is suggestive of the sexual politics of nursing, where sexual politics are the power-structured relations characteristic of a patriarchal society (Millett, 2016). Existing in a patriarchal context, the sexual politics of nursing are both complex and conflicted, linked again to the Victorian understanding of the intimate connection between reproductive biology and gender roles that gave rise to nursing's normative values (Ashley, 1980; Smith-Rosenberg & Rosenberg, 1973). The distinct gendering of nursing and concurrent subjugation to medicine is a function of patriarchal sexual politics. Moreover, naturalizing feminine gender in the provision of emotional labor in nursing "negate[s] the skills necessary for feminine work" (Ruchti, 2012, p. 38), erasing the skilled praxis necessary to cultivate intimacy in nursing care. The naturalization of this kind of skill in nursing erodes boundaries that exist between profession and individual. The naturalization of care work and entitlement to intimacy is in some ways explanatory for the slide from intimacy to sex, suggestive of how sexuality and gender fuse in the popular imagination of nursing.

Stereotypes of nursing are predicated on a patriarchal foundation of gendered expectations constructed by sexual politics. These tropes construct binaries—good/evil, naughty/nice, angel/battle-ax, Madonna/whore—where nurses-as-women must be all things, an impossible tension because inhabiting one side of the dualism definitionally precludes her from inhabiting the opposing side. This doubling is emblematic of sexual politics, an ideology, mythology, religion that is fundamentally impossible to escape, the yardstick by which nurses-as-women are measured but to which they can never quite measure up, an apparatus of patriarchal control (Muff, 1982). Patriarchal assumptions that structure the historiography of compulsory heterosexuality in nursing conceal the possibility of other sexualities throughout history, including the Victorian era that gives root to contemporary nursing episteme (Faderman, 1981).

Scholar of lesbian literature and culture Lillian Faderman asserted that Victorian gender mores often imposed a certain asexuality on women, especially in the British and United States contexts. Women of station and character were understood as and expected to be disinterested in sex, guardians of morality that they were. When these women were interested in sex, the assumption went, it was with the aim of either pleasing their husbands or of fulfilling their reproductive duty (Faderman, 1981). In this context, lesbian existence was erased in the Victorian era that coincides with professional nursing's 19th-century origins, a reality that persists in the 21st century (P. Chinn & Berrey, 2014; P. L. Chinn, 2008; Randall & Eliason, 2012; Searle, 2019). In spite of—or perhaps because of—this erasure, resistance to compulsory hetersexuality was possible in some instances. One example is the so-called "Boston marriage," longterm same-sex pair bonds that allowed women to set up households (Faderman, 1981). This was possible primarily through the absence of the possibility of lesbian romantic and sexual love in the Victorian imagination. In some respects, in order for Victorian women to achieve any kind of professional status, they were required to resist the compulsory heterosexuality that shaped cultural expectations for their time. Nursing was a profession that enabled white women to defy compulsory heterosexuality by avoiding the mandate to marry through financial independence while paradoxically maintaining an appropriately feminine veneer (Stark, 1979, p. 2). Indeed, without making assertions about any of these nurses' sexual identity, many of the nursing heroines recorded in our textbooks never married, including Nightingale, Lillian Wald, and Lavinia Dock. Remaining unmarried meant that these women were able to attend to their professional aspirations in nursing.

Nursing, both in the early days of professionalized nursing and now, afforded women economic opportunity to support themselves, undervalued though it was (Leighow, 1996, pp. 14–15). As with other professions women were able to enter in the early part of the 20th century, most women who were nurses left the profession when they married. Both the limitations imposed on the appropriate professions for women and the expectation that they would leave the workforce once married is reflective of compulsory heterosexuality. Here, the expectations of compulsory heterosexuality demanded women behave certain ways in all settings and, once heterosexually paired, that behavior was oriented toward the reproductive labor of the family rather than wage-earning labor. White femininity here is fused with class expectations. CASSANDRA challenged this narrative.

SEXUALITY AND GENDER IN CASSANDRA

Resisting the gendered dimensions of compulsory heterosexuality that shaped much of nursing, CASSANDRA's efforts connected at radical cultural and lesbian separatist feminist activism to the otherwise sanitary and respectable narrative of Nightingale. This was an act of appropriation that provided an air of legitimacy for CASSANDRA's efforts, a narrative arc for feminist thought (precarious though it may be) in nursing. The aim of CASSANDRA was to "create and develop a group that would truly provide an open forum for feminist nurses from all walks of life and how to avoid the usual male-oriented hierarchy and rigidity of most national organizations" (LaGodna, 1982, p. 1). As mentioned in the introduction, the formation of CASSANDRA was occasioned by founding members' consternation that the American Nurses Association failed to substantively engage with the critical work of the Equal Rights Amendment, part of a longer trajectory of the discipline's refusal to enter women's movements in a formal way. CASSANDRA's founding vision was explicitly woman-identified: "Our primary commitment is to end the oppression of women in all aspects of nursing and health care. We believe that oppression of women is fundamental to all oppressions and affects all women" ("Purposes," 1984, p. 3). First theorized in 1970 by Radicalesbians in a leaflet, the "woman-identified woman" sought to shed the masculine mediation that all too often characterized women's relations to one another. Resisting the notion that "the essence of being a 'woman' is to get fucked by men" (Radicalesbians, 1970, p. 2), woman-identification shifted the focus, emphasizing the "primacy of women relating to women, of women creating a new consciousness of and with each other" (Radicalesbians, 1970, p. 4). In the spirit of avoiding the coercion, seeing the deleterious impact of coercion in compulsory heterosexuality, CASSANDRA was not comprised exclusively of lesbian nurses. However, CASSANDRA was a separatist organization dedicated to creating spaces for nurses who were women to flourish and grow, collectively (Chinn & Wheeler, 1983).

Questions of gender and sexuality were never comfortably settled in CASS-ANDRA's short life. According to some members, CASSANDRA was a balm and respite from the compulsory heteronormativity of nursing and society more broadly (Kagan, 2008c, 2008a). This would prove nourishing and instrumental for many of the lesbian members of CASSANDRA, who reflected on their time with CASSANDRA in both oral history interviews I conducted as well as video interviews recorded by nurse researcher Paula Kagan as part of an unpublished documentary around 2008. But it was also somewhat thorny: some nurses feared publicly associating with CASSANDRA because the link might out them in a hostile environment, a concern raised in Gatherings and the Newsjournal ("REPORT OF THE 1985 CASSANDRA CONTINENTAL GATHERING," 1985). Still other members could not let go of the "what about men" question, which required frequent and tedious justification for the duration of CASSA-NDRA's existence (Kagan, 2008b). While there is little question that CASS-ANDRA was by and for women, the question of sexuality was never really resolved and internalized patriarchal politics frequently mired the organization in hashing (and rehashing) its values. While CASSANDRA was consumed by questions of sexuality, the women of CASSANDRA rarely took up the question of race.

Race and Normative Whiteness

Just as professional nursing inscribes particular expectations around gender and sexuality, the discipline also constructs expectations around race. Echoing the expectations of compulsory heterosexuality, nursing defaults to a normative whiteness, reinforcing a racist hegemony that is insidious and frequently rendered invisible. Nursing mobilizes discourses of white normativity specific to the discipline. For nursing, one dimension of normative whiteness in nursing has been constructed through the alleged conflict between Mary Seacole and Florence Nightingale. In brief, Mary Seacole was a contemporary of Nightingale. Seacole aspired to join Nightingale's nursing ranks but was denied, deemed unfit due to her Creole countenance (Seacole, 2019, p. 57). Seacole went on to establish herself with a hotel near the front at Crimea. The racialized discord between Seacole and Nightingale is not a problem solely of the past, however. Manifest through a white-centered historiographic hegemony, current patterns of normative whiteness in nursing are manufactured in narratives that valorize Nightingale while dismissing Seacole. The vigor with which Nightingale devotees defend and police Nightingale's legacy is both rooted in a nursing imaginary that is white-coded and complicit with white cisheteropatriarchy, entangled products of a shared process.

Though it began, perhaps, in the 19th century at professional nursing's earliest moments, this legacy of normative whiteness persisted (and persists) into the 20th century (and beyond). In the United States, most nurse training programs, as historian Darlene Clark Hine (1989) noted, barred Black nurses, leading to separate schools in the Southern United States and racial quotas for schools in the North. This was part of a project to elevate nursing from its pre-professionalization reputation to a position of respectability. In trading on racialized and gendered tropes of womanhood, early nurse leaders in the United States constructed a white-centered sensibility that necessitated the creation of a parallel "infrastructure of black nursing" to mitigate the threat of white racism in nursing (Hine, 1989). This white sensibility was - and remains - central to the discipline of nursing from its earliest inception in the 19th century. I now turn to the construction of whiteness in CASSANDRA.

RACE AND WHITENESS IN CASSANDRA

If the constructs of gender and sexuality were central to CASSANDRA in ways that both echo and resist the hegemonic expectations of the normative Victorian ethos of nursing, race was afforded little active consideration. While the mission and vision of CASSANDRA pays homage to their openness to nurses from all walks of life ("Purposes," 1984), there is little evidence of active engagement with racial justice in CASSANDRA's newsjournals. When race was treated in the newsjournals, it centered the whiteness of the organization, addressing the racism others might experience using a "we" that consolidated nursing as white, creating distance between the discipline and those who might experience racism, as if the two are mutually exclusive (McDonald, 1987).

There is no evidence that any Women of Color were part of CASSANDRA's polity. Similarly, there is no evidence that race or racism was considered at all during Gatherings or in meetings, based on surviving meeting notes. This kind of silence is quite loud, considering the formation of the National Black Nurses Association and the National Association of Hispanic Nurses less than a decade prior, for reasons parallel to CASSANDRA's - disillusionment that the American Nurses Association could or would address their priorities. And the woman-identfied separatism upon which CASSANDRA was founded further reinforced whiteness, considering the logic of the Combahee River Collective (1978), who rejected lesbian separatism on the basis that it excluded too many and too much, writing

> as Black women we find any type of biological determinism a particularly dangerous and reactionary basis upon which to build a politic. We must also question whether Lesbian separatism is an adequate and progressive political analysis and strategy, even for those who practice it, since it so completely denies any but the sexual sources of women's oppression, negating the facts of class and race. (Combahee River Collective, 1978, para. 15)

Like much of professional nursing past and present, CASSANDRA exercised a kind of unquestioned, uncritical normative whiteness that reinforced the racialized order of nursing, even while carving out radical feminist political space in the disicpline.

Conclusion

The warp and the weft of the contemporary nursing imaginary reside in the discipline's mythology, hagiography, and historiography, which are threaded with Victorian expectations of gender, sexuality, and race. The ideas that structure our present are rooted in centuries-old origin narratives that we choose and keep choosing to tell the stories of what it means to nurse. These narratives are not the only ones that are possible, if we listen and look carefully. There are other points of entry, alternate lines of flight. In some ways, the story of CASSANDRA Radical Feminist Nurses Network is one of these alternate points of entry, a sort of alt-text for the liberal reforms that shaped nursing during the late-20th century. In other ways, however, CASSANDRA, in striving for feminist liberation, actively shored up some of the oppressive dimensions of the discipline of nursing, replicating the normative whiteness of the discipline more broadly. Ultimately, CASSANDRA's voice was quieted, unable to sustain itself as founders (and organizational glue) Charlene Eldridge Wheeler and Peggy Chinn navigated Charlene's ultimately fatal illness (P. Chinn, personal communication, November 25, 2019).

History—including nursing history—is neither singular nor definitive. Interrogating the foundations of nursing's hegemonic narratives can give us different insights into our discipline, its history, and the function of history itself, making alternate stories possible. These alternate stories for the history of nursing may allow folks to see themselves in the discipline, to make it a home. This is the reason to tell the CASSANDRA story. But these stories cannot simply be singular replacement narratives. This risks replicating the same kind of acclamatory myths that anchor nursing history as we know it, albeit with its center shifted. Nursing is messy, complicated, multiple, human. Our disciplinary histories and the stories we tell about this work should reflect this. Rather than dodging that which is messy, uncomfortable, conflicted, problematic, unpacking all of this baggage allows us to see the ways that our present was constructed and maybe, if we can do the work, create a more just, equitable present/future for nurses, for the folks we accompany in care, for the students we teach, for everyone.

Note

1 In a letter quoted in Cook's biography, Nightingale shares her thoughts about her fellow women with Harriet Martineau in 1858, belying an internalized misogyny that undermines those feminist impulses that sparked the authorship of "Cassandra."

References

Anderson, B. (2016). *Imagined communities: Reflections on the origins and spread of nationalism* (Revised). Verso.

Ashley, J. A. (1976). *Hospitals, paternalism and the role of the nurse.* Teachers' College Press. https://repository.library.georgetown.edu/handle/10822/772546

Ashley, J. A. (1980). Power in structured misogyny: Implications for the politics of care. *Advances in Nursing Science, 2*(3), 2.

Carryer, J. (2019). Letting go of our past to claim our future. *Journal of Clinical Nursing,* n/a(n/a). 10.1111/jocn.15016

Chinn, P. (2019, November 25). *Cassandra oral histories (part two)* (J. Dillard-Wright, Interviewer) [Audio recording].

Chinn, P., & Berrey, E. (2014). Cassandra: Lesbian non-presence in nursing. *Sinister Wisdom, 92*(Spring), 50–64.

Chinn, P. L. (2008). Lesbian nurses: What's the big deal? *Issues in Mental Health Nursing, 29*(6), 551–554. 10.1080/01612840802046604

Chinn, P., & Wheeler, C. (1983). Report of the gathering. *Cassandra Radical Feminist Newsjournal, 1*(3), 4–9. Peggy Chinn, personal electronic archive.

Combahee River Collective. (1978). *The combahee river collective statement.* circuitous. org/scraps/combahee.html

Cook, S. E. T. (1914). *The life of Florence Nightingale: 1862-1910.* Macmillan.

D'Antonio, P. (2006). History for a practice profession. *Nursing Inquiry, 13*(4), 242–248. 10.1111/j.1440-1800.2006.00332.x

de Certeau, M. (1988). *The writing of history.* T. Conley (Trans.). Columbia University Press.

Enloe, C. (2021). Femininity and the paradox of trust building in patriarchies during COVID-19. *Signs: Journal of Women in Culture and Society, 47*(1), 3–10. 10.1086/715260

Faderman, L. (1981). *Surpassing the love of men: Romantic friendship and love between women from the renaissance to the present.* Quill William Morrow.

Foth, T., Lange, J., & Smith, K. (2018). Nursing history as philosophy—Towards a critical history of nursing. *Nursing Philosophy, 19*(3), e12210. 10.1111/nup.12210

Foucault, M. (1984). Nietzsche, genealogy, history. In P. Rabinow (Ed.), *The foucault reader* (pp. 76–100). Pantheon Books.

Hine, D. C. (1989). *Black women in white: Racial conflict and cooperation in the nursing profession, 1890-1950.* Indiana University Press.

Hunter, J. (1984). Historical & Resolution; Series II; File 38. *Juanita Hunter, RN & NYSNA Papers [1973-1990].* https://digitalcommons.buffalostate.edu/jhunter-papers/136

Hunter, M., & Times, S. T., the N. Y. (1982, June 25). Leaders concede loss on equal rights. *The New York Times.* https://www.nytimes.com/1982/06/25/us/leaders-concede-loss-on-equal-rights.html

Kagan, P. (2008a). *Interview with carol ashton, tape 1* [Interview]. Unpublished interview transcripts, Paula Kagan's private collection.

Kagan, P. (2008b). *Interview with peggy chinn, tape 2* [Interview]. Unpublished interview transcripts, Paula Kagan's private collection.

Kagan, P. (2008c). *Interview with Sue Dibble and Jeanne DeJoseph, tape 1* [Interview]. Unpublished interview transcripts, Paula Kagan's private collection.

LaGodna, G. (1982). Cassandra: A report of beginnings. *Cassandra Radical Feminist Nurses Newsletter, 1*(1), 1–2. Peggy Chinn, personal electronic archive.

Leighow, S. R. (1996). *Nurses' questions, women's questions: The impact of the demographic revolution and feminism on the united states working women, 1946-1986.* Peter Lang Publishing.

Lerner, G. (1975). Placing women in history: Definitions and challenges. *Feminist Studies, 3*(1/2), 5–14. 10.2307/3518951

McDonald, N. P. (1987). Racism in nursing practice. *Cassandra Radical Feminist Nurses Newsjournal, 5*(2), 20–22. Peggy Chinn, personal electronic archive.

Millett, K. (2016). *Sexual politics.* Columbia University Press.

Muff, J. (1982). Handmaiden, battle-ax, whore: An exploration into the fantasies, myths, and stereotypes about nurses. In J. Muff (Ed.), *Women's issues in nursing: Socialization, sexism, and stereotyping* (pp. 113–156). Waveland Press, Inc.

Nelson, S. (1997). Reading nursing history. *Nursing Inquiry, 4*(4), 229–236. 10.1111/j.1440-1800.1997.tb00108.x

Nelson, S., & Gordon, S. (2004). The rhetoric of rupture: Nursing as a practice with a history? *Nursing Outlook, 52*(5), 255–261. 10.1016/j.outlook.2004.08.001

Nightingale, F. (1968). *Notes on nursing: What it is, and what it is not.* Dover Publications.

Nightingale, F. (1979). *Cassandra: Angry outcry against the forced idleness of victorian women.* Feminist Press.

Peggy, L. C. (1982). What's in our name? *Cassandra Radical Feminist Nurses Newsletter, 1*(1), 3–5.

Purposes. (1984). *Cassandra Radical Feminist Nurses News Journal*, 2(1), 3. Peggy Chinn, personal electronic archive.

Radicalesbians. (1970). *The woman-identified woman*. Atlanta Lesbian Feminist Alliance, Duke University Digital Repository. https://idn.duke.edu/ark:/87924/r3gx1t

Randall, C., & Eliason, M. (2012). Out lesbians in nursing: What would florence say? *Journal of Lesbian Studies*, 16(1), 65–75. 10.1080/10894160.2011.557644

Report of the 1985 cassandra continental gathering. (1985). *Cassandra Radical Feminist Nurses News Journal*, 3(3), 3–12. Peggy Chinn, personal electronic archive.

Reverby, S. (1987). *Ordered to care* (1st ed.). Cambridge University Press.

Rich, A. (1980). Compulsory heterosexuality and lesbian existence. *Signs*, 5(4), 631–660.

Ruchti, L. (2012). *Catheters, slurs, and pickup lines: Professional intimacy in hospital nursing*. Temple University Press.

Seacole, M. (2019). *Wonderful adventures of Mrs. Seacole in many lands*. Dover Thrift Editions.

Searle, J. (2019). Compulsory heterosexuality and lesbian invisibility in nursing. *Creative Nursing*, 25(2), 121–125. 10.1891/1078-4535.25.2.121

Shamas, L. (2011, July 13). Understanding the myth: Why cassandra must not be silenced. *On the Issues: A Magazine of Feminist, Progressive Thinking, Summer 2011*. https://www.ontheissuesmagazine.com/2011summer/cafe2.php?id=163

Showalter, E. (1981). Florence nightingale's feminist complaint: Women, religion, and "Suggestions for Thought." *Signs*, 6(3), 395–412.

Smith-Rosenberg, C., & Rosenberg, C. (1973). The female animal: Medical and biological views of woman and her role in nineteenth-century America. *The Journal of American History*, 60(2), 332–356. 10.2307/2936779

Stark, M. (1979). Introduction. In *Cassandra: Angry outcry against the forced idleness of victorian women* (pp. 1–23). Feminist Press.

Threat, C. (2015). *Nursing civil rights: Gender and race in the army nurse corps*. University of Illinois Press.

3 Madeleine Knows Best: Culture, Race, and Whiteness in the Discipline of Nursing

Cory Ellen Gatrall

In 2017, Facebook user Onyx Moore posted a screenshot of a page from her nursing textbook. A table titled "Focus on Diversity and Culture" contained a bullet-point list of "Cultural Differences in Response to Pain:" "Muslim clients must endure pain as a sign of faith," it stated, and "may not request pain medication but instead thank Allah." "Jews may be vocal and demanding of assistance," and "believe that pain must be shared and validated by others." "Blacks often report higher pain intensity than other cultures," but Native Americans "usually tolerate a high level of pain without requesting pain medication." The text below the table exhorted nurses to "approach each client with cultural competence" (Moore, 2017).

Moore's Facebook post went viral. The internet collectively gasped and expressed shock that such blatant stereotyping in the guise of education could exist in this day and age. Nurses themselves, however, were mostly unsurprised; many had seen similar tables in their own textbooks in nursing school, in whatever course they had that included cultural content. And the chances were excellent that any nurse looking at Facebook in 2017 had had some such course. Since the National League for Nursing published its "Cultural Dimensions in the Baccalaureate Nursing Curriculum" in 1977, "cultural competence" and related concepts such as "cultural congruence," "cultural sensitivity," and "cultural humility" have become increasingly central to US nursing and nursing education.

These related terms are most often invoked in the context of health (in) equity and disparities, as guiding frameworks which will enable the nurse who implements them to provide better care to individual patients and communities. But the concepts themselves have remained elusive. "Cultural competence," for example, is defined variously by the American Association of Colleges of Nursing (2021) as "the ability to effectively work within the client's cultural context;" by the American Nurses Association (2017) as "the process by which nurses demonstrate culturally congruent practice;[1]" and by the Department of Health and Human Services (2013) as "the capacity for individuals and organizations to work and communicate effectively in cross-cultural situations."

There is, to speak plainly, a lot to unpack here. And people have begun to unpack it, with a litany of critiques including the reification of essentialized

DOI: 10.4324/9781003245957-5

definitions of culture, the futility of placing the burden of systemic change on individual interactions rather than structural forces, and the challenges of measuring outcomes (Drevdahl et al., 2008; Drevdahl, 2018; Kleinman & Benson, 2019; Metzl & Roberts, 2014). Scholars have begun to propose alternate models for moving forward, including an increasingly popular iteration called "structural competency" which locates the immediate encounter between patient and clinician in a web of systems, and encourages providers to intervene at macro as well as micro levels (Metzl & Hansen, 2014; Metzl & Roberts, 2014; Orr & Unger, 2020). Yet relatively little attention has been paid to how we arrived at this place, and how so much energy became invested in such an unstable concept. In replacing one approach with another, it is critical to understand not only what is wrong with the current approach, but how it came to be wrong.

All of the definitions of cultural competence given above rely on several implicit assumptions: first, that the nurse and the patient inhabit separate social spheres, separated by an invisible barrier; second, that this invisible barrier is an identifiable, discrete entity called "culture;" and third, that should the nurse navigate this barrier successfully, they will offer "effective" nursing work. Together, these assumptions represent a lopsided amalgam of ideas from academic disciplines and social movements which often used the same words to mean not quite the same thing. The weight given to particular meanings in this accretion was the outcome of racialized power structures and the relative positions held within them by those assigning meaning.

This paper seeks to tease apart the tangled threads of the culture concept in nursing. My tripartite goal is to provide an overview of how (1) "culture" supplanted "race" as the locus of human difference in the early 20th century; (2) "culture" became defined, bounded, and leveraged to center White comfort; and (3) the "culture" concept was then upheld and defended by those in power against efforts to center a different model of culture in nursing—one rooted in anticolonial philosophy and the health activism of the US civil rights movement.

No story is told without a standpoint or a frame. I come to this work as a cisgender, white, queer, Jewish woman; as a former doula and current nurse who has provided care primarily in reproductive health settings, including labor/delivery and abortion, but also in public health during the COVID-19 pandemic; as an activist who has served in the field of reproductive health, rights, and access; and as a scholar whose first degree was in anthropology. These identities and experiences shape both my interest in and my understanding of the story I tell here. I also situate my understanding of this story within theoretical frameworks of racialization, symbolic violence, and Black feminist theory, which collectively direct my attention toward the ways in which individuals and institutions both attain and negotiate their racialized identities within larger systems, which are themselves also racialized (Barbee, 1993; Davis, 2007; Fassin, 2011; Gallagher, 2020; Hall, 2017, 2019; Hill Collins, 1991; Roberts, 2011).

The Prehistory of Culture in Nursing

Madeleine Leininger, chief architect of academic nursing's engagement with culture, first encountered anthropology in clinical seminars with the iconic Margaret Mead at the University of Cincinnati in the late 1950s. Mead, having blown up American ideas about sex and adolescence some 30 years earlier with her best-selling ethnography, *Coming of Age in Samoa*, had just become a Visiting Professor in the Department of Psychiatry, where Leininger was Director of the Child Psychiatric Nursing Program (Leininger, 2010; Wolfskill, 2009). Leininger was impressed at how Mead "superbly challenged" clinicians in the seminars she attended, asking them whether they had considered cultural factors when making their diagnoses. She recalled that a "dead silence" followed such questions, reflecting "a void in professional knowledge to understand the patient's cultural behavior and needs" (Leininger, 1978, p. 6).

Although Leininger was correct that the "culture" framework was not yet comfortably ensconced in either nursing or medicine, professional nursing had been acutely attentive to racialized categories of social difference from its beginning. In 1913, an afternoon session of the very first annual meeting of the National Organization of Public Health Nursing (NOPHN) was devoted to the issues encountered by nurses working with immigrant families. An attendee later reported that "every nurse present ... was convinced that she needs to know more of the background and of the social psychology of our foreign friends in order to do effective work. The emotional Italian, the idealistic Jew, and the stolid Slav must be reached by different paths" (Patterson, 1913, p. 15).

The public health nurse's "effective work" was that of a double agent: while venturing forth to relieve suffering and prevent disease among her "friends," whether foreign-born or formerly enslaved, she also strove to prevent suffering and disease from reaching native-born White people. Presenters at the NOPHN meeting elaborated not only on the social and health problems faced by new immigrants, but also the threat those problems (and, by extension, those immigrants) posed to the non-immigrant communities around them (Mayper, 1913). At the third annual meeting of the NOPHN, dire warnings echoed about the same threat posed by southern Black domestic workers: "[E]ach dish we eat is fraught with danger from their diseases," intoned Dr. Charles E. Terry, who had only recently stepped down as president of the American Public Health Association. "[I]n a multitude of unmentioned and no few unmentionable ways ... are we and our children daily made victims of the most unnecessary exposures" (Terry, 1916, p. 36; Fee, 2011).[2]

Dr. Terry could refer to *they* and *we* without too much regard for nuance in this setting, not least because the field of professional nursing was, per 1920 census records, 97% white (D'Antonio & Whelan, 2009). While Black nurses were a growing and organized constituency[3], they were challenged by white supremacist structures at every turn, from training to licensure to wages to advancement— even by barriers arising from the nursing field's own drive for professionalization (Hine, 1989). In the arena of public health nursing, however, Black nurses negotiated a space in which they could provide care to Black communities (D'Antonio, 2017; Hine, 1989; Roberts, 2009). Ethel Johns, the white Englishwoman who authored the 1925 *Report on the Present Status of Negro Women in Nursing* at the behest of the Rockefeller Foundation, highlighted Black nurses' superior communication skills even as she repeatedly dismissed their authority and intellect, citing their "better psychological approach" and "intuitive understanding of racial characteristics" (Johns, 1925, p. 33).

Johns' perception that Black nurses were *only* suited for community work with Black patients *and* that they could do work white nurses could not in that context—"ferret out information and interpret domestic complications" (Johns, 1925, p. 33)—reflected a contemporary understanding of racial categories as simultaneously biological and social, and, above all, inherently hierarchical. This was in keeping with Enlightenment and 19th-century race science, which had produced a taxonomy of racial categories, supposedly biologically distinct and conveniently ranked to justify existing settler colonialism, genocide, and enslavement (Roberts, 2011).

Race, nationality, language, and religion were conflated, as the 18th-century charts setting Europeans at the top and Africans at the bottom were expanded during the height of early 20th-century immigration to include European groups such as Poles, Italians, and "Hebrews" (Kevles, 1985). The eugenics movement, which claimed it could improve humanity through the scientific management of heredity, was in its heyday. While individual public health nurses may (or may not) have been conflicted as to the merits of eugenics, they could not ignore it: eugenics influenced a range of scientific disciplines, and was classed as natural science alongside biology, zoology, and mathematics (Buhler-Wilkinson, 1989; Pernick, 1996, 1997).

Race was also central to the work of the new social scientists, including social psychologists, sociologists such as W.E.B. DuBois, and anthropologists such as Franz Boas, whose body of work during the early 20th century challenged the scientific basis for racial hierarchies, and contributed to the popular decline of eugenics (King, 2019; Ross, 1991; Stocking, Jr., 1992; Visweswaran, 2010). Through scientific work and popular writings, Boas and other anthropologists of the early 20th century directly challenged the eugenicists, asserting that the important differences between groups of people were social and learned, rather than hereditary—in other words, cultural. Boas and his students, including Ruth Benedict and Margaret Mead, did not discard the concept of race, but sought to defang it, turning it into a purely biological category which they saw as value-neutral. By the mid-1930s, as eugenics began to lose its sheen among many scientists because of its association with Nazism, anthropologists loudly and publicly reiterated the importance of demoting "race" and promoting "culture" (Kevles, 1985; Visweswaran, 2010).

This emphasis on the primacy of culture over race played an important role in delegitimizing scientific racism, and influenced Supreme Court desegregation cases such as *Brown v. Board of Education* (Baker, 1998). But it was hardly the panacea for discrimination that its proponents envisioned. Federal and state sterilization programs continued and, in some cases, even expanded in the decades following World War II, targeting populations based on racialized categories of economic dependency, juvenile delinquency, and high birthrates (Kevles, 1985).

As Kamala Visweswaran has argued, "separating race from racism ... left no means for anthropologists to understand how racism produces the objective reality of race at any given historical moment" (Visweswaran, 2010, p. 60). The inability of anthropology to speak about racism left a void—what Visweswaran calls "relativist outlines ... filled by racist content" (67). This empty space became home to cultural essentialism, the idea that cultures themselves are the source of intractable difference. Race continued to operate beneath the surface of culture—as it had beneath the surface of class, religion, and nationality before; as it would beneath other categories later—functioning as what Stuart Hall names a "floating signifier:" a conceptual signpost without a fixed referent (Hall, 2017). And this mid-century moment, when this culturalist approach was attaining maturity, was the moment when anthropology and nursing were formally introduced.

Social Science and Nursing

The Great Depression, World War II, and the mid-1940s passage of the Bolton and Hill Burton Acts—which poured unprecedented federal funding into nurse training and hospital construction respectively—had drastically reshaped the professional landscape. As nursing leaders strategized about how to both increase their numbers and how to advance their field in terms of professional respectability, they turned their eye on nursing education (National Nursing Council & Newell, 1951).

Shortly after the war ended, the National Nursing Council asked social anthropologist Esther Lucile Brown to conduct a study of the nursing profession, and to make recommendations for how nursing education might meet the predicted needs of a society whose health needs were rapidly increasing and changing in nature. In her influential 1948 report, *Nursing for the Future*, Brown emphasized the necessity of an educational "foundation that permits continuing growth of many kinds," including "cultural patterns that condition human behavior" (Brown, 1948, p. 138). Six years later, Brown conspired with Dean Virginia Dunbar to create an experimental course at Cornell University-New York Hospital School called "Psychosocial and Cultural Aspects of Nursing" (Dunbar, ca. 1953).

The social scientist selected to lead this course was Frances Cooke Macgregor, a sociologist and photographer eventually best known for her work on disfigurement and disability. In 1951, Macgregor had published a photography book with Margaret Mead, who had some years earlier been her teacher; she now asked Mead, who was Associate Curator of Ethnology for the American Museum of Natural History, to contribute to the new course. For each session, from 1954 through 1957, Mead provided guest lectures.

Several themes which appeared in this course laid the groundwork for nursing's ongoing approach to teaching culture. The first of these was the idea that cultural understanding was, perhaps above all, the key to making life simpler for the nurse and increasing patient compliance. Introducing the course, MacGregor framed interaction with patients of "different cultures" as "a potential source of daily problems within the hospital" (Macgregor, 1960, p. 66); in a later article titled "Uncooperative Patients," she addressed the nurse's "frustration of not being able to get patients to do what one wants them to do even when it is for their own good," warning that "unless the nurse learns to think in cultural terms ... she will continue to be baffled, if not exasperated, on such occasions"(Macgregor, 1967, pp. 37–38) Mead similarly counseled that "[c]ultural differences ... may be regarded as complications which do least harm when they are most articulately recognized" (Mead, 1956, p. 260). Works recommending the inclusion of cultural content in nursing education often prioritized this promise of easing the work of nurses challenged by patient diversity even over the goal of improving patient care.

Mead encouraged students to consider not only the cultural construction of such nursing issues as nutrition, birth, and death, but also of their own roles as nurses; the cultural vantage point from which they were to consider this, however, Mead and Macgregor both termed "American." In encouraging "American" nurses to familiarize themselves with particular cultures they might encounter, Mead cited case studies including Italian, Jewish, Puerto Rican, Navajo, and "Southern Negro" patients. If the nurse being addressed was American, then these patients were all implicitly *other than* American; and, by logical extension, people of Italian, Jewish, Puerto Rican, Navajo, and "Southern Negro" culture were excluded from the defined category of "nurse" (Macgregor, 1960; Mead, 1956).

One consequence of this promotion of cultural understanding as a convenience strategy for nurses was the "checklist" approach to cultural diversity. Mead, as guest lecturer, recounted the tale of a nurse who had come to her some years earlier "'to get a chart of racial differences,' which would explain, in one lecture, all that was necessary to know about patients' backgrounds" (Macgregor, 1960, p. 82) As no such chart existed or - she believed - could be feasibly made, she recommended (in a separate but contemporaneous article) that students instead develop an awareness of the sorts of behaviors which might be culturally determined. Such awareness would help the nurse suspend judgment of her patients, and "allow for whimsies and strange requests without becoming resentful" (Mead, 1956, p. 261). While Mead did not advocate the development of checklists, and in fact warned against oversimplification, she and others promoting culture to nursing were not immune to the demands of their target audience; her description of the earlier nurse's request foreshadowed later efforts to produce such quick reference guides for textbooks.

In this course, Mead and Macgregor also established culture as the analytical framework that would save "American" nurses from having to engage with those issues which made them most uncomfortable: race, religion, and class.

Macgregor argued that in the "age when a cult of tolerance has tended to conjure away all sense of ethnic, racial, and religious difference," anthropology would help students to discuss cultural difference without resort to prejudice (Macgregor, 1960, p. 72). Mead, invoking the recent Holocaust in Europe and ongoing struggles against segregation in the United States, held that focus on culture implied a democratic approach, without judgment. "By emphasizing culture ... we then come to realize," she said, "that race is irrelevant" (Mead, 1956, p. 262).[4]

The replacement of the contested and contentious categories of race, religion, and class with culture allowed "American" (white, Christian) nurses access to the social context of their patients' lives without requiring them to acknowledge, much less confront, political and structural systems of oppression. Nonetheless, for the nursing students of the Cornell University-New York Hospital School, this course felt revelatory. "I never realized how little I knew, how much I need to know, and how complex human behavior is," read one anonymous evaluation (Macgregor, 1960, p. 237). Another student, having recognized that her patient "was of Jewish faith," which "might account for some of his outward expression of pain," reported that her changed understanding made the encounter "more pleasant for both of us ... the complaining and the whining were still present, but when properly understood, the patient was no trouble at all" (Macgregor, 1960, p. 227).

Macgregor was also pleased with the outcome of the educational experiment. In her 1960 report, she concluded that "Nurses who plan to teach social science ... should take more advanced courses of the kind offered by the graduate departments of universities" (Macgregor, 1960, p. 305). She did not believe—nor did Esther Lucile Brown—that nurses necessarily required PhDs in social science disciplines in order to reap their benefits. However, as nursing leaders were seeking strategies to increase their ranks, confirmation of the value of social science preparation for nurses provided a compelling opportunity for professional advancement.

"We are crying for teachers," wrote Lucile Petry Leone, leader of the US Public Health Service's Division of Nurse Education, in 1955. "Our line of attack, then, is to increase the number of paid leaves of absence and scholarships for advanced study" (Leone, 1955). Nurse Traineeship grants were made available that same year, which enabled nurses to pursue research and predoctoral study. In 1962, the Division of Nursing additionally created the Nurse-Scientist Graduate Training Grants, which provided funding directly to university departments of social and behavioral sciences to subsidize doctoral study for nurses. By 1967, departments at seven universities were participating in the program; at every one of those schools, nurses were seeking PhDs in anthropology.

Leininger's Two Worlds

Immediately following Macgregor's three-year course, in 1957 Mead took up her position at the University of Cincinnati, where her piercing questions soon inspired Madeleine Leininger to seek further education in anthropology[5]. Leininger received a Fellowship from the Division of Nursing to study with Dr. Kenneth Read at the University of Washington (Abdellah, 1963). Read had been a student of S.F. Nadel, whose lineage of British social anthropology heavily influenced Leininger's 1966 dissertation, an "ethnopsychological comparative study" of two villages in the Eastern Highlands of New Guinea (Leininger, 1966a). That same year, Leininger went to teach at the University of Colorado, where she developed a course called "Cultural Dimensions in Nursing:" her handwritten note on a copy of the syllabus describes it as the "first course on culture and nursing in USA and overseas" (Leininger, 1966b). As Mead had been actively engaged with Macgregor's course immediately prior to her encounter with Leininger, it seems improbable that Leininger was wholly unaware of that course, however such embellishment was typical of Leininger, who throughout her career would fiercely claim ownership of nursing's approach to cultural theorizing.

In her 1970 book, *Nursing and Anthropology: Two Worlds to Blend*, Leininger presented a view of "culture" that aligned with the anthropology of her era. She defined the concept for her nursing audience using the words of anthropologist Melville Herskovits: "the man-made part of the environment" (Leininger, 1970, p. 48). She explained that culture was not biologically inherited, but transmitted intergenerationally through socialization practices. She even noted that labels for "major population groups" were subject to misinterpretation when used to ascribe "racial and hereditary inferiorities or superiorities to different population groups" (Leininger, 1970, p. 10).

Yet Leininger's application of anthropology to the field of nursing highlighted both her own biases and the way in which cultural boundaries could be constructed and adjusted to reify established racialized hierarchies. In this text, she presented a case study of an "Afro-American" nurse from the northern US assigned to care for a southern "Afro-American" patient. The nurse, "Mona," was uncomfortable with the patient and provided minimal care. When the head nurse spoke to her about it, Mona stated, "He appears like me. He belongs to my group, but I think I am different. If I spend time with Alex, the staff will think I am like him." Mona, said Leininger, was experiencing "ambivalent feelings about her own cultural identity," which she eventually resolved over the course of the patient's stay as she "learned that there are subcultural differences between Afro-American groups in the United States" (Leininger, 1970, p. 95).

While Leininger did not use the word "race" in this text—or at all in any of the archival documents that I have reviewed—the utterance she ascribed to (the likely invented) Mona reflected an understanding of racialized identity based in biology: "He appears like me. He belongs to my group." Yet while biology was the unifier, culture was the separator: somehow, Mona's personal understanding of "subcultural" differences removed her from her patient's "group," and thereby solved the problem. Leininger's analysis through the lens of culture obfuscated the experience of racism implicit in her own narrative: after all, why should Mona be concerned about her coworkers' perception that she was "like" Alex, unless she knew such similarity would be held against her?

Leininger doubled down on her acrobatic elision of racism when she posited that nurses from "particular cultural groups which are currently looked down upon by other cultural ... groups" might be challenged in serving patients from shared backgrounds due to self-hate. Just as Mona's "most patient and understanding"—and presumably white – head nurse had walked her through her experience, "listen[ing] to Mona's feelings about herself and the patient as Mona continued her work," Leininger recommended that nurses experiencing similar difficulties "have supervision from qualified nurse-anthropologists" (Leininger, 1970, p. 86). This was the first appearance of a regular theme in her published and unpublished work: distrust of the lived experience of people of color as a basis for authority in engaging with, interpreting, or teaching cultural matters (Leininger, 1980).

While Leininger had been instrumental in founding the Council on Nursing and Anthropology (CONAA) within the American Anthropological Association in 1968, she soon concluded that her path lay elsewhere. In 1974, to the dismay of some fellow nurse-anthropologists who felt she was undermining their efforts to have anthropology taken seriously by nursing, Leininger founded the Transcultural Nursing Society, which became the major force behind the academic study of culture and nursing from that time onward. She quickly established masters and doctoral programs in this new subfield, and within a few years began to publicly assert that a doctorate in anthropology was not enough to teach culture in the field of nursing; only preparation in Transcultural Nursing would suffice.

Providing Safe Nursing Care for Ethnic People of Color

While Leininger avoided naming race or racism, she could not escape the subject entirely in the wake of the 1960s, when dismal health outcomes for people of color were being actively discussed in both elite public health circles and major newspapers. She regularly exercised racialized proxy terms such as "culturally disadvantaged," "culturally deprived," and "the four federally defined minority cultures" in addressing policy matters, such as when she asserted that the public health focus on "'culturally disadvantaged and deprived' groups" was inappropriate. While she did not claim that the health outcomes of these groups were equal to those of non-minority populations, she attributed disparities to the fact that some "economically deprived cultural groups" prioritized other matters over health; presuming that they should do otherwise, she said, was an example of ethnocentrism and cultural imposition (Leininger, 1970, p. 52).

But try as she might, Leininger did not hold a monopoly on the conversation about nursing and culture. In 1976, Marie Branch and Phyllis Perry Paxton published *Providing Safe Nursing Care for Ethnic People of Color*, which named racism as "a factor in disease causation" and called for the validation of nursing textbooks by "ethnic people of color belonging to the particular group under discussion at the time" (Branch & Paxton, 1976, pp. 130, 134). Branch had traveled to China with the Black Panther Party in 1972, and had co-founded the Alprentice "Bunchy" Carter People's Free Medical Clinic in 1969 (Branch, 1973; Nelson, 2011, p. 62). The framework of "ethnic humanism" that she proposed in this textbook drew from the wellspring of Frantz Fanon, the Martinican psychiatrist, revolutionary, and anticolonial philosopher whose work was central to the health activism of the Black Panther Party (Nelson, 2011, p. 65).

Branch and Paxton were not alone in centering matters of culture, race, and racism in health equity. While nursing journals of this period continued to publish articles by white nurses with titles like "Working with others who are not like me" (Kegley & Savier, 1983), a new genre of work began to appear in their pages as well: articles about culture by nurses who, like Branch and Paxton, explicitly identified themselves within their text as members of the group they were discussing. These works collectively deployed culture as a source of community strength and political alliance: a potential resource rather than a deficit. They were adamant that the cultures of people who have experienced structural oppression cannot be fully accessed by those who do not share them, and that the absence of shared culture in the context of systemic racism endangers patients. While authors felt it was imperative to educate white nurses about how to care for Black and other patients of color, they advocated vehemently in these articles and elsewhere for the recruitment, education, and retention of more nurses of color to care for their communities (Branch, 1977; Pegues, 1979; Primeaux, 1977; Rodriguez, 1983).

The degree to which culture, race, and ethnicity were treated as social as opposed to biological varied among—and sometimes within—articles of this genre. "Caring for the American Indian patient" emphasized the "intimacy of religion and medicine" for American Indian families, and went on to focus on values, beliefs, kinship structures, and health care practices—in other words, the social (Primeaux, 1977). "Mexican Americans" addressed social but also epidemiological concerns, specifying that these conditions were related to poverty (e.g., tuberculosis) and stress (e.g., alcoholism) rather than any intrinsic biologic vulnerability (Rodriguez, 1983). Thelma Pegues centered biology, in the form of assessment guidance for darker skin, in "Physical and psychological assessment of the Black patient," congruent with her definition of "Black" as "an ethnic, genetic assimilation of people whose language, behavior and characteristics change ... linked together by a commonality in heritage and identifiable by the color of their skin." Echoing Marie Branch, Pegues drove home an important point early in her piece: "[S]ince ours is a racist society, the effect of race on the health and well being of the client must also be recognized." (Pegues, 1979, p. 4).

This last approach, taken most often by Black nurses, explicitly naming racism and treating race as simultaneously social, embodied, and *political*, deeply unsettled white nursing academics. Anthropologist Noel Chrisman, who taught in a school of nursing, summed up his objections to this "widespread and dangerous set of beliefs" at the time: "in my view, this approach (a) obscures the very different meanings of race (a biological concept) and ethnicity (a cultural concept) and (b) inappropriately reinforces a biological, and potentially stereotypic, view of minority groups in American society" (Chrisman, 1982, p. 125). Notably, Chrisman did not apply this same critique to contemporary works by white researchers which pathologized Black and Brown bodies as intrinsically deficient.

Leininger also responded to what she perceived as an incursion into her territory. She asserted in public speeches that Transcultural Nursing was "not an affirmative action program to retain or recruit a few ethnic groups into nursing. It is much more than that ... Transcultural nursing focuses on all cultures in the world and their nursing and health care practices and not a few Federally defined minority cultures" (Leininger, 1978). She even objected in writing to the American Nurses Association's establishment of an Intercultural Council, which was charged with supporting cultural diversity in nursing curricula. She proposed that the ANA instead institute a Transcultural Nursing Council, and further threatened that if this were not done, she would take her business elsewhere and open such a council under another disciplinary umbrella: anthropology (Leininger, 1978).

The two most progressive textbooks of this era, *Providing Safe Nursing Care for Ethnic People of Color* and *Ethnic Nursing Care: A Multicultural Approach* (Soberano Orque et al., 1983), were both well (if infrequently) reviewed, yet neither was widely adopted into nursing school curricula (Diers, 1984; Evelyn Barbee, personal communication, April 15, 2019; Hudak, 1977). University-based schools of nursing, dominated by white faculty who were teaching predominantly white students, had little incentive to adopt a model of culture which challenged white comfort. And, of course, Madeleine Leininger—university dean, prolific author, journal editor, and founder of two professional organizations—continued her denunciations from the pulpit in the years that followed. In the first issue of her Journal of Transcultural Nursing, she blamed "minority nurses who wanted to control and establish their 'ethnic' teaching programs about 'their culture'" for "limit[ing] progress" of transcultural nursing (Leininger, 1989).

In 1992, the American Academy of Nursing issued a report by its newly formed Expert Panel on Culturally Competent Nursing Care that used "cross-cultural" rather than "transcultural" as its term of art, and centered health disparities and equity in its rationale and recommendations (Davis et al., 1992). Leininger was incensed, firing off a letter to the editor accusing the panel of ignoring her contributions to the field as well as "feminine jealousy, hunger for group image and status, [and] female competition." She claimed that she had coined the term "culturally competent care" years earlier – a claim she would repeat often thereafter – and warned of "real danger and many potential problems with a panel focusing mainly on 'minority populations'" (Leininger, 1993). The panel responded diplomatically but firmly in the pages of the same issue: "It is a fact that in many societies such groups exist, and their health is frequently affected by their relationships with the dominant culture" (Meleis et al., 1993).

Conclusion

It may be tempting to say simply that whiteness became centered in nursing's academic approach to culture because nursing academia has been overwhelmingly white. One could say so, and not be entirely wrong, but it would be far too facile. This centering of whiteness was neither natural consequence nor historical inevitability. Rather it was the aggregation of a thousand moments, of concrete actions by individuals and organizations, accumulating over many years: who hired whom into this and such position, who denied whom a letter of recommendation, whose grant proposal was approved and whose letter of protest went ignored. Whose theoretical construct was enthusiastically embraced, and whose was written off as biased. The story of how whiteness became the central organizing framework of culture in nursing is, like so many others, a story of how white supremacy maintains and reproduces itself.

In telling this story, it is not my intention to rewrite a hero into a villain, nor to attribute to Madeleine Leininger more importance than she actually held. Leininger's multiple roles converged to make her not only a powerful voice but also a powerful gatekeeper, with great influence in shaping the way nursing approached research generally and came to understand culture specifically. Yet just as examining health inequity only through the lens of individual-level racism is insufficient, it is insufficient to view the current state of culture in nursing only through the lens of Madeleine Leininger. We must ask two central questions: why was the discipline of nursing so eager to accept the depoliticized, ostensibly colorblind view of "culture" promulgated by white academics (including Leininger), and why has it stubbornly clung to this view even when offered ample evidence and opportunity for change?

A partial answer may lie in nursing's historical quest for respectability, as both a profession and a discipline closely associated with femininity. Applying the racialized organization theory of Victor Ray (2019), we can see how nursing has contested its gendered devaluation by leveraging its whiteness (1) as a credential for access to resources both within and without, (2) as a legitimizing force to reinscribe racial hierarchy and justify inequitable resource distribution, and (3) to expand the agency of white nurses while constraining the agency of Black and other nurses of color (Ray, 2019). As the discipline has fought to solidify its academic institutions and claim intellectual authority, whiteness remains central to its armament (Tobbell, 2018).

Recognizing the entrenchment of whiteness is not, of course, tantamount to uprooting it. But identifying the warp yarns of race and racism running through the long history of nursing's engagement with ideas of social difference may attune us to how they are functioning in the present moment. Onyx Moore's (2017) Facebook post is just one example of that persistence, and of nursing's vested interest in maintaining the status quo of depoliticized (and therefore deeply political) academic respectability and white supremacy.

Notes

1 "Culturally congruent practice is the application of *evidence-based* nursing that is in agreement with the preferred cultural values, beliefs, worldview, and practices of the healthcare consumer and other stakeholders (emphasis mine)" (Marion et al., 2017).
2 This "race infection" argument was a direct echo from the not-so-distant era of Reconstruction, when segregated hospitals were established for previously enslaved people (Gamble, 1995).
3 The National Association of Colored Graduate Nurses was founded in 1908, and by 1920 had 500 members (Hine, 1989).
4 Fourteen years later, Mead would express regret about this assertion in a recorded conversation with James Baldwin. "I was speaking in those days about three things we had to do: appreciate cultural differences, respect political and religious differences and ignore race. Absolutely ignore race ... This was wrong, because ... skin color can't be ignored. It is real" (Mead & Baldwin, 1971, p. 8).
5 Late in her life, Leininger took credit for having brought Margaret Mead to the University of Cincinnati. I have not been able to either verify or disprove this claim (Pamela N. Clarke et al., 2009).

References

Abdellah, F. G. (1963). *Correspondence* (Folder 1–7). Archives of Caring in Nursing, Christine E. Lynn College of Nursing, Florida Atlantic University.

American Association of Colleges of Nursing. (2021). *The essentials: Core competencies for professional nursing education*. American Association of Colleges of Nursing. https://www.aacnnursing.org/Portals/42/AcademicNursing/CurriculumGuidelines/Cultural-Competency-Bacc-Edu.pdf

Baker, L. D. (1998). *From savage to negro: Anthropology and the construction of race, 1896–1954*. University of California Press.

Barbee, E. L. (1993). Racism in U. S. nursing. *Medical Anthropology Quarterly, 7*(4), 346–362. 10.1525/maq.1993.7.4.02a00040

Branch, M. (1973). A Black American nurse visits the People's Republic of China. In *Nursing Forum* (Vol. 12, No. 4, pp. 402–411). Blackwell Publishing Ltd.

Branch, M. (1977). Catch up or keep up? Ethnic Minorities in Nursing. *Urban Health*, 49–52.

Branch, M., & Paxton, P. P. (1976). *Providing safe nursing care for ethnic people of color*. Appleton-Century-Crofts.

Brown, E. L. (1948). *Nursing for the future: A report prepared for the National Nursing Council*. Russell Sage Foundation.

Buhler-Wilkinson, K. (1989). *False dawn: The rise and decline of public health nursing*. Rutgers University Press.

Chrisman, N. J. (1982). Anthropology in nursing: An exploration of adaptation. In N. J. Chrisman & T. W. Maretzki (Eds.), *Clinically applied anthropology* (pp. 117–140). Springer Netherlands. 10.1007/978-94-010-9180-0_5

Clarke, P. N., Andrews, M. M., McFarland, M. R., & Leininger, M. (2009). Some reflections on the impact of the culture care theory by McFarland & Andrews and a conversation with leininger. *Nursing Science Quarterly, 22*(3), 233–239.

D'Antonio, P. (2017). *Nursing with a message: Public health demonstration projects in New York City*. Rutgers University Press.

D'Antonio, P., & Whelan, J. C. (2009). Counting nurses: The power of historical census data. *Journal of Clinical Nursing, 18*, 2717–2724. 10.1111/j.1365-2702.2009.02892.x

Davis, D.-A. (2007). Narrating the mute: Racializing and racism in a neoliberal moment. *Souls, 9*(4), 346–360. 10.1080/10999940701703810

Davis, L. H., Dumas, R., Ferketich, S., Flaherty, Sr. M. J., Isenberg, M., Koerner, J. E., Lacey, B., Stern, P. N., Valente, S., & Meleis, A. I. (1992). AAN expert panel report: Culturally competent health care. *Nursing Outlook, 40*(6), 277–283.

Diers, D. (1984). Ethnic nursing care—A multicultural approach. *Western Journal of Nursing Research, 6*(2), 245–246.

Drevdahl, D. J. (2018). Culture shifts: From cultural to structural theorizing in nursing. *Nursing Research, 67*(2), 146–160. 10.1097/NNR.0000000000000262

Drevdahl, D. J., Canales, M. K., & Dorcy, K. S. (2008). Of goldfish tanks and moonlight tricks: Can cultural competency ameliorate health disparities? *Advances in Nursing Science, 31*(1), 13–27. 10.1097/01.ANS.0000311526.27823.05

Dunbar, V. (1953). *A proposed plan for the appointment of a full-time social scientist to the School of Nursing Faculty* (Box 8, folder 2, from the Records of the Office of the Dean (Virginia Dunbar) 1923–1970, Cornell University-New York Hospital School of Nursing). Medical Center Archives of New York-Presbyterian/Weill Cornell.

Evelyn, B. (2019, April 15). *Evelyn Barbee interview* [Personal communication].

Fassin, D. (2011). Racialization: How to do races with bodies. In F. E. Mascia-Lees (Ed.), *A companion to the anthropology of the body and embodiment* (pp. 419–434). Wiley-Blackwell. 10.1002/9781444340488.ch24

Fee, E. (2011). Charles E. Terry (1878–1945): Early campaigner against drug addiction. *American Journal of Public Health, 101*(3), 451. 10.2105/AJPH.2010.191171

Gallagher, C. A. (2020). Institutional racism revisited: How institutions perpetuate and promote racism through color blindness. In C. D. Lippard, J. S. Carter, & D. G. Embrick (Eds.), *Protecting whiteness: Whitelash and the rejection of racial equality*. University of Washington Press. https://www.jstor.org/stable/j.ctv1b3qqrj.9

Gamble, V. N. (1995). *Making a place for ourselves: The black hospital movement, 1920–1945*. Oxford University Press.

Hall, S. (2017). Race—The sliding signifier. In K. Mercer (Ed.), *The fateful triangle: Race, ethnicity, nation* (pp. 31–79). Harvard University Press.

Hall, S. (2019). The multicultural question. In D. Morley (Ed.), *Essential essays, volume 2: Identity and diaspora*. Duke University Press.

Hill Collins, P. (1991). *Black feminist thought: Knowledge, consciousness, and the politics of empowerment*. Routledge.

Hine, D. C. (1989). *Black women in white: Racial conflict and cooperation in the nursing profession, 1890–1950*. Indiana University Press.

Hudak, C. M. (1977). Providing safe nursing care for ethnic people of color. *The American Journal of Nursing, 77*(1), 71.

Johns, E. (1925). *A study of the present status of the negro woman in nursing*. Rockefeller Foundation; Rockefeller Archive Center.

Kegley, C. F., & Savier, A. N. (1983). Working with others who are not like me. *The Journal of School Health, 53*(2), 81–85.

Kevles, D. (1985). *In the name of eugenics: Genetics and the uses of human heredity*. Alfred A. Knopf.

King, C. (2019). *Gods of the upper air: How a circle of renegade anthropologists reinvented race, sex, and gender in the twentieth century*. Doubleday.

Kleinman, A., & Benson, P. (2019). Anthropology in the clinic: The problem of cultural competency and how to fix it. In J. Oberlander, M. Buchbinder, L. R. Churchill, S. E. Estroff, N. P. King, B. F. Saunders, R. P. Strauss, & R. L. Walker (Eds.), *The social medicine reader: Differences and inequalities* (3rd ed., Vol. 2, pp. 116–126). Duke University Press.

Leininger, M. (1966a). *Convergence and divergence of human behavior: An ethnopsychological comparative study of two Gadsup villages in the Eastern Highlands of New Guinea.* University of Washington.

Leininger, M. (1966b). *Syllabus: Cultural dimensions in nursing* (The Madeleine M. Leininger Collection on Human Caring and Transcultural Nursing). Boca Raton, Florida, USA: Archives of Caring in Nursing, Christine E. Lynn College of Nursing, Florida Atlantic University.

Leininger, M. (1970). *Nursing and anthropology: Two worlds to blend.* John Wiley & Sons, Inc.

Leininger, M. (1978). *Letter from M. Leininger to M.F. Carroll, Deputy to the Executive Director of the American Nurses Association.* The Madeleine M. Leininger Collection on Human Caring and Transcultural Nursing. Boca Raton, Florida, USA: Archives of Caring in Nursing, Christine E. Lynn College of Nursing, Florida Atlantic University.

Leininger, M. (1978, December 5). *What is transcultural nursing? Keynote presentation.* Second Annual Nurse Educator Conference, New York City. Madeleine M. Leininger Collection, Walter P. Reuther Library, University Archives, Wayne State University.

Leininger, M. (1980, September 24). *Envisioning transcultural nursing into the twentieth century.* Sixth National Transcultural Nursing Conference, Snowbird, UT. Archives of Caring in Nursing, Christine E. Lynn College of Nursing, Florida Atlantic University.

Leininger, M. (1989). Transcultural nursing: Quo vadis? (Where goeth the field?). *Journal of Transcultural Nursing, 1*(1), 33–45.

Leininger, M. (1993). Letter to the editor. *Nursing Outlook, 41*(6), 281–282.

Leininger, M. (2010). *Academic vitae of Madeleine M. Leininger, PhD, RN, CTN, LHD, DS, PhDNSc, FAAN.* The Madeleine M. Leininger Collection on Human Caring and Transcultural Nursing (ARC-008, Folder 1-8). Boca Raton, Florida, USA: Archives of Caring in Nursing, Christine E. Lynn College of Nursing, Florida Atlantic University. https://nursing.fau.edu/uploads/docs/1262/ARC-008_Folder%201-11_Leininger %20CV%2006-20-2010.pdf

Leone, L. P. (1955). Editorial: Where will we find teachers? *The American Journal of Nursing, 55*(12), 1461. 10.2307/3469540

Macgregor, F. C. (1960). *Social science in nursing: Applications for the improvement of patient care.* Russell Sage Foundation.

Macgregor, F. C. (1967). Uncooperative patients: Some cultural interpretations. *The American Journal of Nursing, 67*(1), 88–91.

Marion, L., Douglas, M., Lavin, M. A., Barr, N., Gazaway, S., Thomas, E., & Bickford, C. (2017, January). *Implementing the new ANA Standard 8: Culturally congruent practice.* The Online Journal of Issues in Nursing. https://ojin.nursingworld.org/ MainMenuCategories/ANAMarketplace/ANAPeriodicals/OJIN/TableofContents/ Vol-22-2017/No1-Jan-2017/Articles-Previous-Topics/Implementing-the-New-ANA-Standard-8.html#Implementing

Mayper, J. (1913). The immigrant. *Public Health Nurse Quarterly, 5*(3), 89–98.

Mead, M. (1956). Understanding cultural patterns. *Nursing Outlook, 4*(5), 260–262.

Mead, M., & Baldwin, J. (1971). *A rap on race.* J. B. Lippincott Company.

Meleis, A. I., Davis, L. H., Ferketich, S., Flaherty, M. J., Isenberg, M., Koerner, J. E., Lacey, B., Stern, P., & Valente, S. (1993). Reply. *Nursing Outlook, 41*(6), 282–283.

Metzl, J. M., & Hansen, H. (2014). Structural competency: Theorizing a new medical engagement with stigma and inequality. *Social Science & Medicine, 103,* 126–133. 10.1016/j.socscimed.2013.06.032

Metzl, J. M., & Roberts, D. E. (2014). From virtual mentor special contributors structural competency meets structural racism: Race, politics, and the. *American Medical Association Journal of Ethics, 16*(9), 674–690.

Moore, O. (2017, October 16). *CN: Racism across the board. This is an excellent example of how not to be even remotely culturally sensitive. These [Image attached] [Status update].* Facebook. https://www.facebook.com/photo.php?fbid=10101196457438273&set=a. 637314815613.2097083.177202720&type=3&theater

National Nursing Council, & Newell, H. H. (1951). *The history of the National Nursing Council.* National Organization for Public Health Nursing.

Nelson, A. (2011). *Body and soul: The black panther party and the fight against medical discrimination.* University of Minnesota Press.

Orr, Z., & Unger, S. (2020). Structural competency in conflict zones: Challenging depoliticization in Israel. *Policy, Politics, & Nursing Practice, 21*(4), 202–212.

Patterson, F. (1913). The first annual meeting of the NOPHN. *Public Health Nurse Quarterly, 5*(3), 15–19.

Pegues, T. (1979). Physical and psychological assessment of the Black patient. *Washington State Journal of Nursing,* 4–8.

Pernick, M. S. (1996). *The black stork: Eugenics and the death of defective babies in American medicine and motion pictures since 1915.* Oxford University Press.

Pernick, M. S. (1997). Eugenics and public health in American history. *American Journal of Public Health, 87*(11), 1767–1772.

Primeaux, M. (1977). Caring for the American Indian Patient. *The American Journal of Nursing, 77*(1), 91–94.

Ray, V. (2019). A theory of racialized organizations. *American Sociological Review, 84*(1), 26–53.

Roberts, D. (2011). *Fatal invention: How science, politics, and big business re-create race in the twenty-first century.* The New Press.

Roberts, S. K. (2009). *Infectious fear: Politics, disease, and the health effects of segregation.* University of North Carolina Press.

Rodriguez, J. (1983). Mexican Americans: Factors influencing health practices. *The Journal of School Health, 53*(2).

Ross, D. (1991). *The origins of American social science.* Cambridge University Press.

Soberano Orque, M., Bloch, B., & Ahumada, L. S. (1983). *Ethnic nursing care: A multicultural approach.* C.V. Mosby.

Stocking, Jr., G. (1992). Anthropology as kulturkampf: Science and politics in the career of Franz Boas. In *The ethnographer's magic and other essays in the history of anthropology* (pp. 92–113). University of Wisconsin Press.

Terry, C.E. (1916). Public health nursing: A municipal duty. *Public Health Nurse Quarterly, 8*(3), 29–39.

Tobbell, D. A. (2018). Nursing's boundary work: Theory development and the making of nursing science, ca. 1950–1980. *Nursing Research*, 67(2), 63–73. 10.1097/NNR. 0000000000000251

Visweswaran, K. (2010). Race and the culture of anthropology. In *Un/common cultures: Racism and the rearticulation of cultural difference*. Duke University Press.

Wolfskill, M. M. (2009). *Margaret mead papers and the south pacific ethnographic archives: A finding aid to the collection in the library of congress*. Manuscript Division, Library of Congress; Library of Congress.

Part II

A Critical Understanding of the Present

Thinking about the title of this part, A Critical Understanding of the Present, it is easy to be constrained by the enormity of the challenges we see and feel and carry. Science fiction writer and visionary Ursula LeGuin (2018) wrote, "the wind beats on the drums of my ears and overturns the chairs" (p. 6), rendering attending to anything else impossible. For nurses, especially those doing nursing work during the COVID-19 pandemic, the lived experience of nursing is sometimes inflected with overwhelming despair. After all, how much and what *can* one person possibly *do*? It is completely understandable how nurses get stuck in the here of the present when faced with the enormous precarity of the issues that abound under systems of late stage capitalism, nursing without adequate protective equipment, rampant inequities, climate disaster, rising authoritarianism. As feminist anthropologist Anna Tsing (2015) surmises, realistically and pessimistically while pondering the state of the world in the present, "there may not be a collective happy ending" (p. 21). The four authors in this part tackle the precarious issues of the critical present within the scrim of the Covidicene, confronting planetary injustice, while thinking with and thorough philosophical ideas of nursing identity, power, politics, and art.

Part II begins with a chapter by Burton, Holmes, Jenkins, and McIntyre, titled *For Whom Does the Alarm Bell Toll? On Nursing Identity and Revolution*. In this essay, the authors argue that the ways that nurses identify themselves as individuals and as a group are entangled within complex cultural, political, and historical webs. The threads of thought start with western philosophical explorations of identity, and weave through post structural analyses to critically uncover ideas about how we as nurses arrived at the precarious present. In the later half of the essay, the concept of nurses as *sentinels*, meaning ones who keep watch, always at the front line, ready to call the alarm is explored with analyses and multiple situated discussions of the nurse as sentinel tied up with forces of gender and power. This essay is an example of how to critically think with both theory and philosophy, and it powerfully outlines how nurses can and should reclaim sentinelity in order to affect radical change for patients, communities, and nurses.

The second essay is by Smith and Willis entitled "imagining afFIRMative futures for nursing." Writing from the perspectives of the United Kingdom and

DOI: 10.4324/9781003245957-6

Germany, the authors critique nursing's philosophical groundings in humanism that lead to narrow and individually focused conceptions of (the hegemonically popular) idea of person-centered care. They offer critical posthuman pedagogical perspectives that challenge the received view that white cis-het human, basically the Vitruvian man, is the center of the universe, upsetting assumptions about the nursing self and her role within traditional eurocentric global northern and western views. Smith and Willis introduce the reader to critical posthumanism through explorations of post anthropocentrism entangling Braidotti's (2019) notion of the posthuman convergence which examines vast structural injustices, destruction of species and planet, and robotic and human technological interdependence. Smith and Willis end with a call for affirmative ethics and situated knowledges as a way toward a more critical vision for human, more-than-human and planetary health.

Further investigating themes of nursing identity, the third chapter in this part is entitled "Hypervisiable Nurses in the Covidicene: Reclaiming the Scripts of Personhood and Agency." This essay by Amélie Perron adds an important critical overview and critique of how nurses were made both highly visible and yet remained simultaneously invisible during the COVID-19 pandemic, using analyses of disciplinary power and control. The critical themes and analyses of identity fit well with other chapters in this section focused on the present epoch, building a case for unpacking the politics of nursing in the present. We particularly appreciate the author's call to embodied activism, not just advocacy. Perron gives an unapologetic framing of the politics of nursing practice as this relates to tensions around why nurses are highly valued but remain largely excluded from policy and decision making. This chapter builds on Perron's scholarly work on the sociology of ignorance; a concept that also helps to critically evaluate the history of the present. The author includes connections to tensions in nursing in the United Kingdom and Canada, providing the opportunity for readers to compare and examine the geopolitics of their own situated experiences.

Part II ends with the final chapter, a visual art essay entitled "METASTATIC GROWTH: The Healthcare Industry's Increasing Contribution to the Plasticene." Emmanuel Christian Tedjasukmana is an artist and practicing nurse working in the inpatient hospital setting in the United States. Tedjasukmana's essay and his art is sparked by his own experience of the critical present including a conscientization (Freire, 2018), a critical awareness at the bedside, about the healthcare system's contributions to planetary destruction producing shocking amounts of hospital waste and plastics. His essay outlines the complex paths of plastics in their many forms as they poison the environment and our bodies, exacerbated and compounded further by the waste products of the Covidicene, gloves, masks, PPE, and more. This essay both shows and tells the story embodying the power of aesthetics for knowing, creating deep meaning about how things touch other things in nursing, borrowing a phrase from multi species ecologist Haraway (2016). Tedjasukmana leaves the reader with a nursing care plan highlighting actions nurses can take to reduce waste, helping readers to imagine a praxis for increased planetary health.

Overall, the four essays in Part II balance short term pessimism around our precarious present with long term optimism, and each author or set of writers outlines actions that motivate action toward radical imagination. Radical imagination risks getting trapped within the precarity of critical present, but these essays demonstrate how the critical framework with which you examine issues is the blowing wind that can take us all from *here* to *there*.

References

Braidotti, R. (2019). *Posthuman knowledge*. John Wiley & Sons.

Freire, P. (2018). *Pedagogy of the oppressed*. Bloomsbury publishing USA.

Haraway, D. J. (2016). Staying with the trouble. In *Staying with the trouble*. Duke University Press.

LeGuin, U. K. (2018). *So far so good. Final poems 2014–2018*. Copper Canyon Press.

Tsing, A. L. (2015). The mushroom at the end of the world. In *The mushroom at the end of the world*. Princeton University Press.

4 For Whom Does the Alarm Bell Toll? On Nursing Identity and Revolution

*Candace Burton, Dave Holmes,
Danisha Jenkins, and Jon McIntyre*

Identity as a Philosophical Concept

In the field of nursing, narratives of professional identity are closely tied to the shape(s) of the discipline. How we conceptualize our nursing-selves, individually and collectively, is intimately related to how nurses perceive themselves and their practices; how we compare, contrast, and relate our discipline to others, and widespread, but imprecise popular culture narratives regarding form and functions of nursing. Reimagining nursing identity/identities is thus essential to radical change for patients, communities, and nurses. Refocusing, or perhaps altogether replacing, the conceptual lenses through which we see ourselves, and through which others see us, reaffirms our role in shaping a nursing identity from complex current, historical, social, and cultural relations. Despite its relatively recent rise to prominence in academia and popular politics, the concept of identity has a long history in the Western philosophical tradition (Appiah, 2010; Lewis, 1966; Ricoeur, 1991; Sayers, 1999).

Identity: Seeking Ontological Boundaries

A traditional philosophical understanding of identity is captured in "Liebnez's Law" or "the identity of indiscernibles" (Feldman, 1970; Hacking, 1975). This maxim states that two things without any differentiating properties are indeed the same; they are identical. If we understand identity as complete correspondence of properties (numerical identity) an entity can only share the relation of identity with itself. Anything else with all the same properties is indistinguishable. It is impossible to imagine, for example, two apples which share every property (location in time and space, physical properties, relations to other objects) without thinking of them as identical. The problem is not that things share every property with other things (violating Liebnez's Law), but that they do *not* share every property even with themselves. When looking at what should be a singular thing, we are confronted with innumerable stubborn points of discernment.

DOI: 10.4324/9781003245957-7

The Problem of the Many

In *Many, but Almost One*, Lewis and David (1999) consider human inability to determine that a particular thing is a unique entity separate from those with which it shares physical and/or conceptual properties. The authors present readers with the example of a cloud. If one attempts to define the cloud, to distinguish it from surrounding "non-cloud," it is impossible to pin down internal or external borders. It contains innumerable, shifting fields of more and/or less densely associated water molecules. The line between cloud and non-cloud becomes at best an indistinct gradient. Outside some arbitrarily imposed level of density at which "cloudness" occurs, it is impossible to locate the edge. If we set the required density high enough, less of the "cloud" qualifies. If we set it low enough, surrounding wisps and invisible vapors are included. Clearly, the intuitively perceived cloud entity is actually a much more complicated, and ambiguous, ontological situation. Lewis and David identify this as "the problem of the many":

> ... all things are swarms of particles. There are always outlying particles, questionably parts of the thing, not definitely included and not definitely not included. So there are always many aggregates, differing a little bit here and a little bit there, with equal claim to be the thing. We have many things or we have none, but anyway not the one thing we thought we had (1999, pp. 164–165)

We thus tend to interpret the world in terms of static and discrete entities when, upon dissecting our conceptual schema, we find exceptions, border cases, overlappings, and ambiguities. This is especially true when adding temporal properties to analysis. An apple's progress from seed, to tree, to apple, to food, to biochemical energy and metabolic byproducts, to waste, etc ... hardly reinforces a sense that it has a static or discrete identity. More accurately, we function in terms of partial or "almost-identity." Lewis and David observe how the ontological situation of identity is thus more nuanced:

> We have a spectrum of cases. At one end we find the complete identity of a thing with itself: it and itself are identical, not at all distinct. At the opposite end we find two things that are entirely distinct: they have no part in common. In between we find all the cases of partial overlap: things with parts in common and other parts not. The things are not entirely identical, not entirely distinct, but some of each.
>
> (Lewis & David, 1999, p. 177)

Nursing's Almost-Identity

If we cannot pin down the identity of a *physical* entity, we must recognize the futility of doing so for social and cultural phenomena. If identity is "a spectrum of cases," the ontologically complex entities which emerge from human inter-actions (language, concepts, societies, cultures, etc ...) must fall into partial overlap. "Almost-identity" is thus useful for discussing social phenomena. In the context of a discussion of nursing identity–historical or contemporary–it is important to recognize that what we might call the identity of the field *is* an almost-identity. Ontologically, nursing has a general set of properties not dis-tinct from other entities nor entirely internally consistent. There is no platonic ideal or "big-N" nursing—a social phenomenon, it emerges from interactions among people, material and nonmaterial environments, into an almost-identity of related practices and concepts.

Science and technology studies researcher Annemarie Mol would say that nursing is "more than one, and less than many" (Mol, 2003, p. 84). Nursing does "hang together" or cohere as a thing in this world—but not always a unitary thing. It is conceptually bounded and does not encompass every conceivable property. But those bounds are hazy, porous, dynamic. It may not have unity but has some ontological coherence. In contrast, when we think and talk about something, we typically do so in ways that assume it behaves, at least heuristically, as an individual entity. We speak of "clouds," not variegated banks of suspended water. Why speak in terms of identity, unity, and essence instead of almost-identity, multiplicity, indeterminacy, and complexity?

The predominant answer, from early in Western thought, has been some variation on Platonic idealism. Such essentialist approaches share a belief that the material world is undergirded by primary essences (Lowe, 2008; Oderberg, 2007). Essentialism posits that we encounter entities as immanent objects of perception and, somehow, recognize them as expressions of universal concepts. When we see banks of suspended water droplets, we ostensibly recognize them as cloud-things because they demonstrate essential properties and characteristics of a universal concept.

An alternative explanation denies transcendence of form or meaning from any source external to the world we inhabit and experience. This reverses the direction of the relationship between essence and existence, between the transcendent and the immanent. Messiness, difference, and multiplicity are primordial. We impose identity upon a world of inchoate chaos by draping es-sences and universal concepts over messier extant topology. Concepts, iden-tities, and meanings are our creations, and our tools. There is nothing essential, nothing inevitable, about how we order and understand the world. There is no essential form dictating that we see distinct clouds in indistinct banks of water vapor. Likewise, there is no ideal form of nursing versus which worldly instances are imperfect renditions. Instead, processes, practices, and relations are what give rise to the almost-identities of phenomena such as nursing. Nursing emerges from the contingent specificities of its performance, from what it does in the world, and its relations with other (equally emergent and contingent) entities and concepts.

Almost-Identity

Following this constructivist argument that the almost-identities which populate our experienced reality emerge and are continually transformed (what Deleuze and Guattari (1987) call a process of continual becoming) through actions and interactions of human and non-human entities, we can investigate how nursing, a concept and almost-identity, emerged historically and how it continues to become "more than one but less than many," entangled with multiple social, cultural and economic forces. As explored in the following sections, we make the radical claim that nurses are people(!) and that nursing is a social construction inescapably borne of the thoughts, words, and actions of those people and the structures wherein they labor. Nurses are agentive co-participants in these structures, contributing and subject to the drives and desires inherent therein. The power-relations embodied in systems of governance (state agencies, professional societies, auditing bodies, clinical administration, regimes of technological management and control, finance and resource allocation, etc …) are inextricably entangled with the emergence of historical, contemporary and future practices and narratives of nursing.

Control over the identity of nursing, the power to define who nurses are and what nurses do, has been a central component of this interplay among power, agency, and governance. Both nurses and non-nurses have attempted to speak strategically of a nursing identity, to shape the profession toward political, moral, and/or economic ends. Nurse scholars have illustrated the roles of religion, gender, class, race, technological change, and the dominance of bio-medical epistemological approaches in such dynamics (D'Antonio, 2010; Dingwall et al., 2002; Hawkins, 2010; Reverby, 1987; Sandelowski, 2000). To the extent that such attempts sought to delineate sharp borders and essential qualities for nurses and nursing practices, they portray fictions: unnaturally static, specified, sets of people and practices. Such fictional identities benefit those who would limit the creative power of nurses to *become*: to embrace productive messiness and openness. Thus, instead of striving for one identity, we might speak instead of our almost-identity, not only because it allows us to speak more accurately of those we call nurses and the practices we call nursing, but also because it recognizes our contextualized co-agency in nursing's future. It is time to deny *one* essential nursing identity and fight instead for those almost-identities that embody nurses' desires for ourselves, our patients, and our communities.

The radical analysis that nurses are *people* diverges from the ways in which nurses have been heretofore constructed. Nurse identity (what nurses do, how and when) is constructed by productive value for the institution and dictated by multiple oversights and controls. These systems are so efficiently incorporated into operations that they become a way of life, particularly in productivity and efficiency-based environments such as acute care hospitals. Technology, oversight, and reimbursement models operating under the guise of patient safety influence nursing practice in ways that nurses must assess and address. In the words of Michel Foucault, these mechanisms manifest as significant yet enigmatic political power that "works to incite, reinforce, control, monitor, optimize, and organize the forces under it" (Foucault, 1978, p. 136). These systems of control work to dehumanize the nurse in both practice and personhood and facilitate mortification of self: the dispossession of role, loss of identity, and devolvement of the autonomy that one holds on the "outside." This was seen clearly during the COVID-19 pandemic when nurses were called "heroes," yet deprived of personal protective equipment, autonomy of work, and generally dehumanized into a commodity rather than a working force.

Technology in Identity

Nurses, and therefore patients, are directed by and managed within a powerful panoptic mechanism of technological control (Jenkins et al., 2021). The electronic health record is an easily auditable (read: surveilled) governing mechanism requiring feeding with data mined by the nurse, surveilled from the patient, then regurgitated as algorithmic tasks for the nurse. Data input by the nurse becomes, "... discrete mineable data points that go on a construct map of the patient experience ... and an audit trail for nurses' behaviors, surveillance in absentia [...] a proxy governing forces that are not necessarily present (Dillard-Wright, 2019, pp. 1–2). Order sets, nursing care plans, clinical guidelines, alarms, triggers, and tasks are programmed into the EHR using a privileged hierarchy of so-called evidence-based practices serving the institution. These "best practices" are power regimes that risk exclusion of knowledge and interventions better suited for the patient and eliminate opportunities for innovation. This institutionalized version of "best," or "truth" is a far cry from theoretical and philosophical visions of nursing knowledge, which assert that knowing comes from multiple domains—rather than a singular, empirically and quantitatively fitted to an algorithm (Carper, 1978).

As reporting measures, technology, and artificial intelligence become increasingly ingrained in health care, it is critical that nurses actively engage in asking who is served by the algorithm/data set/care plan/audit. In a profession which exists for care of human beings, nurses must understand whether technology that dictates practice serves those in our care, or if it serves to improve productivity, billing compliance, close CMS loopholes, etc. We must require clear answers about the ramifications and implementation of such structures and processes, including patient harm, loss of autonomous practice, and implications for surveillance and control. Of significant concern to nursing practice is the economic influence of AI that results in a homogenized (read: omnipotent) decision-making body. Because the creation of AI is so complicated, so expensive, there is ample opportunity for those in power (economic elite) to control not only resources, but to dictate a nursing practice that functions for productivity—not for patients or nurses.

In a healthcare system that already survives on profit margins, and therefore necessarily rationed care, AI mainly increases the efficiency, anonymity, and ambiguity of oppressive and harmful control structures that degrade the profession's ability to care.

Patient Safety Oversight

Nursing practice is heavily dictated by regulatory bodies including departments of public health and The Joint Commission®. The policies of such organizations rely heavily upon a Foucaldian governmentality, embedding a vast panoptic system of self-regulation as a mechanism of control. Such regulatory bodies assess certain patient outcomes with utmost severity, and these outcomes (most of which are considered poor), have been designated as "Nurse Sensitive Indicators" (NSIs) in the National Database of Nurse Quality Indicators. The aim of NSIs is to determine whether a nurse has a quantifiable impact on patients. Despite clear evidence that some of the most significant risks for death and disability to patients and communities are social determinants of health and structural violences, nursing quality indicators focus on patient falls, pressure ulcers, restraint use, and nosocomial infections to indicate the value of nursing (Butkus et al., 2020). Each is heavily audited, and significant investment in technology and surveillance used to prevent them. Self-regulation is culturally integrated and enforced: nurses are frequently injured attempting to prevent or cushion patient falls and are significantly more likely to experience occupational injury than other industries. The frequency of these injuries, coupled with certain underreporting, illustrates the extent to which regulatory oversight and control has shaped not only the operational priorities of the nursing workforce, but its willingness to sacrifice physical bodies to institutional interests. When is enough, enough?

Nurses as Sentinels

The previous sections examined the identification of nurses as both inherently amorphous and as almost entirely conscripted, depending upon whether or not there is a necessary element of humanity within the construction of nursing and its execution in practice, science, or education. This is a crucial question in the context of the present historical moment: the throes of a global pandemic in which nursing faces a depleted workforce. How and why we arrived here must be considered via past, present, and future, particularly insofar as the "doing" of nursing is characterized by what is done and who is doing it. What exactly are the sentinel functions of nursing and nurses?

The most basic definition of sentinel is "one who keeps watch," (Oxford Languages, 2022) with the implication that watch is kept to protect someone or something from threat. Presumably, should the threat materialize, the sentinel alerts others in effort to mount a defense. This is a regular aspect of nursing practice: bedside nurses call for a code team, emergency department nurses call for stroke response, school nurses call caregivers for ill students. In many ways, the nursing profession and nurses themselves thus serve as sentinels for health care. It is this state of *sentinelity* that causes the nurse to be almost invariably positioned at the front line of both care provision and the risk zone for injury. In simplest terms, it is the nurse who is almost always first to observe a change in patient status, and therefore the nurse who is forced to bear the message about this change to someone who can direct action to address it. This is not unlike how nurses are often the first to see the dangers of an oncoming issue—a pandemic, a workforce shortage, a crisis of cost and payment—but are largely barred from initiating decision-making to halt the onslaught. Despite the myriad social structures that cast nurses as lesser professionals in healthcare science and practice, the need for nurses to engage in sentinelity is undeniable—absent nurses, much of what is considered healthcare is also absent, as are warnings when circumstances become dire. Yet, while an army sentinel can generally expect a responsive show of force, for many nurses the response to an alert is silence—a page not answered, a caregiver does not pick up, the rest of the staff are busy elsewhere. Worse, the response is some form of, "Well there's nothing we can do about it." What then is the nature of sentinelity in the nursing profession; how and for whom is it enacted?

Sentinelity and Advocacy

Nurses are often described as engaging in "advocacy"—advocating for patients, for policy change, for professional dynamism in science, education, and practice. This is interesting insofar as it implies that nurses are asking for something. To advocate is to press one's case for a particular action, usually on behalf of a less empowered person or group. In some cases this specifically entails supplication: a way of signaling need that tends to inspire cooperative responses (Van Kleef et al., 2010). In acts of advocacy, the nurse is often required to seek cooperation from diverse sectors and work to unite, cooperatively, their combined assets. Doing so may thus invoke supplication to or pleading with a gatekeeper, bringing to bear once again the state of sentinelity: calling for attention to something. Supplication, however, does not connote a responding defense of the supplicant—rather, perhaps due to its use in religious practices, it implies some sacrifice for both supplicant and respondent. What then is sacrificed in the act of making a request or acting as an advocate, in supplication?

In the religious sense, supplication is an act through which an innately inferior being (human) seeks a particular, positive relationship with a superior force (divine) (Tekke & Watson, 2017). Here, the former must necessarily admit inferiority in seeking the help of the latter—in effect, sacrificing individual ego for a chance at unity. At the same time, the superior (divine) is believed to sacrifice some of its superiority in deigning to respond. Whether or not that is a true sacrifice, there is thus an encoded hierarchy wherein the supplicant (advocate, nurse) must prove worthy of the respondent's attention. Determination of this worth is based on how well the supplicant renders themselves appealing, how well they have followed the tenets of the practice—indeed, how "good" they appear. This resonates distinctly with the ethos of the feminine, particularly the divine or angelic feminine, as invoked throughout the history of nursing.

Sentinelity and Gender

The operationalization of the feminine in nursing is neither a novel nor entirely historic occurrence. Of interest here is the parallel development of nursing and feminist social critique, beginning from the moment Florence Nightingale noted that "On women we must depend ... for personal and household hygiene" (1860, p. 79). Historically, this impetus for nursing is also rooted in first-wave feminist ideologies, which foregrounded the presumed "feminine" ideal as a vehicle for tempering society through "incremental and progressive reform" (Brisolara & Seigart, 2012, p. 293). At nearly the same moment, the idealization of the feminine influence as the "angel in the house" seized the public imagination and enshrined acts of caring, sacrifice, and submission as markers of true femininity (Kühl, 2016).

Crucial to this liminality between the angel in the house and Nightingale's "ministering angels" is the consistency of the deified feminine, and how it is fundamentally self-sacrificing. While the angel in the house sacrifices her own agency to sustain the domestic, private household and provide loving, caring supports for husband and children—with attention to the very clear expectations of heteronormativity and motherhood for women—the ministering angel sacrifices her capacity to *be* the angel in the house by going into the public sphere and caring for those in need. The acts of self-sacrifice carried out by both "angels" are thus appropriately noble for female-identified persons. This suggests that regardless of where and in what capacity the feminine is enacted, it has a specific sacrificial and subjugated character.

Appropriate execution of femininity then imputes these qualities to both the female-identified person and the nurse—and requires that nurses engage in performing actualized femininity and sacrifice by the nature of their work (Rivers, 2020). During the COVID-19 pandemic, such sacrifices became almost taken for granted, and nurses were pressured into ever more impossible working conditions in the supposed interest of public health. One organization even sued to prevent nurse employees from leaving positions they had resigned (Heim, 2022). Although it failed, this attempt demonstrates the presumption that a nurse can be reduced from crucial, individual, and agentic professional to "an object existing to serve the establishment" (Jenkins et al., 2021, p. 3). When nurses are thus objectified and othered, sacrifices of their own health and safety become acceptable losses rather than sentinel indicators of system problems.

Silencing the Sentinel

The histories of feminism and nursing continue to be inextricably bound, with the professionalization of nursing standing at the same juncture as the rights of women to be freed from constraining institutions such as coverture and denied suffrage (Burton et al., 2020; Fowler, 2017). Although the first wave is generally construed as ending mid-20th century, this conjugation of nurses' positionality in the professional environment does not. As late as 1967, Stein described how "the nurse is to be bold, have initiative, and be responsible for making significant recommendations, while at the same time she must appear passive. This … (is) to make her recommendations appear to be initiated by the physician" (1967, p. 699). Notably, the nurse in this passage is specifically female, as Stein describes a remarkable gymnastic of sentinality that both serves to alert the physician to a patient issue while preserving what is obviously a façade of appropriately feminine silence and subservience. Clearly then, nurses must accept and actualize themselves as subjugated, sacrificial, and relatively silent to faithfully (intentional use) execute their professional roles. This is quite at odds with the role of the sentinel, necessarily sentient and aware, holding critical responsibility for assessing and warning of trouble.

Nurses have described the silencing of their sentinality in a variety of contexts, those which affect them as practitioners and scientists as well as those affecting patients, families, and communities. Silencing occurs where nurses' complaints about workplace injury risks are not addressed (Kay et al., 2015), when nurses are forced to ignore ethical qualms about workplace issues (Lamb et al., 2019), and when caring for incarcerated patients (Jenkins et al., 2022), among others. In each case, the nurse's ability to serve as the sentinel, calling attention to an encroaching threat is erased—and conditions remain static or worsen.

When sentinel calls receive no response, there can be a sense of having been rendered helpless in or abandoned by the institution—sensations described as moral distress, moral injury, or organizational betrayal (Brewer et al., 2020; Dean et al., 2019; Wocial, 2020). While evocative of negative experiences, these terms are also connotatively emotional and imply that the reaction of nurses to being silenced is a mere matter of managing feelings—not flagrant subversion of what should be the chain of command. This is particularly evident in the flood of responses to burnout among nurses during the COVID-19 pandemic: much attention was devoted not to bettering institutional supports for the work of pandemic nursing but to fostering "resilience," "mindfulness," and other individually-oriented responses to systems-level problems (Schlak et al., 2022). These impute responsibility for remedying the problem to the nurse—in effect, killing the sentinel messenger. A dead sentinel is by definition silenced, but quite effectively transmits the message that speaking out is dangerous. The losses that spawn betrayal and moral injury or distress among nurses are thus also acceptable losses–they are, after all, only feelings and a sacrifice the nurse should be willing by "nature" to endure.

Reclaiming Sentinelity

Clearly, there are numerous social forces that impugn the legitimacy, authority, and capacity of nursing science and practice as sentinels in health systems. Common among them is the consignment of the most fundamental elements of nursing—advocacy, caring, preservation of health, and safety for nurses and patients—to a subjugated status. Advocacy involves supplication to an "authority:" physician, executive, or manager. Provision of care is somehow gendered in the feminine, and characterized as something done sacrificially and by instinct rather than as a product of dedicated professional, scientific study and practice (Burton, 2020). Preservation of health and safety is assigned not to the system designated as "healthcare," but to the individual nurse—turning wholly on individual "resilience" or ability to be "mindful." In each case, nursing is made subservient and its sentinelity muted. This critical diminishment of the professional "space" for nursing also reduces disciplinary influence on science, practice, education, and policy. Moreover, the systems and institutions with which nurses must affiliate are often used as levers to further constrain the profession—in effect, putting the angels back in the house. Here again the entanglement of femininity and its expected attributes with constructions of nursing is manifest, and the liminality of nurse and angel evoked. The professionalism and import of nursing are confounded by systems and influences that constrain and disempower, clinically and philosophically.

These influences are re-created throughout nursing, where power structures remain disproportionately hierarchical, and create systems that inculcate and acculturate new personnel—from day one nursing students to newly hired faculty members—into "good" behaviors required for success. Mainly, this ensures that nurses continue to internalize silence and sacrifice as integral to the profession—and that this internalization is borne out and repeated across education, practice, and science. Where silence and sacrifice are prized as characteristics of the good angel/nurse, determination of the value of the nurse's contributions—how "good" they really are—can only be made *down* a power gradient. Those at the top of the gradient evaluate those below, and thereby enforce these norms. This has been called horizontal oppression but is perhaps more realistically identified as exploitation of power imbalances and hegemonic norm enforcement.

Acting with sentinelity, however, can disrupt hegemony. In the case of the nurses who were sued to prevent resignation, some fascinating and even oppositional dynamics arose. Initially, the nurses rejected their working conditions–effectively eschewing continued sacrifice and ceasing to act in supplication to the constraining system. The system sought to reassert control, utilizing the legal system to prevent resignation and re-establish status quo.

Interestingly, however, doing so elevated the nurses from resource objects subject to the control of system management to personnel so central to system function that their departure became a crisis. The case exemplifies exactly how and when sentinelity is acknowledged: the point at which continued sacrifice is rejected, and the nurse ceases to act in supplication. This requires a fundamental shift from self-sacrifice to self-advocacy, and reasserts nurse agency—dispensing with what Stein called "a transactional neurosis" meant to preserve the status quo (1967, p. 703).

Rejecting the subjugation of nurses' sentinelity into hegemonic power structures that value meekness, nonresistance, and silence may thus be the most radically imaginative professional act. The disruption of such power structures may ironically return nursing to its feminist roots: aligning with more modern, intersectional feminist perspectives centering choice, opportunity, and social justice (Burton, 2020). Critically, however, such an alignment must actively preserve and amplify sentinel nurse voices rather than allowing them to be absorbed into other structures. As an example, nursing represents itself as a social-justice oriented field–throughout the American Nurses Association (ANA) *Code of Ethics for Nurses with Interpretive Statements* are sections addressing environmental health, human rights, and health as a universal right (ANA, 2015). In fact, the document concludes with direct attention to social justice—but emphasizes its pursuance within *structures*: professional organizations, accrediting bodies, health systems. These by nature cannot be radically sentinel, as they are largely based on and fueled by the same hegemonies that claim subjugating authority over the profession.

Reclaiming sentinel voices within nursing is thus no mean feat, and the tendency for small groups to be collapsed into larger and ultimately less nimble organizations will always carry silencing capacity. Nonetheless, approaches such as Walter's (2017) emancipatory nursing praxis, Dillard-Wright's (2022) enactment of mutual aid, or the work of Holmes and colleagues (see Evans et al., 2020; Holmes & Gagnon, 2018; Johansson & Holmes, 2021; McIntyre et al., 2020) on poststructuralist analytics in nursing are inherently disruptive to hierarchical systems that demand supplication and silence from "good" nurses. These approaches reaffirm the critical nature of and need for active, intentional sentinelity in nursing, and allow creativity, visibility, and equity to flourish for individual nurses as well as in public perceptions of nursing.

Concluding Remarks: On the Importance of Critique

In light of what is discussed throughout this chapter, it is clear that political awareness is an attribute all nurses must develop. Poststructural analysis is a powerful vehicle for deconstructing the discourses and practices surrounding nurses (Williams, 2005). The productive aspect of this perspective has been highlighted extensively. This said, we are left with a pressing question: where do we go from here? The solution is not simple, but we believe that whatever the theoretical and political tools deployed, nurses must resort to ongoing *critique* of the discourses and practices that try to shape and domesticate us. We turn again to Foucault, for insights regarding *critique*. For Foucault, critique is both theoretical and practical. In a 1978 talk titled "What is Critique?" given to the French Philosophy Society, Foucault spoke of critique as "voluntary inservitude" (*"inservitude volontaire"*) or "informed unruliness" (*"indocilité réfléchie"*) (Holmes & Gagnon, 2018). The word "informed" is extremely important. Critique must be informed; it must be anchored in a robust approach and account for continuous interplay between knowledge and power (Holmes & Gagnon, 2018). Such a political approach is clearly akin to resistance. The sentinel approach constitutes a good example of Foucauldian resistance. Foucault famously claimed that "the art of not being governed or better, the art of not being governed like that and at that cost" is the "very first definition of critique."

As mentioned, critique and resistance must go beyond theory to become day-to-day practices. Faced with multiple attempts to govern nurses' discourses and practices, critique ultimately takes aim at the various *apparatuses* (*"dispositifs"*) contributing to exclusion and subjugation, exposing the inner workings of power (including violence) to fight them more effectively (Evans et al., 2020; Holmes & Gagnon, 2018; Jenkins et al., 2020; Johansson & Holmes, 2021; McIntyre et al., 2020) Poststructural tools such as deconstruction, genealogy, and archaeology are some amongst many that could be mobilized to subvert the violence that tries to bend nurses to breaking, both professionally and personally (Holmes & Gagnon, 2018).

References

American Nurses Association. (2015). *Code of ethics for nurses with interpretive statements*. American Nurses Association. Retrieved September 18 from https://www.nursingworld.org/coe-view-only

Appiah, K. A. (2010). *The ethics of identity*. Princeton University Press.

Brewer, K. C., Oh, K. M., Kitsantas, P., & Zhao, X. (2020, 2020/01/01). Workplace bullying among nurses and organizational response: An online cross-sectional study [10.1111/jonm.12908]. *Journal of Nursing Management*, 28(1), 148–156. 10.1111/jonm.12908

Brisolara, S., & Seigart, D. (2012). Feminist evaluation research. In S. N. Hesse-Biber (Ed.), *The handbook of feminist research: Theory and praxis* (pp. 290–312). Sage.

Burton, C. W. (2020). Paying the caring tax: The detrimental influences of gender expectations on the development of nursing education and science. *Advances in Nursing Science*, 43(3), 266–277. 10.1097/ans.0000000000000319

Burton, C. W., Gilpin, C. E., & Draughon Moret, J. (2020). Structural violence: A concept analysis to inform nursing science and practice. *Nursing Forum*, 1–7. Retrieved December 29, from 10.1111/nuf.12535

Butkus, R., Rapp, K., Cooney, T. G., Engel, L. S., & Health Public Policy Committee of the American College of Physicians. (2020). Envisioning a better US health care system for all: Reducing barriers to care and addressing social determinants of health. *Annals of Internal Medicine*, 172(2_Supplement), S50–S59. 10.7326/M19-2410

Carper, B. (1978, Oct). Fundamental patterns of knowing in nursing. *Advances in Nursing Science*, *1*(1), 13–23. 10.1097/00012272-197810000-00004

D'Antonio, P. (2010). *American nursing: A history of knowledge, authority, and the meaning of work*. JHU Press.

Dean, W., Talbot, S., & Dean, A. (2019). Reframing clinician distress: Moral injury not burnout. *Federal Practitioner: For the Health Care Professionals of the VA, DoD, and PHS*, *36*(9), 400–402. https://www.ncbi.nlm.nih.gov/pmc/articles/PMC 6752815/

Deleuze, G., & Guattari, F. (1987). *Capitalism and schizophrenia: A thousand plateaus*. B. Massumi (Trans.). Minneapolis: University of Minnesota Press.

Dillard-Wright, J. (2019). Electronic health record as a panopticon: A disciplinary apparatus in nursing practice. *Nursing Philosophy*, *20*(2), e12239. 10.1111/nup.12239

Dillard-Wright, J. (2022). A radical imagination for nursing: Generative insurrection, creative resistance. *Nursing Philosophy*, *23*(1), e12371. 10.1111/nup.12371

Dingwall, R., Rafferty, A. M., & Webster, C. (2002). *An introduction to the social history of nursing*. Routledge.

Evans, A. M., Holmes, D., & Quinn, C. (2020, 2020/10/01). Madness, sex, and risk: A poststructural analysis. *Nursing Inquiry*, *27*(4), e12359. 10.1111/nin.12359

Feldman, F. (1970). Leibniz and "Leibniz'law". *The Philosophical Review*, *79*(4), 510–522.

Foucault, M. (1978). *The history of sexuality, volume 1: An introduction*. R. Hurley (Trans.). Vintage.

Fowler, M. D. (2017, 2017/01/01). "Unladylike Commotion": Early feminism and nursing's role in gender/trans dialogue [10.1111/nin.12179]. *Nursing Inquiry*, *24*(1), e12179. 10.1111/nin.12179

Hacking, I. (1975). The identity of Indiscernibles. *The Journal of Philosophy*, *72*(9), 249–256. 10.2307/2024896

Hawkins, S. (2010). *Nursing and women's labour in the nineteenth century: The quest for independence*. Routledge.

Heim, M. (2022, January 21). What to know about the battle over Wisconsin health care workers now playing out in court. *Appleton Post Crescent*.

Holmes, D., & Gagnon, M. (2018). Power, discourse, and resistance: Poststructuralist influences in nursing. *Nursing Philosophy*, *19*(1), e12200. 10.1111/nup.12200

Jenkins, D., Burton, C., & Holmes, D. (2021). Hospitals as total institutions. *Nursing Philosophy*, e12379. 10.1111/nup.12379

Jenkins, D., Burton, C. W., & Holmes, D. (2022). Gender influences in the intersection of acute care registered nurses and law enforcement: The collision of caring and carceral institutions. *Advances in Nursing Science*. 10.1097/ANS.0000000000000413

Jenkins, D., Holmes, D., Burton, C. W., & Murray, S. J. (2020). "This is not a patient, this is property of the state": Nursing, ethics, and the immigrant detention apparatus. *Nursing Inquiry*, *27*(3), e12358. 10.1111/nin.12358

Johansson, J. A., & Holmes, D. (2021). Abjection and the weaponization of bodily excretions in forensic psychiatry settings: A poststructural reflection. *Nursing Inquiry*, e12480. 10.1111/nin.12480

Kay, K., Evans, A., & Glass, N. (2015, March 1). Moments of speaking and silencing: Nurses share their experiences of manual handling in healthcare. *Collegian*, *22*(1), 61–70. 10.1016/j.colegn.2013.11.005

Kühl, S. (2016). The angel in the house and fallen women: Assigning women their places in Victorian society. *Open Educational Resources, University of Oxford*, 14.

Lamb, C., Evans, M., Babenko-Mould, Y., Wong, C., & Kirkwood, K. (2019, March 1). Nurses' use of conscientious objection and the implications for conscience. *Journal of Advanced Nursing, 75*(3), 594–602. 10.1111/jan.13869

Lewis, D., & David, L. M. (1999). *Papers in metaphysics and epistemology: Volume 2.* Cambridge University Press.

Lewis, D. K. (1966). An argument for the identity theory. *The Journal of Philosophy, 63*(1), 17–25.

Lowe, E. J. (2008). Essentialism, metaphysical realism, and the errors of conceptualism. *Philosophia Scientiæ. Travaux d'histoire et de philosophie des sciences 12*(1), 9–33.

McIntyre, J. R. S., Burton, C., & Holmes, D. (2020). From discipline to control in nursing practice: A poststructuralist reflection. *Nursing Philosophy, 21*(4), e12317. 10.1111/nup.12317

Mol, A. (2003). *The body multiple.* Duke University Press.

Nightingale, F. (1860). *Notes on nursing: What it is and what it is not* (Dover ed.). Harrison and Sons.

Oderberg, D. S. (2007). *Real essentialism.* Routledge.

Oxford Languages. (2022). *Oxford english dictionary.* Oxford University Press. Retrieved February 28 from https://languages.oup.com/google-dictionary-en/

Reverby, S. M. (1987). *Ordered to care: The dilemma of American nursing, 1850–1945.* Cambridge University Press.

Ricoeur, P. (1991). Narrative identity. *Philosophy today, 35*(1), 73–81.

Rivers, B. (2020). Reforming the angel: Morality, language and mid-victorian nursing heroines. *Australasian Journal of Victorian Studies, 8*(1), 60–76.

Sandelowski, M. (2000). *Devices & desires: Gender, technology, and American nursing.* UNC Press Books.

Sayers, S. (1999). Identity and community. *Journal of Social philosophy, 30*(1), 147–160.

Schlak, A. E., Rosa, W. E., Rushton, C. H., Poghosyan, L., Root, M. C., & McHugh, M. D. (2022). An expanded institutional- and national-level blueprint to address nurse burnout and moral suffering amid the evolving pandemic. *Nursing Management, 53*(1), 16–27. 10.1097/01.NUMA.0000805032.15402.b3

Stein, L. I. (1967). The doctor-nurse game. *Archives of General Psychiatry, 16*(6), 699–703.

Tekke, M., & Watson, P. J. (2017, February 7). Supplication and the muslim personality: Psychological nature and functions of prayer as interpreted by Said Nursi. *Mental Health, Religion & Culture, 20*(2), 143–153. 10.1080/13674676.2017.1328401

Van Kleef, G. A., De Dreu, C. K. W., & Manstead, A. S. R. (2010). An interpersonal approach to emotion in social decision making: The emotions as social information model. In *Advances in experimental social psychology* (Vol. 42, pp. 45–96). Academic Press. 10.1016/S0065-2601(10)42002-X

Walter, R. R. (2017). Emancipatory nursing praxis: A theory of social justice in nursing. *Advances in Nursing Science, 40*(3), 225–243.

Williams, J. (2005). *Understanding poststructuralism.* Acumen Publishing, LTD.

Wocial, L. D. (2020). Resilience as an incomplete strategy for coping with moral distress in critical care nurses. *Critical Care Nurse, 40*(6), 62–66. 10.4037/ccn2020873

5 imagining afFIRMative futures for nursing

Jamie Smith and Eva Willis

Our theoretical embeddedness instructs our approach to nursing practice as an affirmative and creative critique to humanistic assumptions in healthcare. In this essay, we propose nursing as a radical pedagogy and move from critique to affirmative practice to (re)imagine a posthuman care that takes the possibilities of relationality into account through affirmative ethics and situated knowledges. We encourage setting boundaries for the profession and individual practitioners who are bound within neoliberal healthcare sectors, being kind but firm and by acknowledging the ever changing places from which we speak. In this text, posthumanism means thinking with the human and the more-than-human, not excluding them or (tacitly) declaring their redundancy (Haraway, 2016)[1]. We inquire about the metaphors that are ascribed in contemporary nursing and embedded by examples such as regulatory frameworks. The inquiry of such examples are not necessarily a call to fundamentally change or abolish such structures such as regulatory frameworks (although such claims could be made elsewhere), but to illustrate with them toward broader systemic challenges that we wish to engage with.

We are practising nurses and nurse educators working in Germany and the United Kingdom (UK). We write from this situatedness and we acknowledge the limitations that this perspective brings. We share migration experiences in Europe, are able-bodied, speak German and English, have a working-class background, hold nationalities that allow us to travel freely at the moment, are cisgendered and white, an agnostic hetero woman, and an atheist gay man.

Nursing Challenges as Global and Ecological Challenges

The main challenge facing nursing and healthcare is meeting the care needs of a globally aging population. The over-60 population is growing faster than any other (Buchan et al., 2019) while the working-age population remains static. This presents the challenge of who will care for people and how humans will care for their elderly if there are fewer working age people. The aging population increases demands on nursing and care, and subsequently contributes to nursing shortages. The political leadership of most high-income countries are issuing calls for more nurses to meet the growing demands on healthcare systems.

DOI: 10.4324/9781003245957-8

With about 28 million nurses in the workforce globally, estimations indicate that 13 million (and more?) nurses are needed over the next decade (Buchan et al., 2022). Where are these nurses going to come from? Birthrates in the Global North are steadily declining (and we are not arguing that this is a bad development) with estimates of the global population to peak in 2064 at 10 billion and a decline to 9 billion by 2100 (Vollset et al., 2020). With around 15% nurses globally born or trained in another country (that is one in eight or 3.7 million) (World Health Organization, 2020b, p. 69), strategies of sourcing nurses from lower-income countries to higher-income countries to plug the nursing shortages is a popular strategy but at the least unethical and unsustainable, as it bleeds nursing from low-income countries (Nolan, 2022; Hossain, 2020). We find it also ethically ambiguous that nurses from higher income-countries temporarily work in low-income countries in a humanitarian effort, grooming these higher-income countries' charitable self-perception (Bauer, 2017; Loiseau et al., 2016; Welling et al., 2010). Besides needing about 13 million more nurses globally in the next decade, other global and economical dimensions must be considered and addressed with regards to nursing care. For example, how much will it cost to train 13 million nurses worldwide? Who will train these nurses? What and where are the budget plans to meet this demand? How will we finance these 13 million nurses once they are practitioners? The COVID pandemic has made the nursing shortage hypervisible and we must pay attention to how many nurses have left the bedside or are considering leaving the bedside due to pandemic stressors. How many nurses have lost their lives or who are unable to work due to Covid? Additional global challenges surround the community-based care work due to nursing shortage. For example, how many laypeople are compensating for the lack of nurses globally by looking after their neighbors, friends, and relatives? What is the value of this unpaid labor, the economic loss of laypeople not being able to contribute to the economy while compensating care work of nurses, and what might be the potential, unintentional damage in care errors caused by systems in which laypeople must compensate for missing resources? We do not presume to have the answers to these questions posed but we understand that affirmative futures require us as citizens and nurses to consider these challenging questions as necessary part of radical imagining, understanding that all things touch other things (Haraway, 2016).

Many (and more) approaches are needed if we aim to handle these global and ecological challenges even rudimentarily. In this essay, we consider these challenges through questioning implied, taken-for-granted philosophies, and theories in nursing and (re)imagining possible shifts. We situate our work with the words of ecological philosopher Tsing: "It is time to turn attention to the non scalable, not only as objects for description but also as incitements to theory" (Tsing, 2015, p. 38). The increasing global demand for care within the challenges of planetary health embeds nursing deeply within the posthuman convergence. With posthuman convergence we mean the confluence "of technological development [...] and environmental depletion"

(Braidotti, 2022, p. 112; Kolbert, 2014; McAfee & Brynjolfsson, 2017). Increasing care demands also raises political and philosophical questions into what more sustainable future configurations of care and society will look like.

In response to global challenges, the World Health Organization (World Health Organisation, 2016; 2020a), highlighted by the general director leadership, has repeatedly made calls to upskill nurses to improve global health. Nurses need to be research-based, addressing and informing advanced technologies, globally focused interdisciplinary, and prepared for radical (and perhaps uncomfortable) change in response to these calls (Rafferty et al., 2019). If we as nurse researchers consider these calls in the context of the posthuman convergence, then this raises the question: how do we upskill nurses in bio-socio-politically changing contexts? Nurse researchers can learn from where we have come from, however, the solutions to the issues of now and the future will not be found solely in the past; we must produce the radical futures we imagine. The next section will imagine nursing future as radical pedagogy while the last section will underpin these imaginings within a theoretical rhizomatic assemblage.

Imagining Nursing Futures

Nursing as Radical Pedagogy

Nursing is a radical pedagogy because it negotiates the multiple and dynamic focal points in a situation. Nursing is not special or different from other parts of how social worlds are made, however in the context of healthcare, nursing has been tasked with being the glue that holds systems together and enacts the continuity of an institution. Nursing as a historically and presently feminized profession is tasked with the labors that have been rendered invisible by patriarchy and capitalism, such as emotional and organizational labors. These invisible labors are how realities are produced and how the materiality of healthcare is enacted. In this way nursing is a radical pedagogy because it works with the liminal boundaries of materiality and creates knowledge through material practices (Taylor & Fairchild, 2020).

Nursing and caring practices navigate multiple contingent, focal, and dynamic situations. Imagine the practice of a nurse in a hospital who is assigned four patients when they arrive on shift. Sometime early in the shift a patient requires assistance with personal care and the nurse begins to prepare for this by bringing fresh linen for the bed, fresh pajamas for the patient and other sanitary items to help the patient change. Just as they are attending the bedside, a patient in the neighboring bed complains of central chest pain. The nurse becomes acutely aware that the patient in the neighboring bed could be having a heart attack and re-prioritises her workload and attends to the patient with chest pain immediately, leaving the patient who needs personal care. A purist approach to person-centered care denotes that both patients have a choice in their care and that the person who needs support with their personal care should have choice in the same way that the person having a heart attack does. In reality, nurses know this is not the case and manage the situation to prioritize according to safety and needs of the patients by navigating available more-than-human and human resources. The needs of patients are subjective and dynamic as they change with the situation. The needs of patients are not limited to being clinical but are also emotional, physical, cognitive, and so forth. Adding to that, patients are not passive recipients or consumers of care but active co-producers in their care (Mol, 2010, p. 18). Nursing practice already acknowledges the dividual (see below), rather than the individual and we underpin this with theory. The dividual operates to define personhood as a social and relational process, where the person can be understood as a porous social being, whilst simultaneously being situated and with agency (Smith, 2012). The patients, the nurse, others in the healthcare team and the institution exist simultaneously but with different priorities and needs, and realities are produced through negotiating these sometimes contradictory positions.

The needs of patients are not the only needs in a healthcare setting. Healthcare systems exist to provide healthcare to more than one person and to continue to care for people; therefore other things should be considered in the sustainability of those systems. There are needs of staff, buildings, institutions, and the materiality of how healthcare is delivered. The staff working in healthcare need to be able to continue to care beyond the individual interactions therefore can not give their all to every patient, as giving one's all would leave nothing left for the next patient or for the person to care for themselves. The needs and resources of the institution should be considered, as an institution giving everything to one patient would leave nothing for the next patient. These needs situate themselves in a critical posthuman new materialist framework as they are fundamentally located in sustainability and the ways in which we continue to exist on a planet constituted of materiality and imagination. Nursing practice perceives these dynamic needs and makes these needs perceptible in the context of their production.

Nursing as a Critical Posthuman Pedagogy

Nursing praxis is critical posthuman pedagogy because it works with materiality and affective assemblages of matters. We have briefly demonstrated how nurse work is (re) configured within environments and produced through affective potentials of relationality. Nursing is critical posthuman praxis because care sprays water on the web of power (Brownlie & Anderson, 2017, p. 1225), and in this context power is understood as the possibility of relationality (Walsh et al., 2021; West et al., 2020). In demonstrating how contemporary nursing frameworks are built on assumptions of the liminal and bounded humans as individuals, not a dividuals, we argue that patient centered care is overly individualistic (and neo-liberal). Autonomous perspectives of the patient, and the "autonomous" practitioner is revered in codes of practice instead of material-discursive, diffracted, negotiated practices of care. Nurse work makes the re-lationality of matter perceptible in ways that are not possible with solely hu-manistic frameworks. A purely theoretical approach to nurse work cannot value nursing because nursing (and teaching and social work!) are practical and theoretical subjects which can not always be planned in advance (Puig de la Bellacasa, 2017); however, nursing is now in the academy and has to navigate the structures of universities.

Nurse work is not special—"nurse work" and care have existed for a long time. Nevertheless, nurse work is a focusing point, a convergence or a point of diffraction in which we can understand relationality from our embedded and embodied human perspective. As discussed in the previous section, care work in nursing is a radical praxis because it is accountable to its dynamic situation and recognises the relationality of the situation. Nursing praxis enables the simultaneous existence of multiple systems of knowledge production. Nursing as a critical posthuman praxis creates a critique of person-centered care. It understands nurse work as always situated and in relation to other things. This approach critiques the absolute independence of an individual (patient or nurse) because it shows how an individual is always reliant and created by their relationality. Individuals exist in multiplicities of contradictions that are not fixed or rational; they are affected and ongoing. This claim diffracts the dominant paradigm of patient centered care; it understands the patient or nurse in their situatedness, and who is produced in their dividuality, not their individuality.

What Our Futures of Nursing Could Look Like

Nursing is not individual but a communal practice that has existed throughout centuries and is not inherently bound to the profession of nurses. The pro-fessionalization of nursing has captured care and feminine histories of care; they are overwritten to create care as a branded commodity, such as the idealized Vitruvian nurse (described below). Imagine if nurses were taught to tell a patient to wait as other care needs might be higher on their priority list to ensure safe patient care for all of their patients. If nurses were to com-municate this, how were they taught to communicate this with their patients to not hurt the patient's fragile individualistic sense of self? If you imagine being a patient, how would you feel if a nurse would communicate the complex navigation of your needs with others and you were aware that at some points you are not in the center of this thinking? Therefore, an irrefu-table future for nurses and patients is predetermined by the narrow philoso-phies of humanistic science; the human (historically cisgendered, masculine and white) as a bound individual is privileged above everything. Then, the Vitruvian nurse is established as the idealized care being. This metaphor ubiquitously is a mechanism to govern care and how care can be imagined because it is misogynistic and reproduces restrictive power relations to keep nurses (mostly women) in their place (Smith et al., 2022).

How Nursing Is Currently Imagined—The Metaphor of the Vitruvian Nurse

Nursing has been built in through the regulatory framework of nurses "as apolitical, devoid of power and agency" (Dillard-Wright & Shields-Haas, 2021, p. 3) with regulatory frameworks as one mode of producing such implications. We have written elsewhere how the metaphor of the Vitruvian Nurse (adapted from Braidotti's (2013) critique of the Vitruvian man) as the collective idea of the perfect nurse is implicated in nursing codes of conduct which contributes to cultivating a framework of a perfect and idealized nurse that is used to serve the neo-capitalist ways in which healthcare systems are produced (Smith et al., 2022). The metaphor of the Vitruvian Nurse then is the collective imagining of the ideal: a uniformed woman, swiftly and joyously attending to the needs of every patient. The idealized human body of the Vitruvian man is used to create the idealized patient and the idealized nurse; a normative blueprint for the ideal patient and perfect nurse. The impossibility of the metaphor of the Vitruvian nurse is actualised when she dissolves her subjectivity in the service of others. The Vitruvian nurse is an axiom that captures the impossible picture of the idealized and infallible nurse in regulatory frameworks, neoliberal capitalism, culture etc. These frameworks have their roots in the Anglo-American traditions but have been exported globally in the context of globalization and colonialism.

Why We Need a Code of Conduct for Nurses

From a legal perspective and considering some of the dark histories in nursing, it makes sense to hold nurses liable as individuals. We agree that the Code of Conduct needs to exist to give structure and for the protection of the public, other professionals, and the organization. Personal responsibility needs to be accounted for. Yet we argue that (without wanting to exclude the importance of personal liability) there is collective and organizational accountability that contributes to preventing the likelihood of shortcomings or sets professionals up to fail more.

Patient-centered care is characterized by a set of principles and activities that work collaboratively between health and social care professionals and the people who use services. Patient-centered care supports people to increase their knowledge, skills, and understanding of their condition in order to make informed decisions about their health. Furthermore, patient-centered care intends to involve patients in their care so they can be treated with dignity and respect.

Nurses—just as any person—have the potential to harm and have not been innocent historically. One of the reasons that code of conducts developed is because of atrocities committed by healthcare workers and systems, such as participation in genocides. There is also evidence of nurses participating in harming vulnerable groups such as the Tuskegee syphilis study where black men were recruited to a syphilis trial but not offered effective treatment (Reverby, 2012). Nurses also participated in the Willowbrook study that intentionally exposed mentally disabled children to Hepatitis to study the disease (Krugman, 1986). Therefore, the code of conduct and the concept of patient-centered care can be understood as a way of preventing further horrors in healthcare by franchising the people being cared for. Nurses also understand that codes serve as a public protector and promoter of professional status (Tadd et al., 2006, p. 383).

We do not argue for a world without a regulatory framework for nursing. If we imagine that nurses are inherently good and therefore no regulatory process is required because nurses can do no harm, then we are repeating the misogyny of nursing where women are there to look after people, and therefore not learning from the past. Lack of regulatory framework leads to the inability to imagine crimes by nurses and hence, prevents accountability and is dangerous. In their book on nurses and midwives in Nazi Germany, Benedict and Shields (2014) state that they were told on several occasions during their research that "nurses would not do those things" (p. 2) with which they refer to nurses who committed crimes during World War II, such as participating in historical genocides. The contradictions of nursing and nursing care practices are highlighted by the following quote:

> Nurses have a history of both upholding oppressive systems that disenfranchise segments of the public, usually poor, often People of Color, and engaging in innovative alternatives to the status quo.
>
> (Dillard-Wright & Shields-Haas, 2021, p. 3)

We as authors critique the metaphor of the Vitruvian nurse because this metaphor influences policies. Instead we advocate for policies that are ethical and affirmative, inviting, and enabling multiple ways of being nurses whilst providing needed structure for patients, the public, and the nursing profession. We argue with standpoint theory (Harding 2004) that everything is viewed from somewhere; therefore, we as nurses must become accountable for our position. If we do not make the ways in which we are implicated in the production of reality perceptible, then we risk being territorialized, overwhelmed and restricted in different ways. Guattari (2005) uses the examples of the canals in Venice becoming overwhelmed with algae to highlight the restrictive potential of not taking a position. Examining regulatory frameworks and the metaphors they create are one way to take a position and represent nurses' work; however, to accept them uncritically or ignore diffractive possibilities is as bad as not taking a position. Taking a position is a contemporaneous and ongoing process. The position is, was, and will never be static or fixed; moreover, it exists with materiality in ratios of motion and rest (Deleuze, 1994). Taking a position is affirmative praxis.

What Futures Are There Then?

We aim to diffract these metaphors in care and nursing by understanding how they became territorialized. The ethics of affirmation and joy as understood by Lloyd's reading of Spinoza, is the process of becoming aware of the conditions of one's own bondage (Lloyd, 1994). Shared understandings of these conditions create the ethics of affirmation and joy. This could mean that care and nurse work is about making the materiality, possibilities and (im)possibilities of a situation, perceptible to each other. What metaphors and imaginations could support nurses to practise affirmative ethics within a code of conduct? How do we negotiate contradicting perspectives with patients and acknowledge long histories of care? When the nurse has a different understanding of what could be best for a patient's health and well-being than the patient, how do we create possibilities where the patient feels acknowledged and sees possibilities for themselves and the nurses' subjectivities and insights are not silenced in this process?

We suggest that future metaphors move away from emphasizing individual responsibility or perfection on nurses or patients. We argue that nurses should be accountable to their position but consider the paradigms of the dividual rather than the individual—that is to say, work with a regulatory framework that acknowledges and supports self-determinacy but not self-sufficiency (Wynter, 1989). Care demonstrates how individuals (both nurses and patients) can be thought of as dividuals (Smith & Willis, 2020); not as isolated entities, rather deeply embedded in and produced through material and social relations (Deleuze & Guattari, 1988). Critical posthumanism sees the bounded self as a site of reconfiguration. Hence, how we conceptualize the self is not as a fixed point but more a dynamic constellation of matter.

Nursing's regulatory frameworks are iterative processes, which is a material benefit to acknowledge the ever-moving ethics of care instead of fixing a moral position. Therefore, future versions of codes of ethics could better acknowledge this affirmative dynamism to include diffractions acknowledging that the production of the self is a dynamic and relational process and nursing education should be world-centered rather (Biesta, 2021) than patient-centered. In addition we encourage nurses (and staff dynamics and organizations) to be afFIRMative and stand firm and accountable by embracing their unique characteristics, such as joy, humor, campness (White, 1993) and feistiness; and others/sometimes none of these. Power relations become perceptible through strong but not pre-defined practices. We encourage nurses (and staff dynamics and organizations) to be afFIRMative and stand firm and accountable by embracing their unique characteristics, such as joy, humor, campness (White, 1993) and feistiness; and others/sometimes none of these. Power relations become perceptible through strong but not pre-defined practices. Also, it is important to recall that humans and more-than humans exist together as dividuals, they are diffracted with and by their environment and form ecologies; this imperative for human and planetary health. Suggestions such as these would begin to create other conditions of possibility for nursing. We imagine that it would create the possibility that the nurse is not responsible for everything, and is at the same time personally implicated in the production of care. Affirmative dynamism begins to diffract away from a neo-liberal model of care, where the patients "wishes" replace others' agency in a situation, because the patient is the "consumer." These suggestions could also create the conditions where a nurse could say no to a patient and not repeat the tropes of a servant or handmaid, whilst still acknowledging the patients and their own personal perspective. However, the nurse and patient should franchise each other in their desires, wishes, and possibilities to co-exist together. Another way to move toward more affirmative nursing futures is to critically examine current philosophical paradigms, which will be addressed in the next section.

Why Do We Need a Critique of Humanism in Healthcare?

Current healthcare in the Global North is embedded in humanism and with it the paradigms of the neoliberal, hyper-individualised subject (Hopkins-Walsh et al., 2022) the focus of person-centred care (Smith et al., 2022). We underpin the assumption of humanism as a permeating philosophy through examining person-centred care exemplarily and argue that assuming humans are the center of the universe is egocentric (Foucault, 2005).

Patient-centered care currently is one of the most eminent paradigms in healthcare. A comprehensive understanding of patient-centered care does not exist (Håkansson Eklund et al., 2019) despite of its prominence on organizational and governmental level (i.e., ICN, 2021). Person-centred care is a collection of principles, rather than a strict definition of a shared decision-making approach (of patient and healthcare provider) to care, that can be used to plan and deliver care. Historically, person-centred care can be understood as a response that emerged in the 1970s to shift from the biomedical model of the patient with its focus on symptoms and illness toward a more holistic understanding, defining a patient as a cultural and social being, privileging the patient's agency in their healthcare (McCormack & McCance, 2010; Wanless et al., 2007; Balint, 1969).

We are not first in criticizing person-centered care (i. a. Arnold et al., 2020). Our critique comes from a posthuman perspective where we argue that a move from the biomedical subject to patient-centered care (the neoliberal subject) is a shift from one narrow understanding of care to another, which coincided with the further neo-liberalisation of societies.

Patient-centredness implies a humanistic philosophy, illustrated through these three principles (see Klein, 2007): Patient-centered care assumes that the person being cared for is a rational agent capable of processing and assimilating knowledge and then making a decision. The concept of who the person is that is described in person-centered care refers back to the person's ability to make decisions therefore decontextualises a person. Patient-centered care emphasizes individualism by promoting an individual's ability to make choices in a situation despite their health status, vulnerability or what options may even be possible.

We argue that a model of care that relies on personal choice over situated realities contains three main weaknesses: An individual is not independent from their environment, therefore, their agency and capacity to produce realities is contingent on their situation, an individual's identity is dynamic and relational, and will change with time and situation, health and vulnerability, and the power relations between people, other people, and things are hidden when assuming that a person can always be in the centre of a situation.

The person-centred care paradigm is ascribed into regulatory frameworks such as code of conducts. Tadd et al. (2006) analyse how nurses in practice from nine European countries understand code of conducts and codes of ethics with many nurses in practice finding them lacking in applications. Nurses think the code is promoted for situations where they would seek guidance from a code, such as resolving ethical dilemmas, finding codes to be "an unworkable ideal ... impossible to adhere to its requirements" (Tadd et al., 2006, p. 385). Nurses also point to the weaknesses that a humanistic reduction of care implies a promotion of the focus on the individual. Nurses describe these contradictions produced: "Patients are more and more aware of their rights and this is good, but sometimes it clashes with performing our duties and our code. They think they are the only people who are sick at the moment" (Tadd et al., 2006, p. 384).

The concept of patient-centered care is a symbolic representation of what we find questionable in an (all too) humanistic perspective on care. It shows how underlying humanism acknowledges and attempts to privilege patient agency while failing to address the interdependence of human and more-than-human entities (Mol, 2002). We also believe codes of conduct can be a valuable document as a protective factor for the public but in order to guide nursing practice, patient-centered care as a paradigm can acknowledge neither the navigation of care work nor the complexity of patients and the ecologies they are embedded in. We argue that critical posthumanism has possibilities (Langton, 2007) to discuss theoretical blank spots:

1   People are interdependent, relational, embodied, and embedded entities (Ferrando, 2019; Mol, 2002; Puig de la Bellacasa, 2017; Theodosius, 2008). Such dependencies (including how patients can make decisions) are: material resources of the hospital, infrastructure, the ability of staff to have time and resources to connect with them so that information is understandable and, in general, to give them the experience of being valued and cared for. Further, mood, education, access to information or knowledge as well as the consequences the decision has for others around them.

2   Patients are an ever-changing dynamic entity, relying more on survival than identity (Rees et al., 2019). Hence, a decision that a patient might make one moment might differ days or weeks later, depending on how they and their circumstances have changed.

3   Power relations between healthcare providers and patients that are embedded with their families, partners, and communities have to be openly discussed. Power relations between nurses/doctors/patients/domestic staff do not stop existing, nor is the existence of such power relations necessarily nefarious.

Advocating for Patients/Nurses/More-Than-Human Perspectives (And, And, And)

We, as healthcare providers, have access to rooms, to private spaces, and to bodies (undressing, washing, examining someone), intimate entanglements of power relations. Delivering care involves negotiating these entanglements and intersections of power, but in the midst of negotiating, power relations do not go away. Patients will most likely still feel vulnerable, nurses will likely be perceived to be lower down the ranks than a doctor. Critiquing patient-centered care does not ignore the fact that patients are very much involved in their care. However, it cannot be central because a ward with 30 patients could never function and benefit the individual patient if 30 centers of care were created on a ward. A ward is a dynamic environment of multiple centers existing at different ratios of motion and rest (Deleuze & Guattari, 1988, Lloyd, 1994). The paradigm shift toward patient-centered care in healthcare has obscured power relations by giving the impression there are choices to be made by an idealized, appropriately advised, and educated patient while often ignoring or silencing those with less power. The opportunity that we perceive here is how to acknowledge and work with power while franchising patients in their care.

Posthuman Convergence—Toward Our Philosophical Understanding of Care

Critical posthuman theory (Braidotti, 2019) acknowledges the histories of feminist movements in influencing nursing and care work (Puig de la Bellacasa, 2017, Rose, 2012) and is relevant to understanding and interrogating care practices. Nursing has undergone a professionalization project over the past 50 years that aimed to create a more educated and self-regulated healthcare workforce. This professionalization coincided with a paradigm shift and meeting of phenomena in economic, political, and cultural production that Braidotti (2013) describes in more detail as the "posthuman convergence." She refers to the posthuman convergence as the current state of the world as the historical position of centering the (white, hetero, male) human a defining feature of the Anthropocene). Braidotti describes the posthuman convergence through three intersections:

> First, at the social level we witness increasing structural injustices through the unequal distribution of wealth, prosperity and access to technology. Second, at the environmental level we are confronted with the devastation

of species and a decaying planet, struck by climate crisis and new epidemics. And third, at the technological level, the status and condition of the human is being redefined by the life sciences and genomics, neural sciences and robotics, nanotechnologies, the new information technologies and the digital interconnections they afford us.

(Braidotti, 2022, p. 3)

The opportunities created by the posthuman convergence for the introspection of the human and what it is to be human is of particular interest to nursing. Braidotti (2013) traces the genealogy of the postanthropocentic shift back to Foucault (2005) who articulates that there is a correlation between an object becoming thinkable and entering a state of crisis, arguing that this is what is currently happening to the "human." Rapid environmental changes and the reduction in biodiversity have forced humanity to consider its mortality in a globalized way. The rapid development and timing of these phenomena create questions both concerning biopolitics (referring to the ways how populations are born and die) and postanthropocentric thought (referring to the individual's position in society and on the planet; Braidotti, 2019). Related to nursing, this means that if we acknowledge that humans exist in dependence within ecologies and not above them, what kind of modes of care do we need to create to account for this dependence and enable cooperative flourishing(s)?

Systems of thought outside the western academic institutions have incorporated thinking beyond the self for much longer than this, for example the philosophy of Ubuntu that attests that I am because you are (Mboti, 2015). Approaching the human in a situated way has again come to the fore because of the man-made existential threats which humanity faces. Braidotti and Bignall (2019) provide examples of how these existential threats are enacted by means of ecological crises, alongside the establishment of new departments at universities which address technology's "threats" e.g., artificial intelligence (the fear of AI overtaking the human). Existential threats to life are framed by humanity's shared existence. However, this is a European cosmopolitan existence. It presumes that humanity and to be human are unified concepts, when in reality, they are a complex network of relationality in which some people never get to be human in the first place (Wynter, 1989).

How the Individual Becomes a Dividual

The approach we take to posthumanism understands culture and actors through the materiality of the human and more-than-human. Nursing is dynamic and multifocal and describes the ongoing relationality of the human and the more-than-human. We use this terminology to acknowledge the ongoing attempts to decentralize the focus of this writing.

Humanism perceives the self as an individual, rational subject, whereas posthumanism questions these discrete categories and asks where the self ends and the other begins (Barad, 2003). The notion of the individual similarly becomes interrogated as the subject in posthumanism is understood as a diffracted self within ecologies, always changing. The person is not an individual "as a single body (...) We no longer find ourselves dealing with the mass/individual pair. Individuals have become "dividuals," and masses, samples, data, markets, or "banks"" (Deleuze, 1992). This does not negate thresholds between the human and more-than-human, but rather reconfigures an understanding of the discrete boundaries of the human. Posthumanism challenges us to think beyond dialectics of the self and others, and to think about the boundaries, which are assumed to be concrete; understanding the human alongside and with the more-than-human as intensities of matter and affective assemblages. This challenge to dialectical knowledge systems therefore requires elaboration. In this chapter, we will provide practical examples from nurse work to illuminate and reconfigure the liminal boundaries of the human, and to situate how a research project can develop from this. We provide examples of care that demonstrate how individuals can be thought of as dividuals; not isolated entities, but rather deeply embedded in and produced by material and social relations (Deleuze & Guattari, 1988).

The posthuman premise that the human is not the center of the universe can be uncomfortable because it challenges contemporary assumptions about the self in the global north and eurocentric western world. All we need to do is think back to when Copernicus proposed that the earth was not the center of the universe, instead revolving around the sun. Posthuman scholars invite us to let posthumanism be a contemporary Copernicus and (re)think the human as not being the center of the universe (Smith & Willis, 2020). Following this, which implications and consequences might the move away from anthropocentric thinking have for the understanding of the self and societies as a whole? Also, which entity/entities (if any) might take the sun's place in this allegory? Posthuman logic encourages decentralization. However, historically in western philosophymuch of our thought builds upon assumptions of central points and stable states. These can now be points of mobilization.

Care Is Ubiquitous

Nursing is everywhere, yet such a broad statement requires context and qualification. It requires us to understand what nursing is as well as how it is understood in different global contexts. Here, if we loosely assume nursing is care, and everywhere is lived human experience, then we begin to understand the intention behind such a statement. Nursing is everywhere because it is entangled with everyone and everything, because care is ubiquitous—that is to say, everyone is born, and everyone dies. These life events are shared by all humans. Birth and death become concepts that create shared points in life. They create a space for shared experiences of care and what care may be, although we may experience all these shared events, they are not one and the same. It is this space of commonality through difference where this project begins and works to establish how nurse work and care are focal points (Taylor & Fairchild, 2020) to interpellate posthuman theory as practical philosophy (Deleuze & Guattari, 1988; Smith & Willis, 2020). As nurses we must begin to look at the politics and philosophies employed to underwrite health systems in order to address challenges in healthcare. The tension that an aging population and a new industrial revolution creates, provides an opportunity for health systems to consider how to do things differently as it becomes clearer that more of the same is not the way to prepare for a changing world. Health systems must face the possibility that they will never be able to train enough nurses to look after the aging population if health systems do not adapt in philosophy and delivery. We must accept the biopolitical shift and work with it to educate and prepare for the future.

How the Individual Becomes a Dividual

In summary, the approach we take to posthumanism understands culture and actors through the materiality of the human and more-than-human. Humanism perceives the self as an individual, rational subject, whereas posthumanism questions these discrete categories and asks where the self ends and the other begins (Barad, 2003). The notion of the individual similarly becomes interrogated as the subject in posthumanism is understood as a diffracted self within ecologies, always changing. The person is not an individual "as a single body [...] We no longer find ourselves dealing with the mass/individual pair. Individuals have become "dividuals," and masses, samples, data, markets, or "banks"" (Deleuze, 1992). This does not negate thresholds between the human and more-than-human, but rather reconfigures an understanding of the discrete boundaries of the human. Posthumanism challenges us to think beyond dialectics of the self and others, and to think about the boundaries, which are assumed to be concrete; understanding the human alongside and with the more-than-human as intensities of matter and affective assemblages. This challenge to dialectical knowledge systems therefore requires elaboration. individuals can be thought of as dividuals; not isolated entities, but rather deeply embedded in and produced by material and social relations (Deleuze & Guattari, 1988).

Similarly to a root system, our essay has no definite end point but many rhizomatic knots. We end by leading into the next chapter of this book with some theoretical thoughts. We have started to imagine futures for nursing through the posthuman convergence. The posthuman convergence is characterized by the coming together of posthumanism and postanthropocentrism. Posthumanism is a philosophical paradigm where what is understood as human is a site of inquiry, where life is considered beyond the self, beyond species, beyond death, and beyond theory (Braidotti, 2013; Hartmann & Gone, 2014). Critical posthumanism is an entry point in to the critique of the humanistic ideal of (able-bodied-cis-hetero-white-european) man as the universal representative of the human. Postanthropocentric thought juxtaposes posthumanism, examining humanity's position in the world from a situated and ecological perspective (Plumwood, 1986). Postanthropocentrism critiques species hierarchy which places humans at the top of any taxonomic tree and begins to imagine realities in which systems of thought do not center on humans. The posthuman convergence, then, goes beyond the terms of a binary structure of human and non-human, them vs. us, to qualitatively describe the constellations of power relations in the production of our worlds. Right now, in our situatedness of the early C21, living with advanced capitalism, human made climate catastrophe, and ongoing fatal armed conflicts, we think as nurses with these two concepts and ponder how and what affirmative care and nursing can mean in the present and future.

Note

1 We use more-than-human as a descriptor for understanding all matter in the universe that is outwith the individual in humanistic approaches to the self (Barad, 2003). How the human and the more-than-human interact and come into being is described by Haraway (2016) as how we make our worlds.

References

Arnold, M. H., Kerridge, I., & Lipworth, W. (2020). An ethical critique of person-centred healthcare. *European Journal for Person Centered Healthcare*, 8(1), 34–44.

Balint, E. (1969). The possibilities of patient-centered medicine. *The Journal of the Royal College of General Practitioners*, 17(82), 269–276.

Barad, K. (2003). Posthumanist performativity: Toward an understanding of how matter comes to matter. *Signs: Journal of Women in Culture and Society*, 28(3), 801–831. 10.1086/345321

Bauer, I. (2017). More harm than good? The questionable ethics of medical volunteering and international student placements. *Tropical Diseases Travel Medicine and Vaccines*, 3, 5. 10.1186/s40794-017-0048-y

Benedict, S., & Shields, L. (2014). *Nurses and midwives in nazi Germany: The "Euthanasia Programs."* Routledge.

Biesta, G. (2021). *World-centred education: A view for the present.* Routledge.

Braidotti, R. (2013). *The posthuman.* Polity Press. http://ebookcentral.proquest.com/lib/ed/detail.action?docID=1315633

Braidotti, R. (2019). *Posthuman knowledge.* John Wiley & Sons.

Braidotti, R., & Bignall, S. (2019). *Posthuman ecologies complexity and process after Deleuze.* Rowman & Littlefield International.

Braidotti, R. (2022) *Posthuman feminism.* Polity Press.

Brownlie, J., & Anderson, S. (2017). Thinking sociologically about kindness: Puncturing the blasé in the ordinary city. *Sociology*, 51(6), 1222–1238.

Buchan, J., Gerschlick, B., & Charlesworth, A. (2019). *Falling short: The NHS workforce challenge.* The Health Foundation. https://www.health.org.uk/publications/reports/falling-short-the-nhs-workforce-challenge

Buchan J., Catton H., & Shaffer F. (2022). Sustain and retain in 2022 and beyond. The global nursing workforce and the COVID-19 pandemic. *ICNM - International Centre on Nurse Migration.* https://www.icn.ch/system/files/2022-01/Sustain%20and%20Retain%20in%202022%20and%20Beyond-%20The%20global%20nursing%20workforce%20and%20the%20COVID-19%20pandemic.pdf, Accessed February 10, 2022.

Cowper, A. (2019). The NHS workforce plan is an off-the-scale fantasy. *BMJ*, *365*, l4036. 10.1136/bmj.l4036

Deleuze, G. (1994). *Difference and repetition*. Columbia University Press.

Deleuze, G., & Guattari, F. (1988). *A thousand plateaus: Capitalism and schizophrenia*. Athlone Press.

Deleuze, G. (1992). Postscript on the societies of control.

Department of Health, UK. (2000). *The NHS plan: A plan for investment, a plan for reform (2000) | Policy Navigator*. https://navigator.health.org.uk/content/nhs-plan-plan-investment-plan-reform-2000

Dillard-Wright, J., & Shields-Haas, V. (2021). Nursing with the people: Reimagining futures for nursing. *Advances in Nursing Science, Publish Ahead of Print*. 10.1097/ANS.0000000000000361

Eklund, J. H., Holmström, I. K., Kumlin, T., Kaminsky, E., Skoglund, K., Höglander, J., ... & Meranius, M. S. (2019). "Same same or different?" A review of reviews of person-centered and patient-centered care. *Patient Education and Counseling*, *102*(1), 3–11.

Ferrando, F. (2019). *Philosophical posthumanism*. Bloomsbury Academic.

Foucault, M. (2005). *The order of things an archaeology of the human sciences*. Routledge. http://www.dawsonera.com/guard/protected/dawson.jsp?name=University%20of%20Edinburgh&dest=http://www.dawsonera.com/depp/reader/protected/external/AbstractView/S9780203996645

Glasper, A. (2015). Can the new NMC code improve standards of care delivery? *British Journal of Nursing*, *24*(4), 238–239. 10.12968/bjon.2015.24.4.238

Guattari, F. (2005). *The three ecologies*. Bloomsbury Publishing.

Håkansson, J., Holmström I. K., Kumlin, T., Kaminsky, E., Skoglund, K., Höglander, J., Sundler, A. J., Condén, E., & Summer, M. (2019). "Same same or different?" A review of reviews of person-centered and patient-centered care. *Patient Education Counselling*, *102*(1), 3–11. 10.1016/j.pec.2018.08.029

Haraway, D. J. (2016). Staying with the trouble. In *Staying with the trouble*. Duke University Press.

Harding, S. (2004). A socially relevant philosophy of science? Resources from standpoint theoryas controversiality. *Hypatia*, *19*(1), 25–47.

Hartmann, W. E., & Gone, J. P. (2014). American Indian historical trauma: Community perspectives from two great plains medicine men. *American Journal of Community Psychology*, *54*(3), 274–288.

Hopkins-Walsh, J., Dillard-Wright, J., Brown, B., Smith, J., & Willis, E. (2022). Critical posthuman nursing care: Bodies reborn and the ethical imperative for composting. *Witness: The Canadian Journal of Critical Nursing Discourse*, *4*(1), 16–35. 10.25071/2291-5796.126

Hossain, F. (2020). Global responsibility vs. individual dreams: Addressing ethical dilemmas created by the migration of healthcare practitioners. *Global Bioethics = Problemi di bioetica*, *31*(1), 81–89. 10.1080/11287462.2020.1773054

International Council of Nurses (2021). Patient centred care. https://www.icn.ch/nursing-policy/icn-strategic-priorities/person-centred-care, Accessed July 18, 2022.

Klein, N. (2007). *The shock doctrine: The rise of disaster capitalism*. Macmillan.

Kolbert, E. (2014). *The sixth extinction: An unnatural history*. A&C Black.

Krugman, S. (1986). The willowbrook hepatitis studies revisited: Ethical aspects. *Reviews of Infectious Diseases*, *8*(1), 157–162. 10.1093/clinids/8.1.157

Langton, R. (2007). Feminism in philosophy. *The Oxford Handbook of Contemporary Philosophy*. 10.1093/oxfordhb/9780199234769.003.0009

Lloyd, G. (1994). *Part of nature: Self-knowledge in Spinoza's ethics*. Cornell University Press.

Loiseau, B., Sibbald, R., Raman, S. A., Benedict, D., Dimaras, H., & Loh, L. C. (2016). "Don't make my people beggars": A developing world house of cards. *Community Development Journal*, 51(4), 571–584. 10.1093/cdj/bsv047

Mboti, N. (2015). May the real ubuntu please stand up? *Journal of Media Ethics*, 30(2), 125–147.

McAfee, A., & Brynjolfsson, E. (2017). *Machine, platform, crowd: Harnessing our digital future*. WW Norton & Company.

McCormack, B., & McCance, T. (2010). *Person-centred nursing*. Wiley-Blackwell. https://www.dawsonera.com/abstract/9781444390490

Mol, A. (2002). *The body multiple ontology in medical practice*. Duke University Press. http://www.ezproxy.is.ed.ac.uk/login?url=http://dx.doi.org/10.1215/9780822384151

Mol, A., Moser, I., & Pols, J. (Eds.). (2015). *Care in practice: On tinkering in clinics, homes and farms* (Vol. 8). Transcript Verlag.

Mol, A., Moser, I., & Pols, J. (2010). Care: putting practice into theory. *Care in practice: On tinkering in clinics, homes and farms*, 8, 7–27.

Nolan, P. (2022). Enlightenment ideas and mental health nursing in the early 20th century. *British Journal of Mental Health Nursing*, 11(1), 1–7.

Nolen, S. (2022, January 29). How rich countries take away poor countries doctors and nurses. *Times of India*. https://timesofindia.indiatimes.com/world/us/us-and-world/how-rich-countries-take-away-poor-countries-doctors-and-nurses/articleshow/89182518.cms

Plumwood, V. (1986). Ecofeminism: An overview and discussion of positions and arguments. *Australasian Journal of Philosophy*, 64(sup1), 120–138.

Puig de la Bellacasa, M. (2017). *Matters of care: Speculative ethics in more than human worlds*. University of Minnesota Press. http://ebookcentral.proquest.com/lib/ed/detail.action?docID=4745533

Rafferty, A. M., Busse, R., Zander-Jentsch, B., Sermeus, W., & Bruyneel, L. (Eds.). (2019). *Strengthening health systems through nursing: Evidence from 14 European countries*. European Observatory on Health Systems and Policies. http://www.ncbi.nlm.nih.gov/books/NBK545724/

Ranisch, R., & Sorgner, S. L. (Eds.). (2014). *Post- and transhumanism: An introduction* (new edition edition). Peter Lang GmbH, Internationaler Verlag der Wissenschaften.

Rees, C. E., Kent, F., & Crampton, P. E. S. (2019). Student and clinician identities: How are identities constructed in interprofessional narratives? *Medical Education*, 53(8), 808–823. 10.1111/medu.13886

Reverby, S. M. (2012). *Tuskegee's truths: Rethinking the Tuskegee syphilis study*. UNC Press Books.

Rose, D. B. 2012. Multispecies knots of ethical time. *Environmental Philosophy*, 9(1), 127–140.

Smith, K. (2012). From dividual and individual selves to porous subjects. *The Australian Journal of Anthropology*, 23(1), 50–64.

Smith, J., & Willis, E. (2020). Interpreting posthumanism with nurse work. *Journal of Posthuman Studies*, 4(1), 59–75. 10.5325/jpoststud.4.1.0059

Smith, J., Willis, E., Hopkins-Walsh, J., Dillard-Wright, J., & Brown, B. (2022, under review) The metaphor of the Vitruvian nurse: A critical posthuman approach to nursing. In *Nursing Inquiry*.

Smith, J. B., Willis, E. M., & Hopkins-Walsh, J. (2022). What does person-centred care mean, if you weren't considered a person anyway: An engagement with person-centred care and Black, queer, feminist, and posthuman approaches. *Nursing Philosophy*, e12401.

Tadd, W., Clarke, A., Lloyd, L., Leino-Kilpi, H., Strandell, C., Lemonidou, C., Petsios, K., Sala, R., Barazzetti, G., Radaelli, S., Zalewski, Z., Bialecka, A., van der Arend, A., & Heymans, R. (2006). The value of nurses' codes: European nurses' views. *Nursing Ethics*, 13(4), 376–393. 10.1191/0969733006ne891oa

Taylor, C. A., & Fairchild, N. (2020). Towards a posthumanist institutional ethnography: Viscous matterings and gendered bodies. *Ethnography and Education*, 1–19.

Theodosius, C. (2008). *Emotional labour in health care: The unmanaged heart of nursing.* Routledge. 10.4324/9780203894958

Tsing, A. L. (2015). The mushroom at the end of the world. In *On the possibility of life in capitalist ruins*. Princeton University Press.

United Nations Population Fund (UNFPA). (2022). State of world population 2022: Seeing the unseen. *The case for action in the neglected crisis of unintended pregnancy.* https://www.unfpa.org/sites/default/files/pub-pdf/EN_SWP22%20report_0.pdf

Vollset, S. E., Goren, E., Yuan, C. W., et al. (2020). Fertility, mortality, migration, and population scenarios for 195 countries and territories from 2017 to 2100: A forecasting analysis for the global burden of disease study. *Lancet*, 396(10258), 1285–1306. 10.1016/S0140-6736(20)30677-2

Walsh, Z., Böhme, J., & Wamsler, C. (2021). Towards a relational paradigm in sustainability research, practice, and education. *Ambio*, 50, 74–84. 10.1007/s13280-020-01322-y

Wanless, D., Appleby, J., Harrison, A., & Patel, D. (2007). *Our future health secured.*

Welling, D. R., Ryan, J. M., Burris, D. G., & Rich, N. M. (2010). Seven sins of humanitarian medicine. *World Journal of Surgery*, 34(3), 466–470.

West, S., Haider, L. J., Stålhammar, S., & Woroniecki, S. (2020). A relational turn for sustainability science? Relational thinking, leverage points and transformations. *Ecosystems and People*, 16(1), 304–325. 10.1080/26395916.2020.1814417

White, A. (1993). *Carnival, hysteria and writing: Collected essays and autobiography/ Allon White*. Clarendon Press.

World Health Organisation. (2016). *Global strategy on human resources for health: Workforce 2030.* WHO, World Health Organization. http://www.who.int/hrh/resources/pub_globstrathrh-2030/en/

World Health Organisation. (2020a). *WHO and partners call for urgent investment in nurses.* https://www.who.int/news-room/detail/07-04-2020-who-and-partners-call-for-urgent-investment-in-nurses

World Health Organisation. (2020b). *State of the world's nursing 2020: Investing in education, jobs and leadership.* https://www.who.int/publications/i/item/9789240003279

Wynter, S. (1989). Beyond the word of man: Glissant and the new discourse of the Antilles. *World Literature Today*, 63(4), 637–648.

6 Hypervisible Nurses in the Covidicene: Reclaiming the Scripts of Personhood and Agency

Amélie Perron

I write this chapter during the late fall/early winter of 2021–2022 (5th wave of the pandemic) as a privileged white Canadian settler, nurse, and scholar in Ontario. Critical and feminist perspectives and the sociology of ignorance guide my work. I study the politics of nursing practice and nurses' participation in the realm of political action, for example, through acts of whistleblowing, refusals to work, and media use. The concepts and theories informing my work are particularly useful to unpack pandemic-related discourses and decisions and to offer an unapologetically political reading of the state of nursing in the wake of the pandemic. Drawing from peer-reviewed articles, media reports, government, and other organizations' texts, this chapter outlines persistent tensions related to nurses' (in)visibility in professional, government, media, and public discourses. While some nursing organizations, nurses, and unions ponder some of these tensions, few situate their analyses within the realm of politics and few discuss what they mean for nursing's relationship with politics. My chapter aims to tackle this issue.

Nurses Made "Hypervisible" during the Pandemic

One would be hard-pressed to find an academic paper or media report that does not extol nurses' contribution to care provision and patient safety during the pandemic. Shortly after the pandemic was declared in early 2020, nurses and other health professionals were positioned as central cogs in public health efforts to curb the effects of COVID-19. Nurses in particular were identified by governments and health authorities as key players in rolling out multilevel measures against COVID-19, rendering them very visible in local, national, and international discourses. Examining more closely what, exactly, made nurses so extraordinarily visible leads me to argue nurses' (hyper)visibility occurred in three main ways, each illustrated by particular nurse figures: nurses as the backbone of pandemic responses; nurses as pandemic heroes; and nurses as pandemic victims.

A clear division of "pandemic labor" emerged when the population was told to "stay home" to "flatten the curve" while nurses and other workers intensified their work hours to sustain essential services. Nurses overwhelmingly expressed their enthusiasm to partake in pandemic efforts, even as disturbing

DOI: 10.4324/9781003245957-9

reports from hard-hit countries cautioned against systemic vulnerabilities (WHO, 2020). Nurses were immediately positioned as pivotal agents in pandemic responses (Jones, 2021). In many jurisdictions, emergency decrees were rapidly issued allowing health authorities to manage human and physical resources as needed, redeploying nurses, and other health workers across care sectors, reorganizing care units into "hot" and "cold" zones, and extensively using overtime to manage staff shortages (mostly nurses). Nurses became widely known as "the front line," providing direct patient care 24/7.

The public response was instantaneous: politicians, pundits, artists, and the public widely lauded nurses' dedication and endurance. Many metaphors emerged, mostly grounded in military jargon (Cox, 2020): nurses were described as "answering the call," "deployed" at "the front lines" to "battle" a "silent enemy" "in the trenches," and "soldiering on" when faced with adversity. Equally powerful discourses also (re)emerged, steeped in religious language praising nurses' "angelic" virtues of selflessness, devotion, vocation, quiet humility, and sacrifice (Bernard et al., 2021). That 2020 happened to be the "Year of the Nurse" provided a fortuitous backdrop for various campaigns furthering the hero mystique of nurses. Over the years 2020–2021, nursing bodies worldwide unquestionably participated in the dissemination of hero discourses. In Canada, the Canadian Nurses Association chose "We Answer the Call" for its 2021 National Nursing Week theme. In doing so, these nursing bodies firmly repositioned and re-cemented hero discourses at the center of nursing identity, reaffirming the desirability of such public visibility.

The substance of nurses' visibility shifted rapidly during the first wave and onward; nurses' initial posturing changed due to critical shortages of personal protective equipment (PPE), serious gaps in public health directives implementation, and healthcare workers worldwide experiencing disproportionate rates of infection and trauma. Health workers (mostly nurses) began to expose how health facilities and authorities mismanaged COVID-positive patients, rationed PPE, disregarded directives, and concealed outbreaks (Gagnon & Perron, 2020). Nurses also disclosed the psychological toll of working short-staffed, unprotected and under-resourced, and witnessing excessive patient mortality, thus disrupting the previous imagery of a cool-headed workforce and challenging officials' claims regarding patients' and workers' safety (Amnesty International, 2020). Nurses, it turned out, were not almighty. Their discourse changed, this time denouncing their treatment as sacrificial lambs and martyrs (Brophy et al., 2021). Nurses' identity as "hero" or "angel" was therefore unsettled (but not eliminated) as reports of victimization surfaced.

Nurses' victimization was manifold, mainly due to bleak working conditions, lack of protections, exhaustion and trauma. Nursing organizations and unions worldwide also warned against inevitable nurse burnout and short- and long-term mental health issues including anxiety, depression, posttraumatic stress disorder, substance use, and suicidality. Furthermore, nurses and other health workers reported hostility, vandalism and assault perpetrated by pandemic deniers and people accusing them of spreading COVID (Amnesty International,

2020). Finally, reports also emerged of nurses suffering reprisals for exposing dangerous care conditions (Amnesty International, 2020).

Victimization stories typically included the following descriptors: *concerned, upset, scared, sad, heartbroken, angry, distressed, exhausted, frightened,* and *burnt out.* Given the widespread use of emotive descriptors pre-pandemic to portray nurses (especially female nurses), I wonder about such depictions reinforcing (and normalizing) the idea of longstanding mistreatment of nurses in health systems, thus (re)producing a familiar discursive relationship between nursing, victim-hood, and powerlessness (Stokes-Parish et al., 2020). I question the reflex up-take of these emotions by media and public commentators as a familiar trope that emphasizes and "chronicizes" nurses' status as powerless victims, thereby excluding other identifiers.

Nurses' visibility might spell a shift in the way healthcare systems, governments, and the public recognize and value nurses and their work, and this was certainly hoped for among ourselves. I argue nurses were made "hypervisible" through the pandemic but in problematic and harmful ways. Their public and media re-presentations as the backbone of healthcare, heroes, and victims constrain their agency because they produce and normalize lopsided and/or untenable identities of, and expectations towards, nurses. The hero discourse, in particular, perpetuates significant harms. Numerous authors underscore negative impacts on nurses' personhood, identity, agency, and sense of self (see, for example, Boulton et al., 2021; Lohmeyer & Taylor, 2021; Mohammed et al., 2021). For instance, they endow nurses with inappropriate roles (e.g., a reassuring, parent-like figure) that inflict the greatest burden of responsibility and risk on them (Einboden, 2020). They create an impression of nurse invincibility and superhumanity, thus nor-malizing unrealistic expectations around the degree of risk nurses should accept as "part of the job." Halberg et al. (2021) further note that these discourses impose a form of "boundless identity" wherein nurses' professional duties overtake all other endeavors (personal, familial, etc.) through which they define their lives, effec-tively rendering them fully subservient to their work, employers, and patients. Finally, hero discourses normalize a "sacrificial mystique" that relieves decision-makers of their responsibilities (Cox, 2020).

To further problematize nurses' visibility, I now explore contrasting examples of how nurses were conversely made invisible through the pandemic. This will allow me to tease out the implications of such in/visibility processes as we en-vision nursing's "postpandemic future."

The Nursing You Don't See

Multiple pandemic discourses and circumstances rendered nurses invisible be-cause they overlooked, neglected, or excluded nursing expertise, experiences, and identity markers. Here, I discuss four invisible figures: nurses as clinical experts and problem-solvers; nurses as policy designers; nurses as media resource; and nurses as humans. I use academic sources more to illustrate this "missing nursing," given official and media reports' role in keeping it "out of view."

Nurses as Clinical Experts and Problem Solvers

To explore how nurses/nursing remained invisible, I ponder "how" and "what" about them remained obscured, and also "who" exactly was missing from government, media, and the public's understandings of nurses. First, I must highlight that, despite COVID constituting a *public health* concern, public health, and community health nurses were surprisingly absent from most official and lay discourses (Bernard et al., 2021; Popoola, 2021). In fact, while nurses seemed to enjoy a high profile in news stories, it was specifically acute and critical care nurses who became the most visible and on whose shoulders pandemic management seemed to rest. Hospitals and ICUs, often overwhelmed with COVID patients, were a focal point of officials reports and decisions, though pandemic management extended well beyond. Interestingly, where pandemic responses were successful and healthcare environments functioned fairly normally, nurses remained invisible just the same. For example, Popoola (2021) notes that New Zealand's limited COVID morbidity and mortality were specifically attributed to government prowess and community engagement, thereby overshadowing nurses' critical role in testing, contact-tracing, vaccinating and protecting long-term care facilities. Opening the black box of "effective government responses" reveals numerous layers of successful interventions, including nursing interventions, that dissolve into imprecise policy and government competence narratives.

Across settings, nurses played multiple roles resting on a coherent, multidimensional knowledge base. Aside from their ongoing (and intensified) responsibilities in direct care, nurses also updated and implemented clinical guidelines (e.g., infection control, PPE use, etc.), performed contact tracing and set up and managed COVID-testing facilities and vaccination clinics (Bernard et al., 2021). They orientated and trained new staff (e.g., redeployed nurses, volunteers, etc.) (Bernard et al., 2021) and also managed staffing shortages and developed workarounds to limit viral transmission and maintain safe care (Jones, 2021). They actively supported the implementation of everchanging directives and care environments reorganization (Nayna Schwerdtle et al., 2020). Many took on *ad hoc* managerial roles without prior training or support. Nurses also stood in as patients' loved ones, communicated with families and assisted dying patients' last conversations with kins (Popoola, 2021). They relayed public health instructions through professional and personal channels. Nursing educators and researchers quickly turned to supporting students' learning and conducting research on pandemic-related topics (Nayna Schwerdtle et al., 2020).

Key elements were needed to achieve the above. First, nurses used extensive expertise, problem-solving, creativity, communication, planning and coordinating abilities, and emotional intelligence. Second, they relied on their well-documented adaptability to manage rapidly evolving situations brought on by the virus and by administrative decisions. Interestingly, these two elements were mobilized in different ways in pandemic-related discourses. Nurses' extensive skillset was seldom described in allusions to nurses' work. Government and media reports did not define nurses' skills despite identifying them as important pieces of pandemic responses (Bernard et al., 2021; Popoola, 2021). In one study on media discourse, Boulton et al. (2021) further noted that nurses were overwhelmingly described as passively providing emotional work (e.g., comforting patients) while physician descriptors were active, assertive, and dynamic. Conversely, nurses' adaptability became overemphasized: being massively redeployed across sectors, nurses from any clinical area could be ordered to work in other sectors or facilities, regardless of their education, knowledge gaps or comfort level. This epitomizes the adage "a nurse is a nurse is a nurse," treating nurses as undifferentiated, generically trained workers with little or no specialized skills, who can spontaneously be moved, and who will "easily" adapt. Finally, nurses' expertise helped identify sources of risk and transmission, and devise solutions to protect patients, scarce resources, and health personnel, yet those solutions were not necessarily appreciated. For example, to address PPE shortages, nurses in some settings garnered masks and visors by their own means or through mutual aid, only to have those confiscated by managers; many nurses were disciplined or terminated as a result (Amnesty International, 2020).

Nurses as Policy Designers

Nurses are minimally present, or plainly absent, from pandemic task forces and working groups. Canada's national COVID-19 Immunity Task Force for example consists almost exclusively of medically-trained individuals and population health experts. Only one of 30 members has a nursing background. In Ontario, the COVID-19 Science Advisory Table has 50 experts, not one of whom is a nurse. This Advisory Table set up four working groups totaling 65 experts and health leaders, only two of whom have a nursing background. In the United States, Trump's White House Coronavirus Task Force did not include a nurse. As president-elect, Biden included one nurse in his transitional COVID-19 Advisory Board only after being pressured to do so; however, upon confirmation as president, he replaced this group with the White House COVID-19 Response Team which does not include a nurse.

Nurses have limited opportunities to participate in policy development despite being the largest group on the implementation end, even when decisions directly impact, as they overwhelmingly do, nurses' work. The widespread decision to bring COVID-positive health personnel (mostly nurses) back to work is just one example of policies that excluded input from nursing bodies, despite clear impacts on nurses' and patients' health.

The lack of nurse involvement in policy contrasts starkly with longstanding calls by nurse academics and leaders to include nurse expertise across policy levels (Rosser et al., 2020). Health policy and directives need input from nurse clinicians, unions, researchers, organizations, managers, and regulatory bodies. Yet when these nursing voices emerge, it is typically after the fact, in reaction to policy announcements with no impact on their design or application. As nurses, we must consider what this chronic exclusion means for nursing's ability to inhabit spaces beyond "the bedside" where decisions are made. This can help rectify inaccurate discourses, including those describing nurses as "the backbone of healthcare systems" when they are more narrowly the backbone of (hospital-based) care settings, away from decision-making structures.

Nurses as Media Resource

Nurses' presence in the media typically hinged on experiences of hardships and distress. Media reports addressed nurses when nurses were the actual topic being discussed (e.g., high workloads, nursing shortage) but not in other respects. Moreover, as noted earlier, the media specifically privileged nurse stories (e.g., distress, victimization) and descriptive language (e.g., fearfulness, powerlessness) with high emotional content. In their media analysis, Boulton and colleagues (2021) noted that nurses only occupied media space when they spoke about emotional labour; other experiences and expertise, including successful care coordination, policy development and crisis management, were not deemed a "good" media story. To discuss nursing-relevant issues (e.g., lockdowns, mass immunization, care delivery, pandemic denial), reporters sought instead expert input from other actors, including epidemiologists, physicians, medical historians, and sociologists (Duncan et al., 2020). Media's tendency to neglect nurses in social, economic, or historical analyses while simultaneously reinforcing their victim status cements a dangerous form of professional socialization and identity centered on cultural norms of invisibility and powerlessness.

Nurses as Humans

Another casualty of the invisibilization of nurses is, plainly put, nurses' basic humanness. Though hero and angel discourses may provide a (short-lived) sense of appreciation, they also induce a perverse sense of obligation, over-compensation for systemic failures, and self-sacrifice, while maintaining a mystique of invincibility and imperturbable self-mastery. Some nurses began rejecting these portrayals during the first wave. Although the public response was initially sympathetic, it shifted in the following waves with the emergence of indifferent, and at times hostile, sentiments: increasingly, nurses were told to stop complaining, that others had it worse (after all, so many people lost their living wages, while nurses kept their "handsomely paid" jobs), that they had signed up for this and that they needed to just do their job. During the second and third waves, nurses worldwide were leaving their positions and profession in droves, accentuating an already existing shortage. This generally led to heightened awareness about nurses' abysmal work conditions but not to policy changes or the inclusion of nurse leadership in decision-making, nor did it disrupt expectations that nurses should power through. It did however lead to hostile reactions. Threads on social media and online forums (e.g., Reddit) emerged, portraying nurses as selfish whiners, quitters, losers, and fake nurses lacking vocation. Some thought that, six months or more into the pandemic, surely nurses would be used to the new reality by now. Others concluded nurses simply lacked resilience and they should "grow a spine." Such hostile reactions have caught nurses off-guard, but they are hardly surprising if one understands the inherently violent ideology underpinning hero discourses. Heroes are barely meant to be celebrated for exceptional feats: their socio-cultural-political purpose is first and foremost to take the gaze away from systemic failures, conceal noxious ideologies governing everyday life and shift accountability away from those in power. Unbeknownst to them, humans-turned-heroes are tasked with the formidable job of safeguarding "a higher being or institution worthy of sacrifice" (Lohmeyer & Taylor, 2021, p. 631)—in this case, the national economy and the public's hope to return to normal—which requires the suspension of their personal rights and agency. When "heroes" question these expectations and attempt to reconnect with their basic humanness, they do not hold up their end of this ideological contract: they are, effectively, traitors to the "great cause" and can therefore be treated accordingly.

While other imposed or rehearsed forms of nurse invisibility exist, the examples discussed hitherto lead me to argue that while nurses were made visible in some (stereotyped) ways, public discourse and governance maintained their otherwise longstanding invisibility, reiterating narrow understandings of nurses' complex and varied knowledge, restricting nurses' subjectivities (hero, generic worker, expendable, defector), and neutralizing their rights to self-determination. Recognizing these processes is critical, as narratives and analyses framing the pandemic as a watershed moment intensify.

The Pandemic: A Turning Point?

Most analyses about the pandemic unquestionably frame it as a health, social, economic, and political crisis. Using a crisis register is powerful because it triggers a sense of suspension, hypervigilance, cautious withdrawal from citizen life, renewed (often uncritical) faith in leaders, and relinquishment of rights and freedoms (Smith & Foth, 2021). In nursing, a crisis narrative has led most commentators to view the pandemic as a catalyst for change that can spell a brighter future for our profession. For example, in the spring of 2020, Howard Catton, head of the International Council of Nurses (ICN), declared that the public's "huge outpouring of positive recognition" worldwide suggested that "we may be seeing some changes in attitude towards nurses" (United Nations, 2020). Many contend that nurses' value, expertise, courage, and hardships are finally recognized, such that they can finally look forward to enhanced prospects in clinical and policy realms (Jones, 2021).

While I cautiously agree the pandemic may create some opportunity for transformation, I cannot overlook the concurrent deepening entrenchment of many issues plaguing nursing. One example is nursing's apparent inability to let go of outdated ideas of vocation and selflessness. There is also continued uncritical and uninformed uptake of problematic ideas in professional discourses despite abundant cautionary literature (for example, see Traynor, 2018 on resilience). And what to make of nursing's continued complicity in perpetuating practices steeped in racism, and its reluctance to fully engage in anti-oppression endeavors (Bell & van Daalen-Smith, 2021)?

Regarding the pandemic, Jones (2020) astutely notes that "Even in the time of this supposed "great equaliser," power relations are still very much alive and well." Entrenched sexism, racism, ageism, and ableism, expansion of police states, the rise of white nationalism and supremacy, and unbridled capitalism govern contemporary individual and collective experiences—including the pandemic—one way or another (Smith & Foth, 2021). Nurses are both subjects and objects of power in these phenomena, in whatever capacity they work. In envisioning our post-pandemic future, we need to genuinely engage with these realities and their implications.

Literature on what we might call post-pandemic nursing however tends to narrowly focus on nurses' clinical world: nurses will need to embrace virtual technologies and telehealth; better integrate infection prevention and control practices; innovate; become leaders; show more kindness; and, of course, develop resilience. While these are relevant endeavours, they considerably restrict nurses' imagination, power and agency because they focus primarily on nurses adapting to existing social and care structures without disrupting them. Nursing literature engaging with the broader ideologies described earlier remains scarce. This is the crux of the issue: if key "pandemic lessons" are not learned, we will not experience a true turning point.

Those lessons are playing out right now. Nurse clinicians, leaders, and scholars have yet to explicitly identify the role of powerful forces such as neoliberalism, capitalism (including disaster capitalism), patriarchy/misogyny (including disaster patriarchy), and white nationalism in our current situation. Nursing guidance documents glaringly neglect such high-level analyses, stifling deeper understandings. A key document by the ICN titled *Nurses: A Voice to Lead* is one example of such inexplicably missed opportunity to politicize conversations and enhance nursing's political consciousness. Evading these notions robs nursing of critically needed insights and language, and significantly undermines nurses' collective agency.

Yet phenomena like neoliberalism, patriarchy, and racism are at the core of disturbing but familiar trends in healthcare. Consider the continued instrumentalization of nurses' minds and bodies to fulfill particular state goals. "Do more with less" is now mundane, trapping nurses in an intractable "deficit discourse" (Wilson et al., 2020). Other examples abound: the enforcement of coercive emergency decrees (with no oversight) in the absence of COVID outbreaks or surges, abusive management practices, unsafe ratios and the sanctioned violation of nurses' labor rights; enactments of institutional violence through managerial strategies (Amnesty International, 2020) and even police interventions (Forgione, 2020); and decisions to lower care standards as we "learn to live with" the virus in order to return to normal (economic) life, ignoring disproportionate impacts on patients (particularly racialized and disabled patients) and nurses.

Furthermore, while elected officials and health administrators worldwide gush and swoon over nurses, they are simultaneously waging a war against them to freeze or decrease their salaries, curtail/suspend their bargaining rights, impede unionization efforts, bypass protections (e.g., whistleblower protections), and curb access to judicial remedies (for example, through increased liability protections for care settings) (for example, in Canada see Ontario Federation of Labour, n.d.; United Nurses of Alberta, 2021; in the U.S. see Brooks et al., 2020; Moskowitz, 2020). It is no coincidence that these efforts often spare sectors dominated by white, male workers (e.g., law enforcement, paramedics, physicians) while targeting workforces where women dominate, such as nursing and teaching (see Ontario's Bill 124 for example). Surely, no amount of handclapping, free donuts, resilience training, and meditation can make up for that.

There is a very real risk the "new normal" will not be so new for nurses. Our obedience to unforgiving socioeconomic ideologies and our willingness to serve "efficient, high-performing" care systems that are demonstrably shortsighted and self-defeating should never form the basis of our social recognition. Performing in such systems does not reflect professional achievement and success, but rather our inclination to defer, neglect, and compromise. In envisioning the pandemic as a catalyst for change, nursing needs to seriously consider how to go about changing a "system [that] does not want to be better" (Smith & Foth, 2021, p. 16) and that benefits immensely from nursing's complacency, readiness to compromise, naiveté or ignorance (Perron & Rudge, 2016).

The pandemic has shown, again, that nurses do not work in a meritocracy. It will not bring health leaders to finally understand nursing's "true" value and modify the system accordingly, because this system is designed precisely around restricted valuing of nurses' work. So what now?

Reclaiming the "New Normal"

I am concerned that current calls to "go back to normal"—the very normal that brought us here in the first place—will pull us into old, detrimental habits. We need to stop "springing into action" and pause, first to assess the deficits of previous/current structures and second to envision more meaningful, equitable, and socially just alternatives. We also need to stop viewing caring and kindness as effective ways forward, and espouse politically charged notions instead, such as solidarity (Porobić Isaković, 2020). To understand our present and imagine our futures, nothing short of a philosophical, critical, and political reading is needed.

Turning one of Milton Friedman's famed argument on its head, Naomi Klein (2020) argues that crises are indeed opportunities to push "unthinkable" ideas, programs and policies forward, but that these must be steeped in justice, the common good and collective wellbeing, not the narrow and predatory interests of elite groups and corporations. The key is to ensure such ideas and programs are "lying around" in the public's, media's, and decision-makers' consciousness such that, as cogent alternatives to failing and corrupt systems, they become seen not only as desirable, but as indispensable and unavoidable.

Developing an alternative and ensuring it "lies around" (in public debates, education settings or workplaces) means reflecting about current issues and their multidimensional origins and consequences; acquiring new tools to think and new language to speak; formulating objectives; normalizing these ideas and socializing others accordingly; articulating related identity elements; nurturing alliances and coalitions; developing strategies for action; and educating the public and elected officials about the need for such programs and policies. The ideas we need lying around must stem from revitalized analyses delineating the historical, political, and philosophical determinants of health, care, and nursing work.

These analyses must imbue all aspects of nurse education and socialization. Nursing curricula mainly consist of teaching clinical competencies with, perhaps, some concepts sprinkled throughout (e.g., care equity, social justice). Curricula should instead be grounded in philosophical, critical, and political perspectives as frames to teach, contextualize, and problematize nursing activities. For example, Feminism—especially post-structural, Black, Global South, post-colonial, and queer feminisms—needs to become more than an uncomfortable "F-word" (Kane & Thomas, 2000) and drive nursing agency. Diverse feminist perspectives reveal the interpenetrating nature of oppression and identity, and foster a coalitional politics (Heywood & Drake, 1997).

Fully engaging with critical, political, and philosophical ideas helps interrupt and deconstruct current systems of thought that pose problems for nurses and the communities they assist. This means confronting taken-for-granted, even "sacred" ideas. For instance, many argue nursing's "caring" narrative needs to shift because it contributes to the systemic disrespect for nurses, it sets them up for exploitation, and it guilts them out of self-advocacy (Granberg, 2014; Wilson et al., 2020). Perron (2013) and Granberg (2014) support the politicization of the concept to eliminate the tendency to pit patient and nurse advocacy against each other. Similar problematization of core nursing ideas, including leadership (Cutcliffe & Cleary, 2015), advocacy (Pariseau-Legault, 2012), and resilience (Traynor, 2018), highlight how their uncritical and individualized interpretations can trap nurses into unrealistic expectations, while concealing collective responsibilities toward the protection of vulnerable persons and the public interest.

Critical, political, and philosophical thought helps identify how certain notions and emotions (e.g., guilt, fear) are routinely weaponized against nurses. This helps avoid reproducing similar patterns of manipulation and violence (against nurses, students, etc.), and better equip nurses to safely respond when they occur. This brings us to another element needed "lying around": normalizing and fully protecting nurses' ability to speak up against wrongdoing, to disobey (Perron, 2013) inappropriate, unjust or dangerous directives, and to protect themselves against unsafe work conditions. This must be further supported by policy and legislative changes that properly balance nurses' duties with their fundamental right to free speech (especially regarding the public interest) and fully protect nurse and other healthcare whistleblowers.

The previous point means also bolstering nurses' ability to speak. Nursing education focuses on extremely narrow understandings of communication, assuming nurses speak only to patients, families, and co-workers. This symbolically reduces nurses' sphere of activity to the immediacy of care units; it restricts the spaces where nurses' interventions rightfully belong and undermines their scope of influence. Besides local collaborators, nurses must also be comfortable approaching upper managers and executives, elected representatives, government officials, ethics committees, human rights officers, privacy commissioners, and the media, and they must know how to strategically navigate these different conversations. They must therefore be trained in influential communication, assertive communication, difficult conversations (including that involving bullying and gaslighting), conflict management, and media training. Importantly, this must be accessible throughout nurses' careers (e.g., undergraduate education, continuing education, professional development). Normalizing and concretely supporting powerful nursing voices is, I believe, an essential part of the alternatives Klein (2020) encourages us to articulate.

Finally, more than advocacy, nurses need to be socialized in the generative powers of activism and militancy. Nursing has a rich and diverse repertoire of activists that illustrate, beyond the sole work of Florence Nightingale, nurses' longstanding combativeness and resourcefulness. Learning activist skills during undergraduate education can cement this disposition in nurses' practices, discourse, and professional identity. Activism, rather than patient advocacy, meaningfully connects nurses to the communities and populations they support beyond the confines of their workplace, and it spells greater engagement, at multiple social and political levels, to exert influence and foster change.

I believe the aforementioned suggestions can help meet Klein's (2020) exhortation that we be ready to articulate, disseminate, and fight for alternative modes of social and health governance when crises crudely expose the harms of current systems. These suggestions also help address the multiple issues identified earlier regarding the paradoxical ways in which nurses can be made hyper- or invisible through various discursive frames. These strategies, though incomplete, help resignify nurses' place in social imaginaries, while fostering a more thoughtful and meaningful sense of agency and identity, well beyond the usual tropes of heroism and victimhood—a critical step to a true "post-pandemic turn."

Conclusion

In this chapter, I have delineated the complex, shifting interplay of nurse (in) visibility during the pandemic and the precarious nurse object/subject positions it generates. The pandemic brings to light the products of obscure calculations regarding the distribution of health and wealth and the divide between worthy and disposable lives. It exposes the limits and, often, the vacuity of laudatory gestures and empathetic discourses that portray nurses as objects of commiseration and/or as "naturally" persevering against all odds. However, the pandemic may also enable shifting norms of dominance and deference, towards another "normality."

Ideas are contagious. I support Klein's (2020) contention that systematically and strategically "laying ideas around" is a key step to shaping what comes next. Nursing's future cannot eschew political education and training. As Nobel peace prize winner Leymah Gbowee argues, we cannot leave footprints that last if we walk on tiptoes. This is not a time to be modest or to run back to old depoliticized notions of "care." Troubling the usual mechanisms of hypervisibility–invisibility, nurses can choose to become visible in militant ways, caring not for noxious ideologies and abusive workplaces, but for those consistently sidelined by economic and political structures as well as fellow nurses and health workers, the sacrifice of whom is casually counted on to strengthen market economies and the social fabric. I hope that critical, emancipatory, and militant consciousness becomes an unshakable feature of nursing identity and agency—but above all, I hope such notions stop being perceived as "radical" by nurses themselves.

References

Amnesty International (2020). *Exposed, silenced, attacked: Failures to protect health and essential workers during the COVID-19 pandemic.* Retrieved December 5, 2021 from https://www.amnesty.org/en/documents/pol40/2572/2020/en/

Bell, B., & van Daalen-Smith, C. (2021). No imagining too radical, no action too disruptive. *Witness: Canadian Journal of Critical Nursing Discourse, 3*(1), 1–3. 10.25071/2291-5796.104

Bernard, L., Bévillard-Charrière, Q., Taha, S., & Holmes, D. (2021). Une revue intégrative de l'identité populaire de l'infirmière durant la pandémie de la COVID-19. *Recherche en soins infirmiers, 145,* 91–103. 10.3917/rsi.145.0091

Boulton, M., Garnett, A., & Webster, F. (2021). A foucauldian discourse analysis of media reporting on the nurse-as-hero during COVID-19. *Nursing Inquiry,* e12471. 10.1111/nin.12471

Brooks, S., Grant, R., & Bonamarte, M. F. (2020). States move to shield LTC facilities from civil liability. *Bifocal, 41*(6).

Brophy, J. T., Keith, M. M., Hurley, M., & McArthur, J. E. (2021). Sacrificed: Ontario healthcare workers in the time of COVID-19. *New Solutions: Journal of Environmental and Occupational Health Policy, 30*(4), 267–281. 10.1177/1048291120974358

Cox, C. L. (2020). "Healthcare heroes": Problems with media focus on heroism from healthcare workers during the COVID-19 pandemic. *Journal of Medical Ethics, 46,* 510–513. 10.1136/medethics-2020-10639

Cutcliffe, J. R., & Cleary, M. (2015). Nursing leadership, missing questions, and the elephant(s) in the room: Problematizing the discourse on nursing leadership. *Issues in Mental Health Nursing, 36,* 817–825.

Duncan, S., Scaia, M., & Boschma, G. (2020). "100 years of university nursing educa-tion": The significance of a baccalaureate nursing degree and its public health origins for nursing now. *Quality Advancement in Nursing Education—Avancées en formation infirmière, 6*(2), Article 8.

Einboden, R. (2020). SuperNurse? Troubling the hero discourse in COVID times. *Health, 24*(4), 343–347. 10.1177/1363459320934280

Forgione, P. (2020, May 15). New patterns of violence against healthcare in the covid-19 pandemic. *BMJ Blog.* https://blogs.bmj.com/bmj/2020/05/15/new-patterns-of-violence-against-healthcare-in-the-covid-19-pandemic/

Gagnon, M., & Perron, A. (2020). Nursing voices during COVID-19: An analysis of Canadian media coverage. *Aporia, 12*(1), 108–112.

Granberg, M. (2014). Manufacturing dissent: Labor conflict, care work, and the politi-cization of caring. *Nordic Journal of Working Life Studies, 4*(1), 139–152. 10.19154/njwls.v4i1.3556

Halberg, N., Jensen, P. S., & Larsen, T. S. (2021). We are not heroes-the flipside of the hero narrative amidst the COVID-19-pandemic: A danish hospital ethnography. *Journal of Advanced Nursing, 77*(5), 2429–2436. 10.1111/jan.14811

Heywood, L., & Drake, J. (Eds.) (1997). *Third wave agenda: Being feminist, doing feminism.* University of Minnesota Press.

Jones, G. (2020). 2020 coronavirus pandemic: A post-structuralist approach. *Sociology Blog.* https://www.sociology.cam.ac.uk/blog/post-structuralist-pandemic

Jones, S. (2021). *"Healthcare heroes"—The change in perceptions of nurses' roles during the COVID-19 pandemic: A critical discourse analysis.* Unpublished Masters thesis, University of Western Ontario.

Kane, D., & Thomas, B. (2000). Nursing and the "F" word. *Nursing Forum, 35*(2), 17–24.

Klein, N. (2020, March 16). Coronavirus capitalism—and how to beat it. *Intercept.* https://theintercept.com/2020/03/16/coronavirus-capitalism/

Lohmeyer, B. A., & Taylor, N. (2021). War, heroes and sacrifice: Masking neoliberal violence during the COVID-19 pandemic. *Critical Sociology, 47*(4-5), 625–639. 10.1177/0896920520975824

Mohammed, S., Peter, E., Killackey, T., & Maciver, J. (2021). The "nurse as hero" discourse in the COVID-19 pandemic: A poststructural discourse analysis. *International Journal of Nursing Studies, 117*, 103887. 10.1016/j.ijnurstu.2021.103887

Moskowitz, P. E. (2020, May 11). One hospital system's response to COVID-19? union-busting. *The Nation.* https://www.thenation.com/article/activism/union-busting-consultants-hospital/

Nayna Schwerdtle, P., Connell, C. J., Lee, S., Plummer, V., Russo, P. L., Endacott, R., & Kuhn, L. (2020). Nurse expertise: A critical resource in the COVID-19 pandemic response. *Annals of Global Health, 86*(1), 49. 10.5334/aogh.2898

Ontario Federation of Labour (n.d.). *Ford government should immediately repeal Bill 124, after manitoba court strikes down similar wage restraint legislation as unconstitutional.* https://ofl.ca/ford-government-should-immediately-repeal-bill-124-after-manitoba-court-strikes-down-similar-wage-restraint-legislation-as-unconstitutional/

Pariseau-Legault, P. (2012). Critique de la responsabilité sociale d'une profession, du potentiel inexploité de sa force collective et de la nécessité conséquente de son éveil. *Aporia, 4*(3), 18–20. 10.18192/aporia.v4i3.3426

Perron, A. (2013). Nursing as "disobedient" practice: Care of the nurse's self, parrhesia and the dismantling of a baseless paradox. *Nursing Philosophy, 14*(3), 154–167.

Perron, A., & Rudge, T. (2016). *On the politics of ignorance in nursing and health care: Knowing ignorance*. Routledge.

Popoola, T. (2021). COVID-19's missing heroes: Nurses' contribution and visibility in Aotearoa New Zealand. *Nursing Praxis in Aotearoa New Zealand, 37*(3), 8–11. 10.36951/27034542.2021.026

Porobić Isaković, N. (2020). *COVID-19: Solidarity as a political tool for radical transformation*. Retrieved November 8, 2021 from https://www.wilpf.org/covid-19-solidarity-as-a-political-tool-for-radical-transformation/

Rosser, E., Westcott, L., Ali, P. A., Bosanquet, J., Castro-Sanchez, E., Dewing, J., McCormack, B., Merrell, J., & Witham, G. (2020). The need for visible nursing leadership during COVID-19. *Journal of Nursing Scholarship, 52*(5), 459–461. 10.1111/jnu.12587

Smith, K. S., & Foth, T. (2021). Tomorrow is cancelled: Rethinking nursing resistance as insurrection. *Aporia, 13*(1), 15–25.

Stokes-Parish, J., Elliott, R., Rolls, K., & Massey, D. (2020). Angels and heroes: The unintended consequence of the hero narrative. *Journal of Nursing, 52*(5), 462–466. 10.1111/jnu.12591

Traynor, M. (2018). What's wrong with resilience. *Journal of Research in Nursing, 23*(1), 5–8. 10.1177/1744987117751458

United Nations. (2020). COVID-19 highlights nurses' vulnerability as backbone to health services worldwide. https://news.un.org/en/story/2020/04/1061232

United Nurses of Alberta. (2021, September 8). *AHS proposal would still include wage cut for Alberta Nurses*. https://www.una.ca/1286/ahs-proposal-would-still-include-wage-cut-for-alberta-nurses-union-concerned-by-ministers-misleading-statement

WHO. (2020). *Shortage of personal protective equipment endangering health workers worldwide*. https://www.who.int/news/item/03-03-2020-shortage-of-personal-protective-equipment-endangering-health-workers-worldwide

Wilson, R. L., Carryer, J., Dewing, J., Rosado, S., Gildberg, F., Hutton, A., Johnson, A., Kaunonen, M., & Sheridan, N. (2020). The state of the nursing profession in the international year of the nurse and midwife 2020 during COVID-19: A nursing standpoint. *Nursing Philosophy, 21*, e12314. 10.1111/nup.12314

7 Metastatic Growth: *The Health Care Industry's Increasing Contribution to the Plasticene*

Emmanuel Christian Tedjasukmana (he/him)

Positionality

My name is Emmanuel Christian Budi Utama Tedjasukmana (he/him/his), and I am a nondisabled, Cisgender, homosexual male. I am a first-generation Asian-American with Chinese-Indonesian ancestry. I entered this Earth on Potawatomi land and currently reside on Abenaki land. Most of the education I received was from private institutions within the United States—most of which were Seventh-Day Adventist—but I no longer identify under this affiliation. I am a nurse, designer, and artist—choosing to view my world through the lens of an environmentalist striving for health equity, environmental justice, and peace (Figure 7.1).

Preface

My preoccupation with environmentalism and health care sustainability first stemmed from my nursing practice and witnessing how much waste is produced through patient care. In throwing so many single-use items away, I became increasingly concerned with how much of it was filling our landfills—and I worried how this waste would ultimately impact our environment. Hospitals operate around the clock, and if care for a single patient during just one phase of care can produce significant amounts of trash within just a few hours, how much waste is made throughout a patient's stay? More notably, how much waste is produced by hospitals annually? I found it paradoxical that the health care industry, whose commitment is to uphold the health and well-being of patients and communities, takes part in practices that harm the environment and contribute to worsening climate change that is negatively impacting us. What's more appalling is that we aren't doing enough to address the issue. What can we, as health practitioners, do to fix this wicked problem? In nursing, there is hardly time left to breathe, hydrate, or even go to the bathroom between caring, medicating, educating, advocating, and charting. Who has the time to try to start environmental initiatives? Despite the difficulty in addressing, solutions to

DOI: 10.4324/9781003245957-10

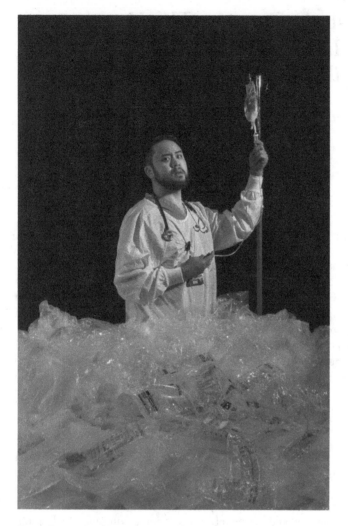

Figure 7.1 Myopia: Harming in Order to Heal #9, 2019. Digital Photograph of Single-use
     Hospital Waste.

Source: Emmanuel Christian Tedjasukmana.

these problems need immediate identification as they directly involve the health
of the Planet and the communities we care for.

   I was slowly able to use any spare time at work to strike up more conversations
about sustainability with my coworkers—and progressively began implementing
unit-based initiatives to deviate items from our waste stream. This process,
however, was painstakingly slow-moving and, unfortunately, not always supported by leadership or the hospital hierarchy. Although it was a good start and
better than nothing, I knew it was not enough. I needed to find other ways to

bring about more attention and awareness of the issue to initiate conversations that could lead to more impactful changes. I knew health care workers were already discussing this issue among themselves—but more public discussions were needed on a hospital-wide, community-wide, nation-wide, and global levels. It took a while, but with some help, I finally realized that I had a unique opportunity as an artist who understood the problem from a medical perspective—and I could take action and raise awareness of the issue in my very own way. I now utilize the power of both my writing and art as an extension of my nursing practice: and use it to process ideas, educate, share stories, create awareness, and disseminate information to a broader audience. I no longer need to wait on the approval of the hospital hierarchy to make the change I want to see. The only person I need permission from is myself.

Introduction

Humans are a dominating force on the face of the Planet. Our utilization of land and its natural resources, the uncontrolled growth of our ever-expanding population, and the rapid development and advancement of innovative technologies provide evidence that we are an assertive—if not domineering—presence on Earth. While our exponential growth, evolution, and advancements are often exciting, we face compelling evidence of how the ramifications of our linear myopic thinking impact our climate. The consequential downfall is that they lack sustainable approaches and subsequently harm the Planet our lives depend on.

Every industry is a contributor to the problem. Many of the largest consumer industries—such as the food and fashion industry—have caught both the attention and critique of the global public and have already begun work to replace their destructive practices with more sustainable ones. Other significant contributors, however, have yet to receive this same attention. The global health care sector, whose climate footprint contributes over 4.6% of net emissions (Watts et al., 2020) and is the second-largest contributor to overall waste (Kwakye et al., 2011), is in dire need of public awareness and critique to catalyze long-overdue improvements and changes to policies. According to Karliner et al. (2019), health care is a significant contributor to the climate crisis, and Watts et al. (2018) cite climate change as the "single biggest health threat facing humanity in the 21st century" (p. 2482). Is it possible to find ways to heal the patient without consequently harming the community in which they reside? How can health care ensure that its current practices cease contributing to climate change and protect the health of future generations? We must fully recognize the root of the problem and break the paradoxical cycle of hospitals extracting and generating harmful pollution to heal. Invoking climate-focused changes will decrease health care's detrimental impact on Planetary health, thus upholding its mission to protect and further health in every way possible. This issue needs the world's attention—and nurses play a crucial role in shifting our current mindset to forge a path forward in resolving our current climate crisis (Figure 7.2).

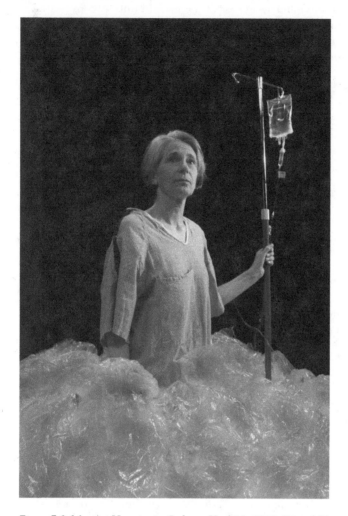

Figure 7.2 Myopia: Harming in Order to Heal #1, 2019. Digital Photograph of Single-use Hospital Waste.

Source: Emmanuel Christian Tedjasukmana.

I. H&P: A History Wrapped in Plastic

Entering the Age of the Anthropocene

In discussing the state of our environment and the causes for its current con-dition, the term "Anthropocene" is frequently referenced. In 2000, scientists Paul Crutzen and Eugene Stoermer popularized the idea that we are situated in a unique geological epoch called the "Anthropocene," a word that stems from the Ancient Greek words *anthropos* meaning "human" and *kainos* or *-cene*, which translates to "new" or "recent" (Carrington, 2016). They chose this term to designate a significant shift in which they—along with the support of many other multidisciplinary scientists—believed that the human race's impact "gradually grew into a significant geological, morphological force" (Crutzen & Stoermer, 2000, p. 17). This human-driven force was so great, and the change was so profound that it was significant enough to take us out of our current post-glacial epoch known as the Holocene—which had been stable and unchanged for the past 12,000 years. In their publication entitled "Anthropocene," Crutzen and Stoermer (2000) called further attention to how the dominance of humankind is playing a significant role in not only shaping its future but also that of the Earth. They wrote, "The expansion of mankind ... [and] exploitation of Earth's resources has been astounding" (p. 17), citing colossal population boom, continual land urbanization, exhaustion of fossil fuels, alterations to ozone and air quality, and increased species extinction as some examples.

Two of the most deleterious impacts resulting from human influence we are faced with today are global warming and the over-abundance of plastic pollution. Accelerated global warming results from continual increases in temperatures due to the overproduction of greenhouse gasses promoted by anthropogenic activities such as extraction, fracking, burning fossil fuels, and increased landfill gas production (Crutzen & Stoermer, 2000). Because energy cannot readily dissipate through this atmospheric build-up of greenhouse gasses, less heat escapes into space and becomes trapped instead—resulting in an accumulation of heat that raises the Earth's overall temperature. This increase sets off a chain reaction that augments catastrophic weather events: ultimately impacting our physical and mental health (Alliance of Nurses for Healthy Environments, 2020).

About 99% of plastic is made from fossil fuels (Seeding Sovereignty, 2021). To attain the durability and plasticity for which they are so coveted, plastics require human alteration to their complex polymer chains. Because of these anthropocentric interventions, they now exceed nature's capabilities and won't readily dissolve, rust, or degrade: ultimately outlasting the humans who have created them (Freinkel, 2011). Because many of the monomers utilized to make common plastics are fossil hydrocarbon-derived and non-biodegradable, these plastics can only be eradicated through combustion or pyrolysis—which add to overall environmental emissions. Without these destructive thermal treatments, plastics stick around and accumulate in landfills or the environment instead of decomposing (Geyer et al., 2017). Plastics, in their various shapes, sizes, and forms—such as microplastics (plastic smaller than 5 mm)—can now be found everywhere. At the present moment, nowhere on Earth is considered free of plastic (Davis & Turpin, 2015). A growing number of studies have also reported the presence of microplastics in our bodies. Not only do they plague the water and food that we consume, but they also invade our lungs (Del-la-Torre et al., 2021), blood (Leslie et al., 2022), stool (Schwabl et al., 2019), and even the placentas that supply nourishment to our unborn children (Ragusa et al., 2021; Figure 7.3).

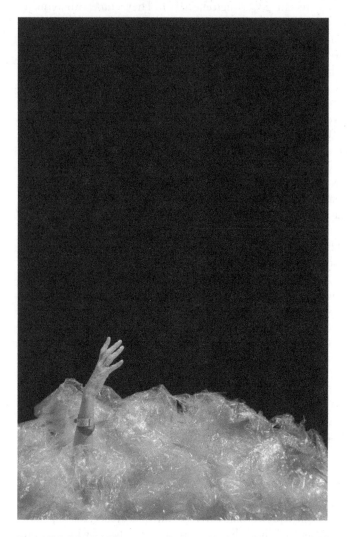

Figure 7.3 Myopia: Harming in Order to Heal #2, 2019. Digital Photograph of Single-use Hospital Waste.

Source: Emmanuel Christian Tedjasukmana.

Plastic: Humankind's Answer to Nature's Limitations

So how did we get so deep into this plastic predicament in the first place? Some may find it ironic that plastic was created to address the scarcity of naturally occurring materials such as ivory, tortoiseshell, amber, and silk to spare nature's resources (Freinkel, 2011). What kind of lifestyle are we now living that has allowed us to have already used over one-third of the Planet's natural resources in just three decades (Leonard, 2007)?

In the first-ever global analysis of all mass-produced plastics ever manu-factured, Geyer et al. (2017) estimated that approximately 8,300 million metric tons (Mt) of virgin plastics had been produced between the 1950s (when large-scale production started taking place) and 2017. The analysis also reported that as of 2015, "approximately 6,300 Mt of plastic waste had been generated, around 9% had been recycled, 12% was incinerated, and 79% was accumulated in landfills or the natural environment" (p. 1). With this in mind, a significant issue that we face today is that we are producing and consuming products in massive, unmanageable quantities and are run-ning out of places to dispose of things. Global plastic production is currently at over 400 million metric tons annually (Schettler, 2020), with over 40% of this amount being utilized solely for single-use packaging (Ragusa et al., 2021). It has become even more problematic for developing countries lacking appropriate waste disposal management systems when developed nations—such as the United States—off-load waste from what Goldberg (2018) de-scribes as "our convenient lifestyle" (p. 6) and impose cleanup on some of the Planet's most vulnerable people. For those living in developed countries with established waste management streams, the actual realization of the amount of waste produced is never fully comprehended—as it is out of sight, out of mind. Because of this, few of us understand the connection between how our consumption habits play a significant role in climate change and how our addiction to a convenient throw-away lifestyle—and dependency on plastic—has dire consequences (Figure 7.4).

Plastic's Roots within the Health Care Industry

Plastic is everywhere. Due to its affordability, durability, versatility, and abun-dance, this material has become a prominent staple in our culture—fueling scientific and technological innovations in every sector possible (Vanapalli et al., 2021). Every industry has found benefits in utilizing its adaptability in one way or another. Of all the various sectors that have benefitted from the in-vention of plastics, the health care sector is "one that has provided enormous PR value. Medicine has long been plastic's indisputable good-news story: the showcase of polymer's benefits. [M]odern medicine owes a huge debt to the advent of plastics, in ways both spectacular and mundane … [as] polymers made possible most of today's medical marvels" (Freinkel, 2011, p. 82). Disposable plastics, particularly with single-use items, have become so deeply rooted in health care that it is now synonymous with safety and sterility: but it hasn't always been this way.

Until the plastics revolution in the late 1940s, it was common practice in health care facilities to process, package, and sanitize their equipment for reuse—either by their staff or processing-sterilizing departments located on-site. Equipment disposal was only considered when items were either im-possible or extremely difficult to re-sterilize. Although a growing hospital supply industry could provide hospitals with pre-packaged sterile items,

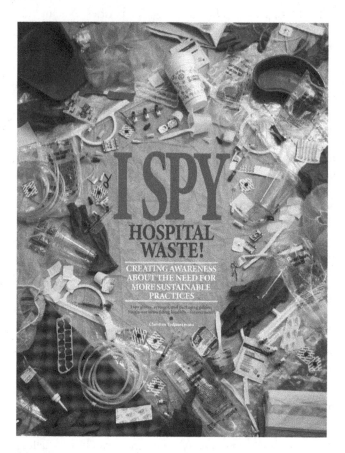

Figure 7.4 I Spy Hospital Waste!, 2018. Digital Photograph of Single-use Hospital Waste.
Source: Emmanuel Christian Tedjasukmana.

the boundary between what was considered reusable (durable) and what was considered disposable (consumable) was always carefully considered. However, this relationship changed shortly after the end of World War II, when the proliferation of plastic products began. Items previously sourced from natural materials that needed time to be carefully produced, maintained, and sterilized were now manufactured in ways that were both cheap and efficient—the primary draw being that the staff no longer had to spend precious time painstakingly sterilizing items. It was now more cost-effective to just throw them out instead. As a result, labor-intensive sterilization practices were phased out, and single-use devices (SUDs) were embraced. Cost and convenience led to this decision—as there was no epidemiologic evidence that hospital sterilizing practices were anything less than adequate (Greene, 1986).

Although these SUDs first became available in the 1950s, it was with the rising prevalence of hepatitis and HIV cases in the United States in the early 1980s that the utilization of disposables and SUDs saw an even more significant surge (Dunn, 2002; Freinkel, 2011). This rise resulted from confusion and fear that rushed forth due to the lack of knowledge about the spread of this outbreak: similarly paralleling the massive uptick for single-use items during the COVID-19 pandemic. While many in the health care industry felt that these devices were a technological godsend during this troubling time of understanding HIV and how it could spread, others held suspicions of the genuine goodwill of these single-use suppliers. Gerwig (2015) proposed that with the appearance of the AIDS epidemic and the growing concerns surrounding infection control, medical device manufacturers "took advantage of the[se] concerns by producing plastic disposable devices and labeling almost everything 'single-use,' even for products that were similar or identical to the previously reusable devices" (p. 121). Gerwig was not alone in noting this. One study found that an estimated 10%–20% of SUDs were mislabeled multiple-use devices (Collier, 2011). Further, it was not uncommon for manufacturers to add plastic components to what would otherwise be a reusable product, making it unsuitable for the autoclave—a form of high-heat steam sterilization—because of this unnecessary plastic element (Stoermer, 1999).

As costs in health care began to climb, hospitals looked to resterilize single-use items as a way to save more money. Manufacturers quickly opposed this idea and firmly took the stance that reuse after resterilization was not proven to be safe. They made it clear that if an institution decided to reprocess their SUDs, they would be exempt from any legal accountability (Dunn, 2002). The FDA, however, has yet to find evidence indicating that reprocessing has caused increased health risks (Kwakye et al., 2011). Chen (2010) points out that the FDA requires reprocessing companies to meet the same safety and quality standards as original manufacturers. The U.S. Government Accountability Office confirmed this in 2008, reporting that "reprocessing has a reliable safety record of excellence identical to that of new equipment" (Chen, 2010, para. 17). While we need more up-to-date research to settle this debate, studies have proven that resterilization saves institutions' money and diverts large quantities of waste from landfills (Kwakye et al., 2011). Moszczynski (2009) states that regardless of stance on reprocessing SUDs, manufacturers need increased accountability toward the environment: stating that companies need to be ecologically accountable in their practices and promote conditions that support the health of both sentient beings and the ecosystem (Figures 7.5–7.7).

II. Diagnosis: The Impacts of Indifference

Myopic Approaches to Health Care

Regardless of one's position toward the use of SUDs in health care, there is glaring evidence of the consequences associated with its ongoing use that

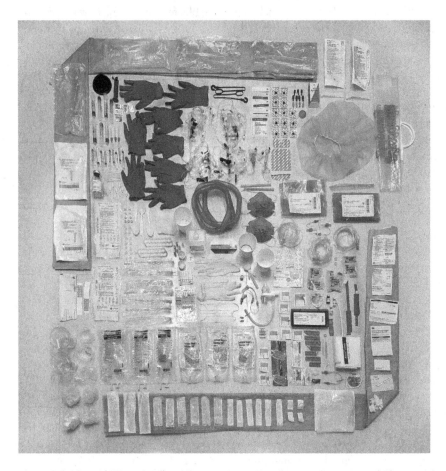

Figure 7.5 Hospital Waste Knolling VI: One Nurse, Five Patients, 2018. Digital Photograph
    of Single-use Hospital Waste.

Source: Emmanuel Christian Tedjasukmana.

continue to be ignored. Although these throw-away items may be more convenient to use during patient care and ostensibly ensure a level of safety and
sterility, the use and disposal of these items adversely influence the patients'
health they are being used to save. As Freinkel (2011) states, "we enjoy plastics-
based technologies that can save lives as never before but … also pose insidious
threats to human health" (p. 10).

In reality, plastic is still a relatively new material—and as a result of its
substantial presence in our daily lives, we are only now beginning to understand
the actual implications of plastic on our health. Because plastic requires mal-
leability for its diverse uses and needs, various chemical additives are mixed with
plastics to give them these unique properties. However, these added pigments,

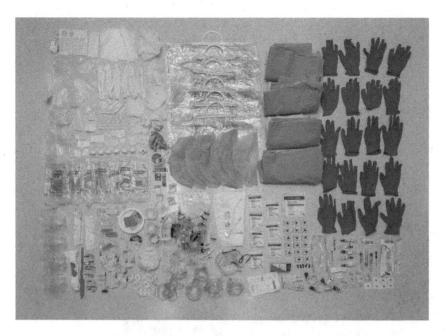

Figure 7.6 Hospital Waste Knolling II: One Nurse, Six Patients, 2018. Digital Photograph
   of Single-use Hospital Waste.

Source: Emmanuel Christian Tedjasukmana.

stabilizers, water repellents, flame retardants, stiffeners, and softeners can then
leach into their surroundings and our bodies. These chemical additives affect
health in ways that range from interfering with the body's hormone functions
and stunting brain development to causing cancer and congenital disabilities
(Royte, 2018).

Phthalates and Bisphenol A (BPA) are two toxins most often associated with
the health risks from plastics in both popular and scientific media. Because these
chemicals readily leach into surrounding environments, they have been linked
to releasing toxins into the food and water that we ingest and the bodies of land
and water that they pollute. This impacts every dimension of our lives, and as
Freinkel (2011) states, "researchers have detected phthalates in blood, urine,
saliva, breast milk, and amniotic fluid, which means people are being exposed to
the chemicals at all stages of life, starting in utero" (p. 98). Phthalates deposit in
the fatty tissues where they act as antiandrogens, and studies suggest that these
phthalates play a role in male reproductive dysfunction and cancer. BPA, which
is often found in food-grade plastic and hospital disposables, has been found to
have an estrogenic side-effect profile and is linked to premature birth, in-
trauterine growth retardation, preeclampsia, stillbirth, and delayed neurological
development. Because BPA, phthalates, and various other chemicals can cross
over to the placenta, they have been linked to growth retardation, neurological

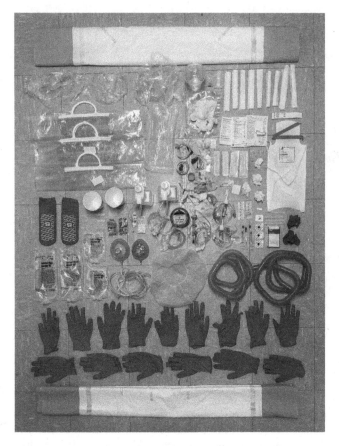

Figure 7.7 Hospital Waste Knolling III: One Nurse, Three Patients, 2018. Digital
Photograph of Single-use Hospital Waste.

Source: Emmanuel Christian Tedjasukmana.

harm, hormonal derangements, and cancers in children—and manifest as adverse health conditions in adulthood (Zaman, 2010).

Polyvinyl chloride (PVC) is a type of plastic associated with health and safety
risks globally and one of the high-volume plastic polymers frequently found
in the hospital setting (Schettler, 2020). A 2002 study by The Nightingale
Institute for Health and the Environment (NIHE) cited PVC as making up
at least 25% of all hospital equipment: and is most typically found in IV bags,
tubing, oxygen masks, catheters, and disposable gloves (Gaudry & Skiehar,
2007). On its own, PVC is both firm and fragile; it requires additional chemicals
to give it plasticity. Because these additives do not fully bond to PVC, they
also tend to leach from the equipment into our bodies—ultimately affecting
the liver, kidneys, lungs, endocrine, and reproductive systems (Freinkel, 2011).

Health issues also arise when medical items are incinerated due to the mercury, lead, formaldehyde, and dioxins released into the air (Gaudry & Skiehar, 2007; Health Care Without Harm, 2022; Muñoz, 2012). Dioxins, a carcinogen linked to reproductive disorders, decreased immunity, diabetes, heart disease, and altered developmental function, add to the high concentrations of particulate matter in the air that have continually risen due to increased fossil fuel combustion. This deteriorating air quality has been implicated as a key contributor to the global burden of mortality and disease and has been responsible for over 8.7 million premature deaths—or about 18% of total global deaths in 2018 (Vohra et al., 2021). It is also essential to point out that these health threats have the greatest impact on already vulnerable populations—such as the low-income and BIPOC communities—who often already have limited access to health care resources and services (Seeding Sovereignty, 2021).

Of increasing concern are the massive amounts of waste generated by the health care industry's increasing use of plastics. By the early 1990s, two-thirds of the United States' landfills were already filled (Zaman, 2010)—and the health care industry is becoming a notable contributor to the world's waste issue. Practice Greenhealth—one of the first organizations to promote environmental stewardship and sustainability within the health care setting—released a report estimating the total amount of waste annually produced by the health care sector to be over 5 million tons. Each occupied hospital bed contributes an average of 29 pounds of waste per day—creating over 14,000 tons of waste per day—with 25% of this waste consisting of plastic (Gibbens, 2019; Practice Greenhealth, 2022).

One study looking to measure the environmental impact of hysterectomies found that a single procedure could produce up to 20 pounds of waste—much of which consists of plastic (Gibbens, 2019). Another study from Canada specifically looked to calculate the waste generated by total knee arthroplasties (TKAs) and found that a single TKA generated an estimated 13.3 kilograms of waste: more waste than an average family of four produces in a week. When multiplying this amount by this hospital's annual total of TKAs performed, they estimated that knee replacements alone would create an estimated 407,889 kilograms (899,241 pounds) of waste (Stall et al., 2013). This waste occupies scarce landfill space and produces methane: a potent GHG that can trap heat more than 25 times that of carbon dioxide. Methane is a significant contributor to global warming, bringing a slew of health-related consequences (United States Environmental Protection Agency, 2021). In addition to methane produced from solid waste contributions, the health care industry also contributes to GHG emissions when delivering care through energy consumption, transport, feeding patients, and manufacturing products. In Health Care Without Harm's first-ever estimate of health care's global climate footprint, they reveal that "if the [global] health sector were a country, it would be the fifth-largest emitter on the [P]lanet"—emitting more than Brazil or Japan. This climate footprint is equivalent to the annual greenhouse gas emissions from 514 coal-fired power plants (Karliner et al., 2019, p. 4).

There has been a dramatic growth of scientific evidence linking human health with environmental health within the last few years. According to Gerwig (2015), "the environment plays a role in nearly 85 percent of all disease" (p. 8), and the impacts on human health concerning climate change can already be linked to the global disease burden. Schroeder et al. (2013) state that the health care sector both "directly and indirectly cause some of the illness and health problems that they try to prevent and treat, so [they] clearly contradict one of the main guiding ethical principles of health care, *primum non nocere—first do no harm*" (p. 73). Increased impact on the environment through global warming is likely to have an even more significant role on human health globally through an increase in heat waves, extreme weather events, flooding, droughts, lack of freshwater sources, sea-level rise, and altered geographical distribution of insect vectors leading to increased communicable diseases. These impacts will subsequently augment global health inequities for vulnerable communities and increase mass migration (Karliner et al., 2019; Figure 7.8).

Impacts Exacerbated by COVID-19

As if long-standing impacts on both environment and health weren't enough to address, the manifestation of the COVID-19 pandemic has further exacerbated our destructive relationship with plastic and its effects on health. The spread of COVID-19 spurred the need for increased personal protective equipment (PPE) for not only health care workers but the public as well—and led to a monthly consumption of over 129 billion face masks and 65 billion gloves globally (Del-la-Torre et al., 2021). Given its high usage paired with its single-use design, one study estimated that if each individual in the United Kingdom wore a single-use face mask every day for one year, an astonishing 66,000 tonnes of unrecyclable plastic waste would be generated (Dean, 2020). In response to this demand for creating more PPE, fracking and petrochemical manufacturing intensified (Ahmadifard, 2020), as did the resulting carbon pollution due to the high demand for both the manufacturing and transport of PPE around the world.

Because PPE was created to be single-use, an overflowing amount of plastic waste is continually introduced into our waste streams. This results in an explosion of plastic refuse entering environmental spaces due to worldwide solid waste management systems that are overwhelmed and overburdened (Del-la-Torre et al., 2021). According to Zhang et al. (2021), if the current disposal patterns continue, "around 75% of plastic PPE waste related to COVID-19 will end up in landfills or ocean environments" (p. 1), and they also estimate that each face mask would take 450 years to fully decompose. If PPE is deemed infectious, it cannot be sent to landfills to decompose and instead must be incinerated. Regardless, our atmosphere is polluted with GHGs, toxins, or other potentially dangerous compounds such as heavy metals, dioxins, and polychlorinated biphenyls (PCBs) (Ahmadifard, 2020; Patrício Silva et al., 2021).

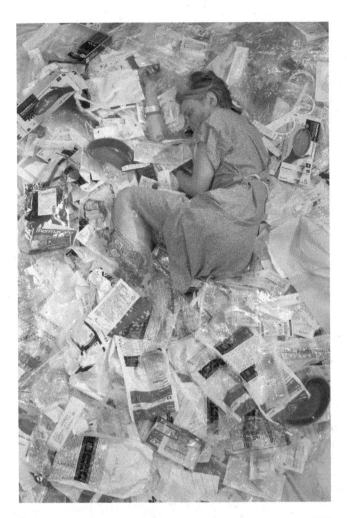

Figure 7.8 Myopia: Harming in Order to Heal #8, 2019. Digital Photograph of Single-use Hospital Waste.

Source: Emmanuel Christian Tedjasukmana.

This growing evidence hastens our need to not only address our dependency on plastic within our lives and within the health care setting but also scrutinize how we respond to global emergencies. As with prior pandemics, the lack of knowledge concerning cause, severity, and transmissibility leads to a severe uptick in waste and single-use items due to uncertainty. But must it continue to be this way? According to Zhang et al. (2021), "although mismanagement of public health crisis is the priority, governments and health care systems must simultaneously implement strategies to mitigate the environmental consequences of the pandemic" (p. 2). It is nonsensical that we address crises with

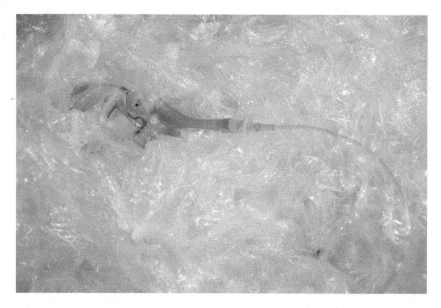

Figure 7.9 Myopia: Harming in Order to Heal #5, 2019. Digital Photograph of Single-use Hospital Waste.

Source: Emmanuel Christian Tedjasukmana.

temporary, quick fixes that will later come back to bite us even harder than before—and allow those with privilege and power to make situations worse for others who already have limited resources. It is vital that we "align our short-term goals of responding to the COVID-19 pandemic with our long term vision for environmentally conscious action" (Ahmadifard, 2020, p. 343). Considering that all the waste created throughout the COVID-19 pandemic will remain with us for an indefinite time, we must prioritize innovation and sustainability in preparation for the next disaster we may face. Referencing our response to crises, Ahmadifard (2020) states that "[it's] important to emphasize that this pandemic is not the problem … Historically, sustainability and environmental quality have not been prioritized in the face of adversity … [they] do not have to be mutually exclusive" (pp. 344–345). We need to form solutions to health crises and global disasters that are circular, sustainable, and support our mission of healing for both the short and long term (Figure 7.9).

III. Plan of Care: Remedies for a Dying Planet

The Nurse's Role in Combating Climate Change

The *2018 Lancet Countdown on Health and Climate Change Brief for the United States of America* calls attention to the fact that "humans need clean air, safe water, and vibrant communities to thrive, and climate change threatens these foundations of health and well-being … [and] is already harming American's health" (Salas et al., 2018, p. 4). The Alliance of Nurses for Healthy Environments (ANHE) recognizes numerous positive health benefits of addressing climate change. These include improved mental health, decreased heart and asthma attacks, healthier lungs in children, less heat stress for workers and vulnerable populations, healthier pregnancies with healthier babies, fewer learning disabilities and incidences of ADHD and autism, and fewer hospital admissions (Alliance of Nurses for Healthy Environments, 2020).

As part of our vital role and commitment to protecting, maintaining, and restoring the health of patients and communities while averting health threats, nurses have both a critical and ethical obligation to mitigate climate change in any way possible. Addressing the climate crisis will not only improve the public health of today's and tomorrow's generations, but it is also "an essential component to addressing the institutionalized racism and health inequities that are amplified in the incidence and death statistics of the COVID-19 pandemic" (Alliance of Nurses for Healthy Environments, 2020, p. 2).

A recent study analyzing nurses' environmental activism revealed that nurses' activism is triggered by threats to human health (Terry & Bowman, 2020). Nurses have always acted as first responders during public health crises, and the current COVID-19 pandemic is the latest example of our continual presence, resilience, and dedication to our communities (Morin & Baptiste, 2020). Around the world, nurses have historically been influential changemakers in advocating for improvements in public health. We are recognized for our roles as political activists, influencers for health policy changes, public educators, and advocates advancing positive changes within our communities. With a global workforce of around 28 million nurses (Woods, 2020) and as "America's Most Trusted Profession" for the 20th consecutive year in Gallup's annual "Most Honest and Ethical Profession's Poll" (Senior, 2022), nurses have rapport and deep connection with communities. As a result of this connection, and because nurses have always been skilled in distilling complex and vital information and making it more accessible, understandable, and relatable in every way possible (Alliance of Nurses for Healthy Environments, 2016), we have crucial opportunities in educating the public and raising awareness on how negative impacts on climate have direct implications on our physical and mental well-being (Gallagher & Dix, 2020).

This essential information needs to continue beyond just the education of our patients and urgently needs to extend to the public sector. We need to educate the heads of hospitals, health care industry leaders, local policymakers, governments, and international leaders that influence the policies that directly influence global health outcomes (Brokaw, 2016). To achieve this, nurses should be heavily involved in politics as the decisions made in legislation affects the various aspects of health for every community member—including our own. Because of this significant influence, experience, and knowledge, we as nurses should be educated, trained, and supported to be involved in politics and policies involving health. We should be invited to influence decisions and sit in places of power. Furthermore, our employers must allow us to vote—even while on the job (Brokaw, 2016). Because we are a diverse group with one of the largest workforces, nurses of every type should also hold positions on boards, committees, design teams, advisories, and councils—and maintain offices at the local, state, and federal levels.

There are so many ways to revolutionize and rebuild our toxic health care system and restore the health of our Planet—and I believe that education and awareness are essential to making this change. Just as continuing education and community involvement are necessary experiences for established nurses, this knowledge and practice should also be incorporated into our nursing curriculum from day one. Nursing students need to be aware of their capabilities to protect health in ways that extend well beyond the bedside. Curriculum and practice should also include health care policy education (Brokaw, 2016; Nash, 2021), history of nursing activism, nursing politics, climate justice, and environmental education that directly links the Planet's health with human health and well-being. Students should be taught that nursing scope of practice includes being stewards of the environment, advocates for its protection, and leaders in transforming health care. We need to empower our nurses from day one and show our students what change, ingenuity, and impact we are capable of. As experienced faculty, preceptors, and mentors, we need to be living examples of this if we are to ever radically change the way we practice and how we view health (Figure 7.10).

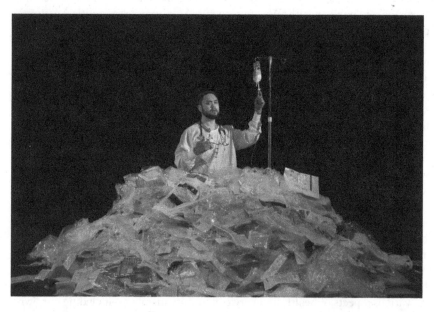

Figure 7.10 Myopia: Harming in Order to Heal #10, 2019. Digital Photograph of Single-use Hospital Waste.

Source: Emmanuel Christian Tedjasukmana.

A Radical Imagination for Health Care

Will it ever be possible for health care to fulfill its mission of providing safe care without further harming the environment and negatively impacting the health of future generations? Our plight with global warming is incredibly complex and complicated by various influences—including the health care industry's continual contributions. Because of our indifference and delay in intervention, we have pushed the limits of polluting and extracting for so long that we are teetering on the point of no return (Harvey, 2022). Regardless of how wicked this problem is and how daunting it may be to solve it, we know that we can no longer afford to push these issues aside. The life of every living thing—including the very Planet we reside on—depends on it. We are well beyond the point of temporary quick fixes: we require everyone's involvement to halt further damage to our health and the health of the Planet. Climate change has to be addressed on every level: every individual, community, corporation, industry, governing body, and country on the Planet. To begin this vital process, however, we must start with significant shifts within our frame of thinking. Our current systems are created to exploit, extract, and profit off problems. They are not set up to be changed and uprooted, and solutions conceived to fit within these pre existing systems are often too limiting. To achieve a world in which we want to live, we must allow ourselves to radically imagine solutions that aren't restricted to the confines of our current systems. With radical imagination, "the idea is not to devise a plan that would work under current systems—but to use the tools of oppression to shape a utopian future" (Atmos, 2022, slide 6).

One change in mindset that would act as a significant catalyst for addressing health care's environmental impact would be to repair our relationship with Mother Earth. As health practitioners, we desperately need to reorient and reorganize our priorities by holding our Planet's health first and foremost. Our twisted view of owning the Planet and doing whatever we please with it is severely deranged, and we can no longer pretend that Earth is ours to misuse. No longer can we act as parasites if we are to survive for more than a few generations. We must live symbiotically, in harmony, and with full respect for nature. Given the data correlating climate change with health, it is blatantly evident that the health of all living things is directly linked to that of the Earth, and we "draw spiritual sustenance from nature in all its beauty and diversity" (Schroeder et al., 2013, p. vii). As a result, care of the Planet is now regarded as preventative health (Schroeder et al., 2013)—and it is our utmost duty to prioritize and lobby for policies, laws, research, innovation, and funds that protect our land, air, and water. To be clear, our goal is never to compromise the quality of care but instead to drive the industry to become net-zero in its emissions and impact—all of which will enhance health (Cohen, 2021).

Furthermore, the health care industry needs to be exemplary leaders of this movement for other sectors to follow, and we need to collaborate on all fronts to achieve and promote this (Karliner et al., 2019). It is hypocritical to vow to uphold the tenets of health and then support practices that extract, exploit, pollute, abuse, and irreversibly damage our Planet's well-being. We must prioritize the health of the Planet and factor this within our health praxis. We must resist ecocide. Gone are the days when our health care industry can consume large amounts of energy and natural resources while simultaneously generating harmful waste and emissions in return. We must espouse sustainable thinking: a view that "meets the needs of the present without compromising the ability of future generations to meet their own needs" (Schroeder, 2013, p. 17) with circular economy: one that "instead of consuming and polluting, it regenerates and restores" (Karliner et al., 2019, p. 29). This collective mindset must be at the core of how our industry functions: continually questioning and focusing on how our care will affect the Planet and its patients. Being that consumption of fossil fuels is at the center of health care emissions (Karliner et al., 2019), we are led to the idea that to be of a circular and sustainable mindset, the divestment from fossil fuels by health institutions is a crucial step. Doing so would make substantial strides toward counteracting our negative impacts on the environment. Through this, we can fulfill our mission of promoting health equity and climate justice: and it is well within our power to do so.

Gary Cohen, president of Health Care Without Harm and Practice Greenhealth, states that "health care is one of the few industries that has the economic clout, the scientific expertise, the public credibility, and perhaps most important, the motivations and mission to 'do no harm' and to change practices that may cause harm not only within its sphere of operations, but through pressure on its supply chain, on a national, economy-wide scale" (Gerwig, 2015, p. 14). With the global health care sector spending over $7.2 trillion annually— close to 10% of world gross domestic product—"the health care industry as a whole has a great deal of economic power in directing policy changes and demanding that their suppliers utilize circular, sustainable, and green approaches that find innovative alternatives that are climate smart" (Karliner et al., 2019, p. 8). With this powerful influence, the health care industry undoubtedly can drive us toward a sustainable culture in which health, equity, renewable energy, and circular innovation are built-in into our core and how we function. In setting this precedent, we also lead the movement of breaking free from fossil fuel dependency—and we can finally show the world what genuine commitment to the Planet, health, and our future looks like (Figure 7.11).

Conclusion

The need to disrupt this ongoing paradox of harming in order to heal is an urgent one. We are far from being in an ideal state. We need to change how we practice and provide health care in radical ways. My hope is that through all the data, research, words, and art, something profoundly connects with

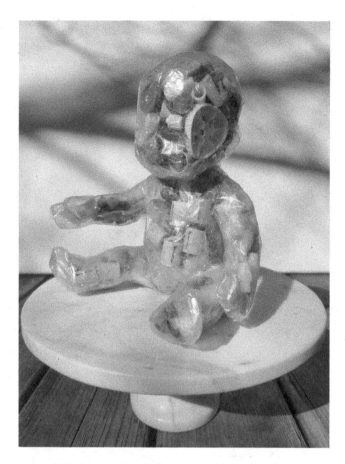

Figure 7.11 We Are the Children of the Future, 2019. Mixed Media Sculpture: Tape, Hospital Waste.

Source: Emmanuel Christian Tedjasukmana.

you and inspires you to view the meaning of health—and the health of the Planet—differently. I hope it changes your relationship with the Earth. I hope some part of it changes how you view your practice, capability, influence, and power as a nurse. We need to step up and intervene if we are to truly support environmental health, preventative health, equity, and climate justice. We have the power to be the drivers of the change we want to see and fight for the future of the Planet. Let us never underestimate our ability to provoke change and protect this tiny blue dot we all inhabit and call our home. Let us band together as a connective tissue that works together to create bodies of movement and resonant action. In doing so, we collectively move toward a more fantastic, brighter, and just future (Figure 7.12).

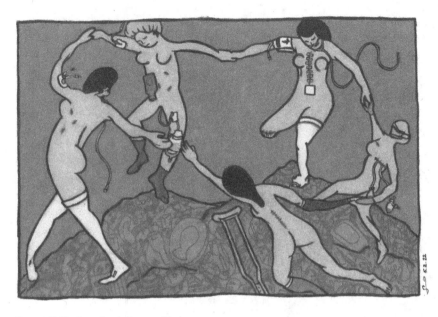

Figure 7.12 Sacrificial Dance (I).

Source: Emmanuel Christian Tedjasukmana.

References

Ahmadifard, A. (2020). Unmasking the hidden pandemic: Sustainability in the setting of the COVID-19 pandemic. *British Dental Journal*, 229(6), 343–345. 10.1038/s41415-020-2055-z

Alliance of Nurses for Healthy Environments. (2016). *Environmental health in nursing*. Alliance of Nurses for Healthy Environments. https://envirn.org/e-textbook/

Alliance of Nurses for Healthy Environments. (2020). The ANHE nurses' guide to what the science teaches us about common solutions to climate change and family health problems. *Alliance of Nurses for Healthy Environments*. https://envirn.org/wp-content/uploads/2020/09/AddressingClimateChangeforBetterHealth_Final.pdf

Atmos [@atmos]. (2022, March 19). It's time for radical imagination. *Instagram*. https://www.instagram.com/p/CbSUuAlLnV2/

Brokaw, J. (2016, September 22). *The nursing profession's potential impact on policy and politics*. American Nurse. https://www.myamericannurse.com/nursing-professions-potential-impact-policy-politics/

Carrington, D. (2016, August 29). *The anthropocene epoch: scientists declare dawn of human-influenced age*. The Guardian. https://www.theguardian.com/environment/2016/aug/29/declare-anthropocene-epoch-experts-urge-geological-congress-human-impact-earth

Chen, I. (2010, July 5). *In a world of throwaways, making a dent in medical waste*. The New York Times. https://www.nytimes.com/2010/07/06/health/06waste.html

Cohen, G. (2021, September 15). *Health care's responsibility at the intersection of climate, health and racial equity* [Webinar]. MGH Center for the Environment and

Health & MGH Institute of Health Professions Center for Climate Change, Climate Justice, and Health. https://mghihp.zoom.us/rec/play/nfxEPGwRyAd0G5 n7rnf4DmIxzYK_WA5jLfx2MnhqAEheE3ZhWCPwNTBlBHYVypOoRg3oXFAcYt ufjDGn.ME9WMQqcIzArvuLD?continueMode=true&_x_zm_rtaid=WqUW7sJcQt C8W4wWPG_X3w.1632513050150.62ea8cc69957fc5d263beb9aac85bf05&_x_zm_ rhtaid=262

Collier, R. (2011). The ethics of reusing single-use devices. *CMAJ: Canadian Medical Association Journal*, *183*(11), 1245. 10.1503/cmaj.109-3907

Crutzen, P., & Stoermer, E. (2000). The anthropocene. *The International Geosphere-Biosphere Programme Newsletter*, *41*, 17–18.

Davis, H., & Turpin, E. (2015). *Art in the anthropocene: Encounters among aesthetics, politics, environments and epistemologies*. Open Humanities Press.

Dean, R. (2020). PPE: Polluting planet Earth. *British Dental Journal*, *229*(5), 267. 10.1038/s41415-020-2130-5

Del-la-Torre, E., Pizarro-Ortega, C., Dioses-Salinas, D., Ammendolia, J., & Okoffo, E. (2021). Investigating the current status of COVID-19 related plastics and their potential impact on human health. *Current Opinion in Toxicology*, *27*, 47–53. 10.1016/j.cotox.2021.08.002

Dunn, D. (2002). Reprocessing single-use devices–the ethical dilemma. *AORN*, *75*(5), 989–999. 10.1016/s0001-2092(06)61462-2

Freinkel, S. (2011). *Plastic: A toxic love story*. Houghton Mifflin Harcourt.

Gallagher, R., & Dix, A. (2020). Sustainability 1: Can nurses reduce the environmental impact of healthcare? *Nursing Times* [online], *116*(6), 29–31. https://cdn.ps.emap.com/wp-content/uploads/sites/3/2020/08/200826-Sustainability-1-can-nurses-reduce-the-environmental-impact-of-healthcare1.pdf

Gaudry, J., & Skiehar, K. (2007) Promoting environmentally responsible health care. *The Canadian Nurse*, *103*(1), 22–26. PMID: 17269580

Geyer, R., Jambeck, J., & Kaw, K. (2017). Production, use, and fate of all plastics ever made. *Science Advances*, *3*(7), 1–5. 10.1126/sciadv.1700782

Gerwig, K. (2015). *Greening health care: How hospitals can heal the planet*. Oxford University Press.

Gibbens, S. (2019, October 4). *Can medical care exist without plastic? National Geographic*. https://www.nationalgeographic.com/science/article/can-medical-care-exist-without-plastic

Goldberg, S. (2018). The plastic apocalypse. *National Geographic*, 6.

Greene, V. (1986). Reuse of disposable medical devices: Historical and current aspects. *Infection Control*, *7*(10), 508–513. 10.1017/s0195941700065140

Harvey, F. (2022, April 4). IPCC report: "Now or never"if world is to stave off climate disaster. *The Guardian*. https://www.theguardian.com/environment/2022/apr/04/ipcc-report-now-or-never-if-world-stave-off-climate-disaster

Health Care Without Harm. (2022). *Waste management*. Health Care Without Harm. https://noharm-uscanada.org/issues/us-canada/waste-management

Karliner, J., Slotterback, S., Boyd, R., Ashby, B., & Steele, K. (2019, September). *Health care's climate footprint: How the health sector contributes to the global climate crisis and opportunities for action*. Health Care Without Harm & Arup. https://noharm-global.org/sites/default/files/documents-files/5961/HealthCaresClimateFootprint_092319.pdf

Kwakye, G., Brat, G., & Makary, M. (2011). Green surgical practices for health care. *Archives of Surgery*, *146*(2), 131–136. 10.1001/archsurg.2010.343

Leonard, A. (2007). *The story of stuff: Referenced and annotated script*. Film script. The Story of Stuff Project. https://www.storyofstuff.org/wp-content/uploads/2020/01/ StoryofStuff_AnnotatedScript.pdf

Leslie, H., Velzen, M., Brandsma, S., Vethaak, A., Garcia-Vallejo, J., & Lamoree, M. (2022). Discovery and quantification of plastic particle pollution in human blood. *Environment International*, 1–8. 10.1016/j.envint.2022.107199

Morin, K., & Baptiste, D. (2020). Nurses as heroes, warriors and political activists. *Journal of Clinical Nursing*, 15–16. 10.1111/jocn.15353

Moszczynski, A. (2009). Is once always enough? Revisiting the single use item. *Journal of Medical Ethics*, 35(2), 87–90. 10.1136/jme.2008.025643

Muñoz, A. (2012). Reducing health care's carbon footprint—the power of nursing. *Workplace Health & Safety*, 11(60), 471–474. 10.1177/216507991206001102

Nash, C. (2021). Time to act: What nurses can do to reduce the environmental burden of PPE. *Nursing Times*, 117(8), 18–20. https://cdn.ps.emap.com/wp-content/uploads/sites/ 3/2020/08/200826-Sustainability-1-can-nurses-reduce-the-environmental-impact-of- healthcare1.pdf

Patrício Silva, A., Prata, J., Walker, T., Duarte, A., Ouyang, W., Barcelò, D., & Rocha-Santos, T. (2021). Increased plastic pollution due to COVID-19 pandemic: Challenges and recommendations. *Chemical Engineering Journal*, 405, 126683. 10.1016/j.cej.2020.126683

Practice Greenhealth. (2022). *Waste*. Practice Greenhealth. https://practicegreenhealth. org/topics/waste/waste-0

Ragusa, A., Svelato, A., Santacroce, C., Catalano, P., Notarstefano, V., Oliana, C., Papa, F., Rongioletti, M., Baiocco, F., Draghi, S., D'Amore, E., Rinaldo, D., Matta, M., & Giorgini, E. (2021). Plasticenta: First evidence of microplastics in human placenta. *Environment International*, 146, 1–8. 10.1016/j.envint.2020.106274

Royte, E. (2018). A threat to us? *National Geographic*, 84–87.

Salas, R., Knappenberger, P., & Hess, J. (2018, November 28). *2018 Lancet countdown on health and climate change brief for the united states of america*. The Lancet. https:// www.apha.org/-/media/files/pdf/topics/climate/2018_us_lancet_countdown_brief. ashx

Schettler, T. (2020, March 3). *The plasticene: Age of plastics*. Science & Environmental Health Network. http://www.trailblz.info/ScienceEnvironmental/doc/MgA2AD MAOAA0ADgANgA1AC0AMQQAwADMANwAxAA2/The_Plasticene_Age_of_ Plastics.pdf

Schroeder, K., Thompson, T., Frith, K., & Pencheon, D. (2013). *Sustainable healthcare*. Wiley-Blackwell.

Schwabl, P., Köppel, S., Königshofer, P., Bucsics, T., Trauner, M., Reiberger, T., & Liebmann, B. (2019). Detection of various microplastics in human stool: A pro- spective case series. *Annals of Internal Medicine*, 171(7), 453–457. 10.7326/M19-0618

Seeding Sovereignty [@seedingsovereignty]. (2021, July 9). Why plastic is intersectional. *Instagram*. https://www.instagram.com/p/CRHDW3orTYq/

Senior, R. (2022, January 12). *Numbers don't lie: Nurses most trusted profession again*. *American Nurse*. https://www.myamericannurse.com/numbers-dont-lie-nurses-most- trusted-again/

Stall, N., Kagoma, Y., Bondy, J., & Naudie, D. (2013). Surgical waste audit of 5 total knee arthroplasties. *Canadian Journal of Surgery*, 56(2), 97–102. 10.1503/ cjs.015711

Stoermer, W. Jr. (1999, October 1). *Reprocessing single-use devices: Why does the debate continue? Medical Device & Diagnostic Industry Magazine.* https://www.mddionline.com/components/reprocessing-single-use-devices-why-does-debate-continue

Terry, L., & Bowman, K. (2020). Outrage and the emotional labour associated with environmental activism among nurses. *Journal of Advance Nursing, 76*(3), 867–877. doi: 10.1111/jan.14282

United States Environmental Protection Agency. (2021, June 30). *Importance of methane.* United States Environmental Protection Agency. https://www.epa.gov/gmi/importance-methane

Vohra, K., Vodonos, A., Schwartz, J., Marais, E., Sulprizio, M., & Mickley, L. (2021). Global mortality from outdoor fine particle pollution generated by fossil fuel combustion: Results from GEOS-Chem. *Environmental Research, 195,* 110754. 10.1016/j.envres.2021.110754

Vanapalli, K., Sharma, H., Ranjan, V., Samal, B., Bhattacharya, J., Dubey, B., & Goel, S. (2021). Challenges and strategies for effective plastic waste management during and post COVID-19 pandemic. *Science of The Total Environment, 750.* 10.1016/j.scitotenv.2020.141514

Watts, N., Amann, M., Arnell, N., Ayeb-Karlsson, S., Belesova, K., Berry, H., Bouley, T., Boykoff, M., Byass, P., Cai, W., Campbell-Lendrum, D., Chambers, J., Daly, M., Dasandi, N., Davies, M., Depoux, A., Dominguez-Salas, P., Drummond, P., Ebi, K., ... Costello, A. (2018). The 2018 report of the lancet countdown on health and climate change: Shaping the health of nations for centuries to come. *The Lancet, 392*(10163), 2479–2514. 10.1016/S0140-6736(18)32594-7

Watts, N., Amann, M., Arnell, N., Ayeb-Karlsson, S., Beagley, J., Belesova, K., Boykoff, M., Byass, P., Cai, W., Campbell-Lendrum, D., Capstick, S., Chambers, J., Coleman, S., Dalin, C., Daly, M., Dasandi, N., Dasgupta, S., Davies, M., Napoli, C., ... Costello, A. (2020). The 2020 report of the lancet countdown on health and climate change: Responding to converging crises. *The Lancet, 397*(10269), 129–170. 10.1016/S0140-6736(20)32290-X

Woods, A. (2020, April 09). *WHO: State of the world's nursing 2020.* Lippincott Nursing Center. https://www.nursingcenter.com/ncblog/april-2020/who-state-of-the-worlds-nursing-2020

Zaman, T. (2010). The prevalence and environmental impact of single use plastic products. *Public Health Management & Policy: An Online Textbook, 11th edition.* Retrieved November 23, 2011.

Zhang, E., Aitchison, L., Phillips, N., Shaban, R., & Kam, A. (2021). Protecting the environment from plastic PPE. *British Medical Journal, 372*(109). 10.1136/bmj.n109

Part III

A Radical Imagination for Nursing

If section one concerned itself with histories of nursing and how they shape the order of things and section two attended to the realities of the present, section three marks a shift toward something more speculative, namely a radical imagination for nursing. Radical imagination, following the collective vision of radical scholar-activists Haiven and Khasnabish (2014), is simply "the ability to imagine the world, life, and social institutions not as they are but as they might otherwise be. It is the courage and the intelligence to recognize that the world can and should be changed. The radical imagination is not just about dreaming of different futures. It's about bringing those possibilities back from the future to work on the present, to inspire action and new forms of solidarity today" (2014, p. 4). Learning from the past, imagining the future, building in the present. Radical imagination is as palpable as it is ephemeral, both visionary and pragmatic.

For this section, we invited authors to conjure what is possible, setting aside what is current or what is likely. Here we were also inspired by Angela Davis' admonition that "You have to act as if it were possible to radically transform the world. And you have to do it all the time" (Davis, 2014). In bringing this kind of ethos to nursing, we acknowledge that without imagination, we are resigned to reinscribing the status quo, over and over and over again in ways that harm us as nurses and in ways that harm the folks we accompany in care. We decline to accept the way things are because we see things that should - and can - change. And we see radical imagination as innate to the project of nursing, should nursing choose liberation. This section comprises three chapters, which include provocations for thinking about what might be in a future that centers practices of decoloniality, harm reduction, cultural safety, and ethics.

The journey in radical imagination begins with nursing education scholar Blythe Bell, who invites readers to imagine what nursing might look like, should it engage in practices of what Bell calls "settler harm reduction." Examining the harms of white-normative assumptions in nursing, Bell acknowledges that widespread anticolonial and antioppressive efforts are in their infancy and teases out the tensions created when nursing purports to value de- and anticolonial efforts but fails to create spaces that are safe for Indigenous, Black, and Brown peoples. In imagining what might be necessary conditions for all comers to grow

DOI: 10.4324/9781003245957-11

and flourish within nursing education, Bell offers generativity, a noncompetitive and collaborative approach to nursing episteme, as a remedy to the harmful and combative methods that have characterized nursing education thus far. In embracing generativity and noncompetition, it is possible to understand nursing educators as part of community subjectivity - nonhierarchical - interrogating the legitimacy of grading amongst other hierarchical practices rooted in consolidation of power. Bell concludes with teachings from the Coastal Salish peoples, situated and contextual as local to Bell's work, reminding us that "there is no conclusion to work that is unending."

From thinking about what it takes to reduce the harm imposed by nursing education - and thus by nurses on the folks in their care - Ruth De Souza's essay, "Using Arts Based Participatory Methods to Teach Cultural Safety," moves to ensuring safety through arts-based methods in Chapter 9. Sharing her reflections on teaching Cultural Safety in undergraduate nursing in Australia, articulating the colonial history of Australia and outlining the development of Cultural Safety, a framework developed by Maori nurses to transform the health impacts of settler colonial systems and practices. De Souza positions herself within this milieu, problematizing her own location within the academy as both outside whiteness and also complicit with the colonial project. De Souza excavates her efforts at unsettling whiteness in nursing through two case studies wherein she partnered with First Nations and racialized artists to bring arts-based pedagogy to nursing as a praxis of critical reflection. She concludes with a call to transformation for nursing, building Cultural Safety while interrupting the reproduction of violent and white supremacist norms, beginning with nursing education.

Chapter 10, parts I and II are a master class for nurses thinking with technology. Here, nurse inventor Rae Walker introduces an essential lexicon for nurses in Chapter 10, part I, "Artificial Intelligence for Health and Care Is Not Inevitable: Introduction and Critical Vocabulary," attending to concepts including artificial intelligence, medical gaslighting, matrix of domination, technochauvanism, algorithmic exceptionalism, abolition, and communities of practice, situating these concepts in the context of nursing. This serves as an introduction, an opening to Chapter 10, part II, entitled "Artificial Intelligence for Health and Care Is Not Inevitable: Ten Commitments to New Futures." Here, Walker outlines ten critical agreements necessary to imagine technologies that can support health and care. These commitments are far-reaching and engage concerns raised by Bell and De Souza regarding harm reduction, anticolonialism, antioppression, and safety. Walker's expansive vision for artificial intelligence (AI) in new futures for health and care includes attending to the sociopolitical realities of technology and the matrices of domination that shape reality. This requires critical perspectives to minimize harm and foster safety for those who are most likely to be harmed by technology (or its uneven application). Doing AI, Walker contends, demands that we prioritize human relations while interrogating the harms and biases that may proliferate in AI and big data. To move toward just futures for nursing, Walker suggests that we embrace a queer, feminist politics of refusal while attending to the planetary impact of the technologies we develop. Ultimately, Walker notes that AI for health is neither intrinscially good nor intrinsically bad, no more certain than the futures yet to be built, all the more reason to engage a radical imagination to lean into liberatory futures and "break shit along the way."

References

Davis, A. (2014). *Lecture at Southern Illinois University.*
Haiven, M., & Khasnabish, A. (2014). *The radical imagination.* Fernwood Publishing.

8 "Settler Harm Reduction" in Nursing Education: Generativity Not Hierarchy

Blythe Bell (she/her)

In this chapter, situated in this particular anthology, I take the liberty to assume rather than argue for an anticolonial and anti-oppressive future for nursing and nurses. From this perspective, we see that nursing education acts as a colonial enterprise, that it is in need of decolonization, and that decolonization as of yet has been taken up only metaphorically (Tuck & Yang, 2012). Decolonization is described as "[...] a position of intelligent inquiry that is meant to unsettle and disturb, which when synthesized transforms" (Dei, 2016, p. 38), or an "intelligent, calculated, and active resistance to the forces of colonialism that perpetuate the subjugation and/or exploitation of our minds, bodies, and lands [...]" (Wilson et al., 2005, p. 223 in McGibbon 2014, p. 4). A nonmetaphorical decolonization requires an abolition of colonial systems of domination in terms of land ownership, Indigenous sovereignty, and epistemological and ontological validation, dissemination, and development (Dei, 2016; McGibbon et al., 2014; Tuck & Yang, 2012). Dr. Eve Tuck and Dr. K. Wayne Yang (2012) argue for the acknowledgement, at least, that any imaginings of settler futurities are incommensurable with true decolonization, even if such imaginings radically subvert power systems. They warn against resting in a radicalism that does not engage with settler colonialism through the de-occupation of lands and thus dispossession of settlers and displaced people of all histories, lest we silently re-inscribe a colonial entitlement and subvert our own radicality. And so I introduce this chapter, written from my White[1] settlerhood[2], with the caveat that it will not go far enough, and the acknowledgment that privileging decolonial imaginings from my standpoint is inherently problematic. Nevertheless, I attempt to engage with notions of anticoloniality in terms of epistemic justice, dismantling hierarchy and processes of exclusion, and abandonment of conventional assessment and evaluation practices; perhaps what Tuck and Yang (2012) name *settler harm reduction*, for the betterment of nursing education and the safety and well-being of nursing students. I do so out of commitment to developing anti-oppressive nursing environments and I intend to tread with care into necessary engagement without invoking White supremacy nor imposing entitled Whiteness. I embrace being accountable to the certain gaps in my perspective. A second caveat; since this writing is an exercise in radical imagination, it does not claim methodological rigor nor exhaustive articulation of

DOI: 10.4324/9781003245957-12

nuances or structural realities that contribute to nursing's present. It will surely offend some with its generality, some who do not, or do not wish to see themselves as part of harmful education, and some who are entrenched in the *ilusio* of nursing science and status.

A Critique of the Status Quo

In this writing, we humbly accept that anticolonial nursing knowledge, theory, and praxis are in their infancy. Since the foundations of Euro-American professional nursing are race, class, and sex and gender elitism (McGibbon et al., 2014) aimed at attaining societal status through fictional hierarchy (Bell, 2021), our anticolonial and anti-oppressive growth and development must not rely on any foundations of nursing that have not been robustly dissected and digested. This leads me to the first of two reasons for the proposition of this chapter; we are in a place of unknowing. There is not a formula or model yet of what nursing should look like in a decolonized reality. This is not to say there isn't guiding anticolonial, decolonizing, Indigenist, anti-oppressive, abolitionist, and post-humanist scholarship (see Bearskin et al., 2021; Dei, 2016; Dillard-Wright, 2021 and many more), but that nursing has clung to its biomedical, racist, and exclusionary roots (McGibbon et al., 2014), and has remained trapped in extractive capitalism via its willing participation in colonial institutions of education and healthcare, rather than transform to be of and for the people. Where there is no formula, when we do not know where we are going or what we are headed to, is not a position of humility the most authentic and integrous path forward? This is arguably not the case in much of contemporary nursing education. I don't believe we have been brave or humble enough to approach students from this unknowing, and yet it is apparent that students can clearly see it. In my experience, students are frustrated with the piecemeal and often superficial social justice rhetoric, and with the stark absence of information about the historical and present-day complicity of nurses in colonial violence in their education beyond discrete and isolated courses or learning experiences (S. Jungwirth & M. Louie, personal communication, October 19, 2021). Further, today's nursing student is not ignorant to the faces of oppression. They can see the racial makeup of nursing departments, can feel the heteronormativity and the ableism, and can hear the absence of a critical appraisal of gender(s). Which brings me to the second reason for the idea I am about to propose; many nursing students are not okay in our care. That nursing education is situated in both extractive capitalist and colonial structures significantly impacts students and the quality of education every day (Valderama-Wallace & Apesoa-Varano, 2019). Where the (barely) hidden curriculum is positivism, white supremacy, and capitalism couched in terms like validity, rigor, excellence, disciplinary knowledge, evidence-based practice, and professionalism ... where students compete against each other for admission, for awards, for clinical placements, for mentorship, and for visibility ... where they are consistently gaslit by faculty and administration through discourses of professionalism and accountability: our students are not okay. The educational environment we are providing nursing students is not one of trust or growth or genuine inquiry; it has historically harmed, and continues to harm students, especially those who live in and with marginalized identities. The education we are providing nursing students reproduces Eurocentric, colonial ontologies of White supremacy, humanism, classism, ableism, sexism, and compulsory heteronormativity by avoiding robust critique of nursing foundations, and by treating anti-oppression and Indigenization as discrete, encapsulated special considerations. This education models how to harm people even while it claims to produce professionals that help people. That nursing school is often not an environment of trust, though we demand our students be trustworthy, and not an environment of supported growth, though we demand that our students support the growth of their clients, and that we teach our students that racism and xenophobia have no place in health care, but have not corrected our White dominance or compulsory heterosexuality, defies the intention of liberatory education and imposes a profound cognitive dissonance as we model a "do as we say, not as we do" ethic.

This chapter aims to radically address the incongruence between claiming a critical social justice education, but not providing a just environment toward the health and wellbeing of nursing students, and our communities broadly. And more specifically the incongruence between claiming to value decolonizing efforts but not maintaining an environment in which it is safe to be Indigenous, Black, queer, or radical and disruptive. The proposition at long last is that while, but not only while, anticolonial nursing frameworks are in their infancy, nursing education will be theoretically emergent and structurally noncompetitive. We will stop reiterating and reinstating the nursing canon, many theories of which were developed through privilege and exclusion (McGibbon et al., 2014), and we will support the development of a nursing future that might not look anything like nursing's present or past. Nursing students will self-direct and self-evaluate their personal and intellectual growth through processes of critical inquiry. Nursing education will be action research, if you will, while we collaboratively and creatively, with and in community, re-shape nursing. This chapter makes a case for imagining an educational exchange that subverts capitalist and colonial hegemony, values the wellbeing of the humans who are nursing students as much as the theoretical healthcare recipients, and trusts these humans to be invested in their own development. I explore the possibility of nursing education as generativity rather than conformity, and nonhierarchical epistemically and structurally.

Nursing Education as Generativity

Dr. George Sefa Dei (2016) explains that decolonizing the academy will require an "epistemic community to develop and nurture hope, dreams, and aspirations, and to transmit energy for this work" (p. 37). They also name the process of

disrupting dominant knowledges as "intellectual combat" (p. 37). I see generative nursing education as dwelling uncomfortably, but necessarily and
hopefully, in this space of collaborative building and simultaneous deconstruction. To face a radical future authentically and not symbolically, nurse
educators will need to disengage from our nursing identities as constructed
through the existing nursing canon to invite a thorough deconstruction of
nursing thought and disciplinarity; to engage in combat with our own developed
intellect. This radical imagining does not include trying to save or patch up
nursing theory to make it more suitable to a decolonial metaphor. It does
however include critical inquiry into the development and reproduction of
nursing thought and disciplinarity toward a critical consciousness from which to
grow. Dr. Kylie Smith (2019) implores us to transform by taking account of
nursing history and present because though we aim to step outside of this un-
broken (colonial) system (K. M. Smith & Foth, 2021), we must maintain an
acute awareness of the sociality and political economy (Dillard-Wright, 2021)
that White supremacist nursing was born of, lest we reproduce an astounding
lack of self-awareness and self-interrogation such as, I argue elsewhere, nursing
performs with gender (Bell, 2021). Dr. Linda Tuhiwai Smith (2013 in
Shahjahan, 2005) explains that the tools of knowledge production used in
academia are those that have been used to legitimize colonization, and as such
"have no methodology for dealing with other knowledge systems" (p. 226). They
are tools for epistemicide not plurality, and as such, clinging to them for validation reinforces a knowledge hierarchy and communicates a disregard for
epistemic justice. A recommendation of Dr. Dei (2016) is interdisciplinary and
institution-wide introductory university courses that ground students in
critical perspectives toward deconstructing rather than re-inscribing knowledge
hierarchies, problematic histories, and social and institutional power relations.
While there are certainly many educators committed to introducing critical
perspectives and developing analytic potential in first-year nursing students,
I contend that the conventional nursing indoctrination agenda mobilized
in introductory nursing courses broadly, acts as a significant barrier to this end.

Generativity

I argue here for a commitment to emergent nursing knowledge and praxis in
nursing education based on principles of deep humility, collective epistemologies and contextualized ontologies, and mutual aid, as recently proposed by
Dr. Jess Dillard-Wright (2021). By deep humility, I refer to the willingness of
nurse academics to dis-associate from encultured nursing norms and cede the
position of authority over nursing knowledge development. A commitment to
collective epistemologies invokes a plurality and a commonness of knowledge
possession. "In Indigenous epistemology, knowledge is not a commodity that
some have while others do not; it cannot be possessed or controlled by educational institutions or academics as it is a living process meant to be absorbed
and understood" (Battiste, in St. Denis et al., 2009, p. 82). Locating knowledge

within communities privileges relevance and inherent validity over the reproduction of standardized ontologies, especially those constructed as *universal*.

I wish to extend Dr. Dillard-Wright's (2021) path to mutual aid of rejecting the power-over and outside-of dynamic of nurse to patient and nurse to community, to the power-over dynamic of educator to student. I will take up the negative construction of *student* more later, but here I draw attention to the generative possibilities that lie dormant when we (educators) exclude students from the community of knowledge holders we assume ourselves to be. Read from a slightly different angle, I wish to invoke Dr. Dillard-Wright's (2021) statement that "the way we set ourselves outside the community to legitimize authority is also the mechanism by which we martyr ourselves" (2021, p. 6). While we scramble to re-fresh our curricula to an "Indigenized" shine, or add stock images of people of color to our slide decks in order to maintain an image of currency and expertise, we are in fact digging ourselves deeper into irrelevance. It will never be enough to Indigenize a colonial curriculum in a colonial structure because the incongruence screams insincerity. In fact, Dr. Ali Drummond (2020) contends this sprinkling of Indigenous ontology or perspective is itself extractive capitalism since the result benefits the institution and not Indigenous people. As educators and nursing leaders, we must be willing to admit that in our current educational structures and epistemologies that are dominated by Whiteness and the spectrum of exclusive normativities, we cannot educate people safely to care for people safely. Dr. Sefa Dei (2016) prescribes a radical inclusivity in the academy to invite marginalized and historically excluded perspectives, standpoints, and ontologies, and the humans they live in, to challenge the hegemony and demand more. Leaning again on Dr. Dillard-Wright (2021), it bears considering what is deemed radical in an environment, and in this case where it means to extend humanity and dignity to all people, radical is absolutely elementary. The point being, however, that neither the curriculum nor the environment of a hegemonic nursing education can be fixed before we dismantle the systems of exclusion that hold it up. And so, humility and collaboration, mutuality and reciprocity, as people and community members, is necessary toward generating relevantly supportive nursing frameworks.

Nursing Education as Noncompetitive

Suggesting that nursing education exists in a noncompetitive structure is not different than suggesting nursing education be generative; these ideas work together to create an environment of growth very different from what I see and participate in today. To be clear, I do not speak for nursing students when I say they are not okay. Perhaps more important is that my claim not come across as condescending or infantilizing. I hope to communicate the opposite in fact, that the construction of *student* in our hierarchical environments is often negative, detrimental to their development, and at worst violent. The people who are nursing students are often treated as unknowers, as if their lived experiences before nursing school were irrelevant. They are often constructed as disengaged, irresponsible, and dishonest, especially if we consider the energy nursing schools put into surveillance technology at the onset of the COVID-19 pandemic (Darbyshire & Thompson, 2021; Walker et al., 2020). Further, their family and social lives, responsibilities, and cultural and structural needs are regularly dismissed as superfluous. Students are socialized into nursing's hierarchical ontology and domineering approach upon entry when they are told that *school needs to come first*, and that if they don't abide (as if it were optional), they likely are not cut out for the discipline. Dr. Philip Darbyshire and David Thompson (2021) invoke Apple's (2016) "epistemological fog" as a mechanism by which educators claim to not understand the context students exist in, and by which they can remain distrustful of students' values and intents. My claim then that many nursing students are not okay is grounded in this construct of power-over and disrespect that is mobilized in a colonial and thus fundamentally exclusionary and oppressive environment, and not at all in any notion of deficit on their part.

An impact of the marketization of higher education is the expectation that learning strategies and resources will be delivered in a service model of engagement, rather than an embodied development (Darbyshire & Thompson, 2021; Serrano et al., 2018). This marketization also results in a primacy of grades over learning; a focus on success rather than process (Serrano et al., 2018). This, in combination with prescriptive education in the form of rigid learning outcomes, frames knowledge as a discrete object that is bought, paid for, and transferred from university to student. The longstanding and dire nursing shortage alongside a wider recognition that contemporary education is colonizing and oppressive puts baccalaureate nursing education into an "ontological crisis" (Serrano et al., 2018) where we are paralyzed by a trifecta of demands to: quickly produce bodies with skills to service the health care industry; decolonize and thus transform the hegemonies in nursing education; and maintain societal and (Western) scientific legitimacy to not lose our share of status or of the health care market. These are just some of the conditions the people who become nursing students are entering the profession in and are responding to, and so a tendency to criticize their academic comportment generally ought to be more thoroughly contextualized. Is it really just the students behaving badly? Or is there (so much) more to that story? Just as nurses deny themselves the subjectivity of community member and care-receiver (Dillard-Wright, 2021), so too do we deny nursing students from occupying these positions. It's as if once people become nursing students, they are in purgatory; no longer community members with lived experience, but also not yet professionals with sanctioned knowledge; at once unknowing and untrusted.

What I did not articulate in the aforementioned section about the construction of *student* is the diversity among how the people who are nursing students may be constructed based on their identities, real or perceived. In speaking generally about nursing students, I do not mean to imply they are all affected similarly by the hegemonic colonial environment. So, despite my argument that nursing students are cast as unknowers, certainly some bodies, and thus their embodied knowledges, are more respected than others. Namely those knowledges that reflect back colonial values and scientific rationalism, and are housed in bodies with cultural capital in a Western academic setting. Dr. Dei (2016) says that "decolonizing the academy is about subversion, putting a critical gaze on structures and processes of educational delivery that continually create and reproduce sites of marginality and colonizing education for learners" (p. 28). The structures and processes I imagine dissolving are those of grading, educator-led evaluation, and prescriptive learning outcomes. The evaluation and grading schemas of higher education are designed to reproduce hierarchy, to discriminate, and to create margins. Importantly, they are neither independent nor objective as they are tools designed by a system that defines its own parameters of validity (Dei, 2016) and are employed by the people who are educators. People who are seasoned with their own complex socialization, motivations, and subversive and/or cooperative relationship with the academy. Dissolving these apparatuses dissolves some of the oppressive hierarchies among students and dissolves the potential for these tools to be weaponized, intentionally or unintentionally, by educators.

Ungrading

The legitimacy and value of grading is certainly contested and I make a case here for abandoning grading altogether. Literature on ungrading lives predictably in educational scholarship, where there is more explicit commitment to investigating and critiquing pedagogies, and andragogies more specifically. Nursing, and other disciplines, have to contend with andragogical theory, skills, and approaches as supplementary to what is of interest, and of benefit to be of interest, to the discipline. The whole grading schema of formal education is so entrenched that it can feel inevitable. Dr. Darbyshire and Thompson (2021) explain that an ideology of inevitability frames "alternative perspectives as idealistic, naïve, elitist or frankly threatening" (p. 3). They also name a "fetishisation of metrics" (p. 3) that in part accounts for a reliance on measurement in nursing education. Nurses and nursing are measured against the dominant epistemological and ontological norms of the Western academy, namely biomedicine and quantitative measurement as truth. So when the perennial battle over nursing's legitimacy is considered, does a departure from measurement in learning elicit significant fear of reprisal? The real discord here though is that the measurements of learning that we employ throughout nursing education that we purport maintain rigor and define excellence are not at all scientific. Are we clinging desperately to constructs that are only symbolically scientific in order to prove our legitimacy through adherence to science? Assumptions that grading provides objective evaluation of knowledge, motivation for student learning, or constructive feedback operate as rhetoric rather than evidenced reality (Schinske & Tanner, 2014).

Another curiosity in the measurement of nursing learning is that in the practice environment where students have hands-on patients and their pharmaceuticals, we often employ pass/fail evaluation, forgoing the opportunity to establish hierarchy or margins in the actual practice of nursing. To be clear, I am not suggesting this should be otherwise, but drawing attention to the fact that in nursing pass/fail evaluative structures are already legitimated, and in the highest risk learning environment at that. That we already use pass/fail systems of evaluation in practice and lab settings also indicates that the application of grading schema in other courses is unnecessary and is done out of compliance and complicity with a colonial ontology that seeks to legitimate privileging the privileged and gate-keeping the rest.

A structural piece of this privileging system that keeps it in place is merit-based financial awards. Students are literally competing against each other for material support and so will value the grade and the effort required to achieve it, regardless of whether it is otherwise meaningful. These arbitrary numbers assigned through the undeniable subjectivity of their educators dictates who is worth supporting and who is not. Knowing that the people who find it easiest to perform the requisite "learnerism" (Macfarlane, 2013 in Darbyshire & Thompson, 2021) are those with significant cultural capital and/or those who have fewer competing demands on their time, the people who are deemed worthy of material support are often those who are already privileged. "Perhaps if the tyranny of grades and the competition to 'outperform' peers were removed, students could experience learning, disappointment, excitement, discovery and improvement without the artificial attribution of a score" (Darbyshire & Thompson, 2021, p. 3). Distributing available capital resources according to financial need rather than subjective metrics of human value would in and of itself changes the landscape of competitive and perhaps performative learner engagement.

Self-directed Learning

An ungraded educational environment in this imaginary engages in constructive evaluation methods that aim to develop the knowledge-bearing person in ways that are relevant to them. This can include self-, peer-, and educator-led evaluation, but to remain aligned with the ethic of student as *embodied knower* and community member, I suggest that evaluative primacy rests with the person as student themselves. Dr. Kevin Kumashiro (2000) discusses the unknowability of the educational exchange in his work on anti-oppressive education. An educator can never know how a teaching has been heard, received, interpreted, and integrated by a learner, and it is perhaps insincere to assume that a learner can ever exactly communicate to an educator what has been learned or embodied by them through the process; each individual's complex web of self and world understandings projected onto the communication. The learning really ought to be evaluated then by the bearer of that knowledge, and not from an outside perspective.

In keeping with this valuation of self-assessment, and of student as community member, the development of contextually appropriate nursing knowledge may well rely on students also developing their learning aims. If we understand curriculum as a political text (Keesing-Styles, 2003) and accept the unknowability of individual students' social politic, then we cannot presume, as educators, to know the specificity of relevant learning for them. The people who are nursing students "are capable of generating assessment strategies and criteria that have immediate applicability and validity in relation to the context of their work and everyday life" (Keesing-Styles, 2003, p. 15). Andragogical strategies of social learning such as poverty or intercultural simulations may provide fundamental learning for some students but also risks harming the students who live the content of these simulations. A student with lived experience of poverty will know whether such a learning opportunity would be of use to their development or not. Maintaining a universal nursing education that is made up of mandatory components for all students either exposes an assumption that the marginalized *Other* does not exist in the program, or that the presumed learning needs of the dominant student body are prioritized over mitigating harm to individuals. Further, ceding power over the specific educational path toward comprehensive nursing knowledge could mitigate potentially harmful conditions where the people who are nursing students are required to evidence their marginality and its ensuing embodied knowledge, in order to be excused from harmful learning experiences. What if students were supported to explore the landscape of nursing knowledge and construct an educational path that was individualized in terms of their holistic learning needs toward becoming a nurse that is prepared to engage in the generation of health and wellbeing alongside community members?

Coast Salish Teachings

I have suggested throughout this chapter that nursing knowledge should rest on community priorities and local contexts. I have also throughout the writing leaned on Indigenous scholars (and others) from across Turtle Island and beyond. In order to resist the reproduction of a pan-Indigeneity, and to honor the knowledge of the people and land that I occupy, this writing needs to be grounded in local knowledge. For this, I engage with the teachings shared by Coast Salish Elders, Knowledge Keepers, and community members with the University of Victoria for the development of their Indigenous plan (University of Victoria, 2016). The principles or teachings shared in this public document are intended for all students, faculty, and staff to engage with as a framework for our work toward an anti-racist environment where Indigenous people can thrive through processes of decolonization and Indigenization. As both a current student and faculty member at this institution, I believe I am engaging appropriately with the four teachings in applying them here to my work, to the depth I am able in absence of relationship to the knowledge holders.

Heʔkw səl'elexw'tala sčeláŋen's—Remember Our Ancestors

This teaching guides us to acknowledge and honor the stories, the people, and the knowledge of the land we occupy, and also those of our own histories. In the context of an anti-colonial nursing education, this teaching guides us to engage with local communities and epistemologies. It also guides us to honor the cultural knowledge that students arrive with rather than encouraging or demanding epistemological and ontological conformity.

Nəə māt gwens čey'i—Work Together

"While individual strands of cedar are strong on their own, they are stronger when braided together" (University of Victoria, 2016, p. 10). This principle models collaborative learning and practice, identifying the strength in relationship and cooperation. In the context of this chapter, I understand this teaching to address the individual nature of academic evaluation, where students' knowledge is assessed in isolation rather than in collaboration. Nurse educators know very well that nurses do not practice in a knowledge vacuum. We continuously lean on each other and on professional resources to guide our practice, and yet accept individualizing knowledge in our educational system.

New'ews sn ʔeyʔ šweleqwəns—Bring in Your Good Feelings

My understanding of this teaching centers authenticity and respect in all relationships. As an educator, I understand this guides me to show up with humility and a genuine desire to be supportive in my teaching relationships, and to trust that students are also arriving with good intentions. Relationships of power-over are normalized in colonial educational structures in that educators have the legitimated authority to gate-keep and to surveil. Trust itself feels disruptive to an educational system and environment with prescriptive learning, and that is designed to "weed out" that which is deemed to not belong. So bringing in our good feelings, our trust in each other has the potential to transform the landscape of higher education.

ə'sacʔəy'xw meqw tə'sa tečel—Be Prepared for All Work to Come

This teaching prepares us for the marathon of cultural and institutional change. It is not as difficult to write about upending the theoretical inculcation and hierarchical evaluation schemas of higher education than it is to persist in an environment of resistance and incremental change. Checkbox change is not enough. One diversity hire or preferential admission, one anti-racism reading, one critical learning outcome, is not enough. This teaching identifies the responsibility for a commitment to good work for the long term.

There Is No Conclusion to Work that Is Unending

> If it costs more money, takes more time, and cares for more people, it's decolonial ....

(Nahanee, 2021)

Are we able to care more when we are cared for? Do we trust when we are trusted? Does confidence and ability grow where they are watered or weeded? Do we create anew with bandages or compost? Can anticolonial thinking be housed in the university? Can anticolonial theorizing be done in Western academic language and literature structures (Shahjahan, 2005)? What I likely have done here is flex a White colonial language all over this attempt to theorize an anticolonial nursing environment, which is a contradiction for me to resolve in future engagements.

A radical transformation of disciplinary culture and educational structures is no small feat, especially in the construct of colonialism and its entrenched epistemic supremacy. It is certainly easier to dismiss these ideas as naïve, or conversely to adopt micro changes and call them radical. Undoubtedly, what is missing from this conversation are the structural "how's." Critique without constructive direction is admittedly self-limiting and yet this work is infinitely broader than this chapter and my perspective. There is so much work to be done.

Acknowledgments

I would like to thank Dorothea Harris (Good) for her friendship and guidance in how to respectfully tie these ideas to local knowledge and Christina Chakanyuka for her loving encouragement.

Notes

1 I elect to capitalize White to formalize and identify this structural position.
2 I write from Whiteness and many other positions of privilege. I am a sixth generation White anglo-European settler in the Canadian colonial state. I was born and raised in the traditional lands of the Tsuut'ina First Nation and the Blackfoot Confederacy. I am writing now, and benefit from, White settlerhood on the traditional, unceded, and occupied lands of the W̱SÁNEĆ and ləkʷəŋən people.

References

Bearskin, L. B., Kennedy, A., Poitras Kelly, L., & Chakanyuka, C. (2021). *Indigenist nursing: Caring keeps us close to the source.* Springer Publishing Company. http://connect.springerpub.com/content/book/978-0-8261-3603-9/part/part03/chapter/ch16

Bell, B. (2021). Towards abandoning the master's tools: The politics of a universal nursing identity. *Nursing Inquiry, n/a*(e12395), 1–12. 10.1111/nin.12395

Darbyshire, P., & Thompson, D. R. (2021). Can nursing educators learn to trust the world's most trusted profession? *Nursing Inquiry, 28*(2), e12412-n/a. 10.1111/nin.12412

Dei, G. (2016). Decolonizing the university: The challenges and possibilities of inclusive education. *Socialist Studies/Études Socialistes, 11*(1), 23–23. 10.18740/ S4WW31

Dillard-Wright, J. (2021). A radical imagination for nursing: Generative insurrection, creative resistance. *Nursing Philosophy, n/a*(n/a), e12371. 10.1111/nup.12371

Drummond, A. (2020). Embodied indigenous knowledges protecting and privileging Indigenous peoples' ways of knowing, being and doing in undergraduate nursing education. *The Australian Journal of Indigenous Education, 49*(2), 127–134. 10.1017/ jie.2020.16

Keesing-Styles, L. (2003). The relationship between critical pedagogy and assessment in teacher education. *Radical Pedagogy.* https://radicalpedagogy.icaap.org/content/issue5_ 1/03_keesing-styles.html?iframe=truewidth=100%&height=100%

Kumashiro, K. K. (2000). Toward a theory of anti-oppressive education. *Review of Educational Research, 70*(1), 25–53.

Learning Knowledge Centre, & Canadian Electronic Library (Firm). (2008). *Reclaiming the learning spirit: Learning from our experience.* Aboriginal Education Research Centre, University of Saskatatchewan. https://go.exlibris.link/DRVFLckm

McGibbon, E., Mulaudzi, F. M., Didham, P., Barton, S., & Sochan, A. (2014). Toward decolonizing nursing: The colonization of nursing and strategies for increasing the counter-narrative. *Nursing Inquiry, 21*(3), 179–191. 10.1111/nin.12042

Nahanee, T. M. (2021, October 8). *If it costs more money, takes more time and cares for more people, it's decolonial.* https://www.instagram.com/p/CUxM7W8lyg1/

Schinske, J., & Tanner, K. (2014). Teaching more by grading less (or differently). *CBE Life Sciences Education, 13*(2), 159–166. 10.1187/cbe.CBE-14-03-0054

Serrano, M. M., O'Brien, M., Roberts, K., & Whyte, D. (2018). Critical pedagogy and assessment in higher education: The ideal of "authenticity" in learning. *Active Learning in Higher Education, 19*(1), 9–21. 10.1177/1469787417723244

Shahjahan, R. A. (2005). Mapping the field of anti-colonial discourse to understand issues of indigenous knowledges: Decolonizing praxis. *McGill Journal of Education, 40*(2), 213–240.

Smith, K. M. (2019). Facing history for the future of nursing. *Journal of Clinical Nursing.* 10.1111/jocn.15065

Smith, K. M., & Foth, T. (2021). Tomorrow is cancelled: Rethinking nursing resistance as insurrection. *Aporia, 13*(1), 15–25. 10.18192/aporia.v13i1.5263

Smith, L. T. (2013). *Decolonizing methodologies: Research and indigenous peoples.* Zed Books Ltd. St. Denis, V., Canadian Council on Learning, University of Saskatchewan. Aboriginal Education Research Centre, Adult Learning Knowledge Centre, Aboriginal

St. Denis, V., Silver, J., Ireland, B., George, P.N., & Bouvier, R. (2009). *Reclaiming the learning spirit: Learning from our experience.* University of Saskatchewan, Aboriginal Education Research Centre, First Nations and Adult Higher Education Consortium, & Adult Learning Knowledge Centre. https://canadacommons.ca/artifacts/1228409/ reclaiming-the-learning-spirit/1781482/

Tuck, E., & Yang, K. W. (2012). Decolonization is not a metaphor. *Decolonization: Indigeneity, education & Society, 1*(1), Article 1. https://jps.library.utoronto.ca/index. php/des/article/view/18630

University of Victoria. (2016). *Indigenous plan 2017–2022.* https://www.uvic.ca/about-uvic/about-the-university/indigenous-focus/index.php

Valderama-Wallace, C. P., & Apesoa-Varano, E. C. (2019). "Social justice is a dream": Tensions and contradictions in nursing education. *Public Health Nursing, 36*(5), 735–743. 10.1111/phn.12630

Walker, R., Dillard-Wright, J., Rabelais, E., & Valdez, A. M. (2020, December 21). Surveillant #EdTech harms nursing students, the profession, and the public. *Medium.* https://rachelkwalker.medium.com/surveillant-edtech-harms-nursing-students-the-profession-and-the-public-6b225c57a7b3

Wilson, W. A., Wilson, A. C., & Bird, M. Y. (2005). *For Indigenous eyes only: A decolonization handbook.* School for Advanced Research

9 Using Arts-Based Participatory Methods to Teach Cultural Safety

Ruth De Souza (she/her)

I acknowledge that I am writing this on the unceded lands of the Kulin Nations and that Aboriginal and Torres Strait Islander peoples are the oldest continuing cultures on the planet. This land always was and always will be Aboriginal land.

Cultural Safety: Interrogating the Culture of Healthcare

Cultural Safety is both a process and the outcome of excellent care that fore-grounds difference as something to be *regardful* of (Ramsden, n.d.). It reverses the gaze from the othered and different, to instead interrogate the culture of health. Practising in a culturally safe way demands the nurse or health professional to understand themselves as a culture bearer, and of the health system having a culture. It is a deliberate intervention in subverting the so-called neutrality and universalism of a health system that was never designed to accommodate the needs and preferences of First People and other marginalised identities. Birthed through Māori nurses in Aotearoa to counter the assimilatory logics of the legacy colonial health system, it has gained traction in settler colonies and beyond health services to be considered in art (De Souza & Higgins, 2020) and other contexts. While in Aotearoa, New Zealand the scope of Cultural Safety has expanded to also encompass other axes of difference including ethnicity, disability, class, sexuality, and so on. In Australia, it has a particular focus on Aboriginal and Torres Strait Islander peoples. In this chapter, I focus primarily on First Nations and People of Color experiences acknowledging the complexity and limitations of terminology.

Setting the Scene

Whiteness in the Lucky Country

Whiteness is central to nursing practice and education in Australia. Even as it is invisible for "those who do not inhabit it (though not always, and not only)" (Ahmed, 2012, p. 3). In common with other settler colonial nations, Australia was founded on Indigenous genocide and dispossession. One of the first acts of the newly federated Australia of 1901 was to enshrine the White Australia

DOI: 10.4324/9781003245957-13

policy by passing the Immigration Restriction Act of 1902 (Jakubowicz, 2002). Non-Aboriginal Registered Nurses have a long history of caring for Aboriginal people from the early 20th century through missionary work in rural and remote Australia (Forsyth, 2007). Even while seemingly sympathetic to Aboriginal communities they were complicit in racist policies including segregated "native wards," sterilization postpartum without consent, and the removal of Indigenous children from their families, making them an untrustworthy professional group (Forsyth, 2007).

These histories are ever-present, their traces remain and are a reminder that colonisation is not a historical event but a structure that continues to define who can flourish (Kauanui & Wolfe, 2012). Histories of genocide, dispossession, brutality, and attendant racism have made services culturally unsafe for Aboriginal and Torres Strait Islander people who experience significant health disparities compared to non-Indigenous Australians (Australian Institute of Health and Welfare, 2016). Consequently, the lack of Cultural Safety in healthcare is an inter-generational problem, for which health professionals in Australia have received inadequate preparation in their undergraduate education (Delbridge et al., 2021). Universities in Australia thus have a moral imperative to better educate future generations of health professions. Developing appropriate and effective curricular and pedagogical strategies for preparing students for this profound and long-term work is challenging (Browne & Reimer-Kirkham, 2014; Rieger et al., 2016). In particular, preparing nurses to simultaneously address the macro in the form of the political, policy, and structural, while enacting social justice at the point of care with its associated demands and constraints is challenging (Browne & Reimer-Kirkham, 2014).

The White Australia policy was only reversed in 1975, inaugurating a period of multiculturalism, and a shift from its post-war policy of assimilation. However, the 1996 election of John Howard reversed these and many other advances ushering a new social agenda to counter a perceived "political correctness" (Jakubowicz, 2002). Likewise, people from culturally and linguistically diverse (CALD) backgrounds (a term used in Australian context to refer to people born overseas, or with parents who were born overseas or speak languages other than English) (Chauhan et al., 2021) experience significant health inequities and are under-represented in health research and engagement (Woodland et al., 2021). This group is significant as one in four people in Australia (26%) were born overseas, and Australians come from nearly 200 countries, and represent more than 300 ethnic ancestries (Australian Bureau of Statistics, 2017).

Introducing Cultural Safety

The Australian Nursing and Midwifery Accreditation Council (ANMAC) inaugurated Cultural Safety into curricula in 2009. Australia's nursing and midwifery education regulator added the requirement for "Aboriginal and

Torres Strait Islander peoples' history, health and culture and … the principles of Cultural Safety to be included in Australian undergraduate nursing accreditation standards" (ANMAC, 2009, p. 12). Then the Aboriginal and Torres Strait Islander Health Curriculum Framework was developed by the Congress of Aboriginal and Torres Strait Islander Nurses and Midwives (CATSINaM) outlining standards for culturally safe practice in undergraduate nursing and midwifery curriculum (CATSINaM, 2017). In 2018 the Australian Code of Conduct requiring Nurses and Midwives to practice in culturally safe ways with people from Aboriginal and Torres Strait Islander backgrounds was introduced (NMBA, 2018). In Australia, Cultural Safety is mandated in the Code and viewed as central to achieving Indigenous health equity, whereas in Aotearoa, New Zealand Cultural Safety has broadened to encompass other forms of difference that may render a person unsafe. In Australia, Indigenous nurse academics have challenged non-Indigenous nursing academics about their ability to teach Aboriginal and Torres Strait Islander Health and Cultural Safety. The inability to understand and teach Cultural Safety is compounded by a lack of knowledge of Aboriginal culture or history, and Indigenous leadership and an institutional commitment to tackle racism are badly needed (Doran et al., 2018). Doran et al., (2018) argue that this political curriculum must also engage with central concepts such as "decolonisation," "racism," "whiteness/white privilege," and "critical reflection."

Developing a nursing student's understanding of Cultural Safety must be a deliberate, consciousness-developing, transformative experience. It must open students up to the potential of doing things differently. It cannot be left to chance, something that can be acquired as a graduate in clinical practice. Furthermore, if a student is able to experience this powerfully, then they might be capable of recognising it in practice or attempting to recreate it. This capability honed as an undergraduate must be supported by critical thinking, reflective practice, and parrhesia (Perron, 2013) so that it can become a central practice by the time the student graduates.

Nursing Education: Reproducing Coloniality or Transformative?

Universities are both colonial sites and places of transformation (Susana Caxaj & Berman, 2014). The neoliberal university is exemplified by reduced funding, audit culture, competition for research findings, and increased workforce precarity challenging the capacity to do much other than reproduction (Harrowell et al., 2018). Nursing degree programs located in Universities experience all the strictures of the neoliberal University and are implicated in reproducing colonial legacy inequalities in the curriculum factory (Allen, 2006). Nurses internalise and then reproduce the norms and culture of the profession unless interrupted (Bell, 2021). Hence how nurses are socialised into the profession (through the curriculum) has critical implications for how they later practice as graduates (Canales & Drevdahl, 2014). Particularly if nursing is committed to holding open the possibility of transformative practices.

Barriers to a Culturally Safe and Transformative Curriculum

There are barriers to implementing the transformative potential of Cultural Safety. These include conservatism, multiple stakeholder demands, techno-managerialism, surveillance, precarity, conservatism, a lack of skills, and un-examined whiteness.

Utilitarianism at the Expense of Deep Thinking

The expectations of nursing graduates are infinite. Health services want "work ready" graduates (C. Holmes & Lindsay, 2018). There is an emphasis on filling the timetable with content which results in an over-crowded content-focused curriculum (Jenkins et al., 2021). The time pressures of a three-year degree program mean acceleration at the expense of process-driven subject areas requiring slower thinking and immersion. Having a utilitarian curriculum can prevent risk-taking and experimentation, and more damagingly prevent the interrogation of oppressive structures or ways of thinking such as white supremacy, capitalism, and heteronormativity.

Techno Managerialism Leading to Conservatism

Utilitarianism and instrumentalism are compounded by the acceleration in digitisation and datafication in both clinical services and education settings. Students and academics are expected to be digitally and information literate, conversant with digital health technologies including telehealth, electronic health records, wearables, and the like (C. Holmes & Lindsay, 2018). These digital health innovations have been accompanied by the proliferation of educational technologies, which some argue have constrained teaching, creativity, innovation, and autonomy (C. Holmes & Lindsay, 2018). The resulting standardisation and regulation of teaching, learning, and course materials have imposed the micromanagement of managerialism which in turn has bred conformity and compliance.

Apolitical/Depolitical

Instrumentalisation, standardisation, and conservatism have made more political subjects contentious to teach. The purportedly neutral frameworks of biomedicine and liberalism limit the ability of the profession to challenge oppression as they leave intact colonial and racist structures implicated in inequities (Tang Yan et al., 2021). Often, the apolitical language of diversity and inclusion is invoked (De Souza, 2018) preventing deep and challenging engagement with concepts such as race and racism, oppression, power, and privilege (Van Bewer et al., 2021b). Rather than a linear form of awareness raising of difference and invoking "diversity" strategies, the complex work of considering institutional racism is more challenging (Kowal et al., 2013).

Staff precarity in the neoliberal University, make it risky to teach differently, leading to criticisms of nursing curricula being "politically soft" and color blind. However, there have been calls to challenge oppressive norms, and enact social justice and Cultural Safety in nursing, as seen by the challenges to whiteness (Allen, 2006; Bell, 2021; Puzan, 2003; Valderama-Wallace & Apesoa-Varano, 2020) liberalism (Browne, 2001) and colonialism (Browne et al., 2005; Holmes et al., 2008). Consequently, there is a need for "leadership, resources, and institutional support to integrate Cultural Safety" (Bourque, 2020, p. iv).

"Manufactured Blindness" That Allows Faculty to See Themselves as Unmarked and Neutral

White supremacy in nursing needs to be dismantled. Whiteness dominates academic nursing spaces in settler colonial nations (Bell, 2021). It shapes how nurses are socialised, the social and political contexts in which they live and work and their identities as racialised or white. It is evident in the racial hierarchies in nursing leadership and management. Cultural Safety can make white nurse educators accountable for supporting the reproduction of whiteness in health systems by confronting their own positionality, whether race blind or convinced of "reverse racism." Although many groups experience the violence of settler colonialism, many nurse educators can move through life without being conscious of the deleterious effects which are then magnified or replicated within nursing education settings in particular for Indigenous nurse educators and those who are racialised who experience structural violence.

Lack of Training and Reflexivity

Unexamined whiteness and a lack of pedagogical training and capacity to sit with discomfort can prevent "constructive dialogue" when issues arise in class (Van Bewer et al., 2021a). Dialoguing or teaching Cultural Safety as an ally or committed anti-racist can be challenging, requiring working through anxiety, discomfort, uncertainty, guilt, anger, and defensiveness (Smith et al., 2017), particularly when navigating the gap between internalised ideals and internalised racist norms (Kowal et al., 2013). Reflexivity can be a way of preventing the classroom from becoming a site for the reproduction of broader dominant discourses and violences (Van Bewer et al., 2021a). Kowal et al. (2013) propose a dual strategy of "reflexive antiracism" requiring a reflexive stance about one's own and others' responses while attempting to have equanimity in one's own identities and emotions. However, the anxieties of feeling poorly prepared, out of one's depth, incompetent, and out of control (Bell, 2021; Smith et al., 2017; Van Bewer et al., 2021a), can be compounded by institutional challenges. For example, work security might be a concern for staff who might be new to academia, precariously employed, or in a process of tenure review.

Positioning Myself: Teaching Safety While Being Unsafe

Preparing nursing students to interrogate and challenge normative or purportedly neutral systems and structures that reproduce colonial violence, exacts a cost for Indigenous and minoritised scholars who are already under-represented in neo/liberal nursing environments (Van Bewer et al., 2021a). Where racialised staff inhabit institutional spaces without being given residence (Ahmed, 2012, p. 176). The experiences of discrimination and isolation working in schools of nursing which are largely white, Eurocentric environments, can result in stress and ill health (see Bell, 2021). Even if racialised educators are structurally powerful, they can still experience racism from non-racialized students which reflects broader societal hierarchies and power relations resulting in silencing from enduring anti-racist pedagogical resistance (Hassouneh, 2006). In promoting critical, reflexive, engaging methods, rather than traditional didactic instructional strategies, student evaluations and promotions for minority faculty might be compromised. Scholars of color teaching about racism in class may be met with responses ranging from "polite indifference to open hostility" from students (and colleagues). Exhaustion from classroom encounters and poor students' course evaluations may be the result (Smith et al., 2017). Resistance or derision can be directed to the racialised educator unless there is an internal culture committed to doing the uncomfortable work of anti-racism.

Case Studies: Trying to Change Pedagogical Practices

In this section I outline two activities I introduced to a School of Nursing. This involved inviting artist collaborators to create spaces for reflection with staff and students. These interventions were intended to develop collective and relational pedagogical spaces that moved away from individualised forms of learning through content acquisition to more embodied forms of engagement that were collectively experienced. The first activity had two connected aims. The first was to interrogate the culture of the department by making whiteness visible. The second was to gain collegial support by challenging the epistemic biases of nursing and placing Aboriginal culture and expertise in a position of strength through Possum skin bracelet making. In the second activity, which used Theatre of the Oppressed/Forum Theatre, the aim was to move beyond didactic faculty–student teaching to an embodied experience of reflexivity to engage students in practice dilemmas around Cultural Safety.

Activity One: Possum Skin Bracelet Making

The academy fulfils a role in the colonial project to dispossess Indigenous people from their own knowledge production (Mukandi & Bond, 2019, p. 261). In nursing, this is also evident. Ali Drummond (Drummond, 2020) a sovereign Wuthathi and Meriam nurse describes an absence of content or pedagogical approaches reflecting Indigenous ways of knowing, being, and doing. In his experience, this devaluing and erasure was matched by an enforced dissociation from his own Indigenous thought and practice, aligned with the racialised logics of invasion and colonisation of dispossession. Facilitating time for an Aboriginal-led relational space to challenge the epistemic biases of our nursing curriculum during a staff retreat was an attempt to recentre Indigenous ways of knowing, being, and doing.

To that end, I invited the artist Vicki Couzens, a descendant of the Gunditjmara and Kirrae Whurrong clans of western Victoria, to facilitate a workshop for staff, in advance of a new unit on Cultural Safety that I was developing for students. Hassouneh (2006) suggests that having white allies is crucial if the aim is to transform inequities. White or racially privileged educators need to teach or engage in Cultural Safety in order to support the socialising of white students as allies in anti-racism (Hassouneh, 2006 as cited in Bell, 2021). Bringing Vicki in meant that the space was Aboriginal-led, and Aboriginal culture and expertise were put in a position of strength. Vicki has been instrumental in the regeneration of possum skin cloak making in the state of Victoria. Possum skin cloaks had been an important aspect of Aboriginal life prior to colonisation and were used for trade, ritual, ceremony, warmth, and for sleeping and carrying infants. In 2005–2006, Vicki brought local artists, community, and traditional owner groups together to create possum skin cloaks which were worn in the Opening Ceremony of the Commonwealth Games. This led to a renaissance of this cultural practice and the largest gathering of Aboriginal people in cloaks in over 150 years. Since then, Possum skin cloak making has been taken up by other groups in other states.

Moving From Damage to Desire

Non-Indigenous colleagues in the School were invited to paint or burn designs onto possum skin representing their culture. Hence, this activity allowed for a period of reflecting on themselves as culture bearers, a tenet of Cultural Safety (DeSouza, 2008). Making bracelets from possum skin moved away from the anthropological acquisition of Aboriginal cultural knowledge or "damage-centered" inquiry as a way of correcting oppression, to having an Aboriginal organising structure that could invite reflective self-assessment on power, privilege, and biases, and create a foundation to enable the work of anti-racism more broadly in the department. This Aboriginal relational, fun space of making could promote openness and curiosity that in turn might enable critical dialogue and collective analysis. Broadening Cultural Safety as being wider than an individual practice to rather an opportunity to focus on organisational and systemic enablers (Curtis et al., 2019).

The workshop created space for both academic and professional to experience other ways of knowing, and to let go of being cultural experts and instead be individuals in a culture that was not theirs. McLaughlin and Whatman (2007) contend that much work needs to be done to decolonise how Indigenous people are imagined. An arts-based participatory project like this one recentred Aboriginal voices and stories which were formerly displaced by colonisation. In this space, the usual dynamic for staff to learn **about** was shifted into learning **from** (Mukandi & Bond, 2019). This was made more poignant as the site of the workshop was adjacent to Coraanderk, an important site for Aboriginal resistance, justice, land rights, and self-determination (Nanni & James, 2013). A significant place of resilience, activism, and the engagement of non-Indigenous allies (Cruickshank, 2017). It was hoped that through this Indigenous-led, artistic, and participatory process, a space was opened up for staff to both explore their own identities and open them up to other histories (Van Bewer et al., 2021a).

A critique of "damage-centered" research and pedagogy with regard to dispossessed communities is the tendency for dominant discourses of pathology, deficit, defeat, and brokenness to be mobilised without taking into account racism and colonisation (Tuck, 2009). As Tuck explains, citing hooks (hooks, 1990, p. 152) this framing asks that the oppressed "only speak from that space in the margin that is a sign of deprivation, a wound, an unfulfilled longing. Only speak your pain." Instead, the workshop was conceptualised to centre desire, foregrounding complexity, contradiction, and self-determination, not only pain but also hope.

Activity Two: Forum Theatre

Following the staff workshop, I developed and trialed a unit for students in the final year of their three-year Bachelor's degree. The aim of the unit was to provide students with resources to understand their own culture, the culture of healthcare, and the historical and social issues that contribute to differential health outcomes for particular groups in order to discern how to contribute to providing culturally safe care for all Australians. The unit examined how social determinants of health such as class, gender, race, sexual orientation, gender identity; education, economic status, and culture affect health and illness. Students were invited to consider how politics, economics, the social-cultural environment, and other contextual factors impacted Aboriginal and Torres Strait Islander and negatively racialised (known in Australia as Culturally and Linguistically Diverse (CALD)) communities. Students were asked to consider how policy, the planning, organisation, and delivery of health and healthcare shaped health care delivery.

The unit was offered online but a workshop was offered at the start of the semester. I worked with two experienced practitioners Azja Kulpińska and Tania Cañas who were trained in Forum theatre developed by Augusto Boal. Forum theatre is focused on promoting dialogue between actors and audience members and promotes transformation for social justice in the broader world. Here, it differs from traditional theatre which involves monologue. Simulated practices like Forum theatre allow students to address topics from practice within an educational setting, where they can safely develop self-awareness and knowledge to make sense of the difficult personal and professional issues encountered in complex health care environments. This is particularly important when it comes to inter-cultural issues and power relations. Such experiential techniques can help students to gain emotional competence, which in turn assists them to communicate effectively in a range of situations.

For the one-day-long workshop, students were invited to identify a professional situation relating to culture and health that was challenging and involved power relations and cultural differences. They then directed this "scene" and showed the scene with student volunteers to their fellow classmates. They were asked to critically reflect on the event/incident focusing on the concerns they encountered in relation to the care of the person. Through the forum theatre process, their fellow students were invited to offer to intervene in any part of the scene and become a character. Students were asked to consider alternative understandings of the incident, and critically evaluate the implications of these understandings for how more effective nursing care could have been provided.

Through the workshop, it was hoped that students could then review the experience in depth and undertake a process of critical reflection in a follow up written assessment by reconstructing the experience beyond the personal. They were encouraged to examine the historical and social factors that structure a situation and to start to theorise the causes and consequences of their actions. They were encouraged to use references such as research, policy documents, or theory to support their analysis and identify an overarching issue, or key aspect of the experience that affected it profoundly. Concluding with the key learnings through the reflective process, the main factors affecting the situation, and how the incident/event could have been more culturally safe/competent. Students were asked to develop an action plan to map alternative approaches should this or a similar situation arise in the future.

Facilitating Collective Reflection

Forum theatre has been used in nursing and health education to facilitate deeper and more critical reflective thinking, stimulate discussion and exploratory debate among student groups. It is used to facilitate high-quality communication skills, critical reflective practice, emotional intelligence, and empathy and appeals to a range of learning styles. Being able to engage in interactive workshops allows students to engage in complex issues increasing self-awareness using techniques including physical exercises and improvisations (Middlewick et al., 2012).

Furthermore, forum theatre is a way of facilitating collective reflection for students where they can learn from each other. The process allows them to consciously reflect on their roles as actors. Bringing creative mechanisms into the classroom where students can practice critical reflection and interrogate power relations can connect nursing inquiry with the broader sociopolitical context of practice in order to transform it (Thorne, 2017). Helping students to develop power analyses and understand multiple axes of discrimination (intersectionality) can help students transform the health system rather than perpetuating harmful structures (Kagan et al., 2014). Creating spaces where embodied collective reflective practice (Duffy & Powers, 2018) is encouraged allows students to be curious, experiment safely, make mistakes and try new ways of doing things. Didactic approaches impart knowledge and provide students with declarative knowledge but don't always provide the opportunity to practice communication techniques or to explore in depth the attitudes and behaviours that influence their own knowledge.

The Forum theatre process allowed for challenging clinical experiences to be replayed in the classroom and allowed for students to playfully engage and experiment. In the process, they developed a collective repertoire of problem solving that they could take with them into their careers. However, I felt like I failed as the evaluations for the course came through and students were unhappy. This was not just because of the Forum theater process but the remainder of the course was online with lectures and this and the critical reflection were new, potentially transformative, and disruptive territory for students.

Drama and theatre are increasingly being used to create dynamic simulated learning environments where students can try out different communication techniques in a safe setting where there are multiple ways of communicating. A problem-based learning focus allows students to reflect on their own experiences and to arrive at their own solutions, promoting deep learning as students use their own experiences and knowledge to problem solve. An added benefit is that forum theatre provides opportunities for collaborative learning, where students "learn with and from each other" (Boud, 2001).

What Lessons Were Learned?

Reflexivity in research must be matched by reflexivity in pedagogical practices within neoliberal education systems (Harrowell et al., 2018). As I reflect on my attempts to undertake anti-racist work using creative methods as a person of color in academia, I'm reminded of the powerful work of friends Watego and Mukandi who ask what it would "look like were our governing socio-political structures to undergo such democratic transformation that Black people were freed from the imperative to constantly confront whiteness, to positing that transformed state of affairs as an ethical norm?" (Mukandi, 2019).

Teaching into a Headwind

In the academy, people of color are meant to know their place while Indigenous people are not supposed to even be present (Mukandi, 2019). Teaching an always already marginalised subject, using disruptive approaches while a minoritised scholar is like teaching into a headwind (Anderson et al., 2020). I could blame a compressed time frame for production and delivery of the unit within an accelerated work context (Mountz et al., 2015) or the lack of time to build a network of allies. But this is disingenuous. Attempting to "out-teach" the imposition of racialised ideas is impossible (Mukandi & Bond, 2019). Undoing racism is slow, painstaking inter-generational work. However, looking back I am proud of my courage and attempts to create pockets where reparative and healing work could happen even as they were seen as interruptions (Mukandi & Bond, 2019).

Lying to Myself

In the time before the unit began when I was doing preparatory work, I was told by a colleague who was going to teach the unit at a different campus that he considered the concept of Cultural Safety "reverse racism." That this was even uttered should have given me a clue about the resistance and lack of support that lay ahead for me. So, perhaps I was lying to myself (Mukandi & Bond, 2019) in thinking I could undo anything or change the culture of the school as one of only two people of color. The painful learning from this experience was that there needs to be a shared commitment and accountability for developing an anti-racist praxis and transforming whiteness. However, there needs to be courageous decision making, resource allocation, and capacity building within nursing departments to allow this to happen. My experience showed me that these environments are few and far between.

Conclusion

> For a long time, I had been trying to find the way to get beyond the veil – to outperform and outsmart racism. But I have resigned myself to the fact that the academy, as a world in which we are longing for a place, is theirs, not ours
> (Mukandi & Bond, 2019, p. 261).

So how do we make sure that the future of nursing is collectively "ours" when the responsibility for the work of Cultural Safety is unevenly distributed, devalued, and displaced onto those who are fighting with both armory and weapons to survive in whiteness? Those who are struggling with the work of fitting in or disappearing, who are tasked with being there without really being there? (Mukandi & Bond, 2019). High-quality academic work including teaching is slow work, time is needed to try things, to engage and innovate, to facilitate curiosity and creativity in students (Mountz et al., 2015). None of which can happen effectively in accelerated and precarious work contexts. If we want to deliberately teach students to not only be capable and competent but to fight for equity, anti-racism, and social justice, we must make time to challenge or experiment, otherwise we risk reproducing a depoliticised "what's already there" future workforce, fixated on the useful, the commodified and utilitarian. A workforce that reproduces structural violence, joining generations who have done much the same. As Cultural Safety becomes tamed and domesticated, into University curricula, we must ensure it does not lose its critical edge. I am unconvinced that we can shift whiteness in nursing. But maybe, just maybe by making this contribution, "being part of a collection [in this book] can be to become a collective"(Ahmed, 2012, p. 13). This is my hope.

References

Ahmed, S. (2012). *On being included: Racism and diversity in institutional life*. Durham, NC: Duke University Press.

Allen, D. G. (2006). Whiteness and difference in nursing. *Nursing Philosophy: An International Journal for Healthcare Professionals, 7*(2), 65–78. 10.1111/j.1466-769X.2006.00255.x

Anderson, L., Gatwiri, K., & Townsend-Cross, M. (2020). Battling the "headwinds": The experiences of minoritised academics in the neoliberal Australian university. *International Journal of Qualitative Studies in Education: QSE, 33*(9), 939–953. 10.1080/09518398.2019.1693068

Australian Institute of Health and Welfare. (2016). Australia's health 2016. Australia's Health Series No. 15. Cat. No. AUS 199.

Australian Bureau of Statistics. (2017). Australian demographic statistics, Mar 2017. Cat No. 3101.0. Canberra: ABS.

Australian Nursing and Midwifery Accreditation Council (ANMAC). (2009). Registered nurses standards and criteria for the accreditation of nursing and midwifery courses leading to registration, enrolment, endorsement and authorisation in Australia – with evidence guide, Canberra, Australia.

Bell, B. (2021). White dominance in nursing education: A target for anti-racist efforts. *Nursing Inquiry, 28*(1), e12379. 10.1111/nin.12379

Boud, D. 2001. Introduction: Making the move to peer learning. In D. Boud, R. Cohen, & J. Sampson (Eds.), *Peer Learning in Higher Education: Learning from and with each other* (pp. 1–17). London, UK: Kogan Page.

Bourque, D. (2020). *The integration of Cultural Safety in nursing education: An Indigenous inquiry of nurse educator experiences* [Masters thesis, McMaster University]. https://macsphere.mcmaster.ca/bitstream/11375/25238/2/Bourque_Danielle_Finalsubmission2020January_Degree.pdf

Browne (2001). The influence of liberal political ideology on nursing science. *Nursing Inquiry, 8*(2), 118–129.

Browne, A. J., & Reimer-Kirkham, S. (2014). Problematizing social justice discourses in nursing. In *Philosophies and Practices of Emancipatory Nursing* (pp. 21–38). Routledge. 10.4324/9780203069097-2

Browne, A. J., Smye, V. L., & Varcoe, C. (2005). The relevance of postcolonial theoretical perspectives to research in Aboriginal health. *The Canadian Journal of Nursing Research = Revue Canadienne de Recherche En Sciences Infirmieres, 37*(4), 16–37.

Canales, M. K., & Drevdahl, D. J. (2014). Social justice: From educational mandate to transformative core value. In P. N. Kagan, M. C. Smith, & P. L. Chinn (Eds.), *Philosophies and Practices of Emancipatory Nursing* (pp. 153–174). Routledge. 10.4324/9780203069097-12

Caxaj, S. C., & Berman, H. (2014). Anti-colonial pedagogy and praxis: Unraveling dilemmas and dichotomies. In P.N. Kagan, M.C. Smith, & P.L. Chinn (Eds.), *Philosophies and practices of emancipatory nursing* (pp. 175–187). Routledge. 10.4324/ 9780203069097-13

Chauhan, A., Walpola, R. L., Manias, E., Seale, H., Walton, M., Wilson, C., Smith, A. B., Li, J., & Harrison, R. (2021). How do health services engage culturally and linguistically diverse consumers? An analysis of consumer engagement frameworks in Australia. *Health Expectations: An International Journal of Public Participation in Health Care and Health Policy*, 24(5), 1747–1762. 10.1111/hex.13315

Congress of Aboriginal and Torres Strait Islander Nurses and Midwives. (2017). The Nursing and Midwifery Aboriginal and Torres Strait Islander health curriculum-framework: An adaption of and complementary document to the Aboriginal and Torres Strait Islander health curriculum framework Canberra. Retrieved January 30, 2022. https://www.catsinam.org.au/static/uploads/files/nursing-midwifery-health-curriculum-framework-final-version-1-0-wfffegyedblq.pdf

Cruickshank, J. (2017). Bringing history to life: Coranderrk as history, performance and curriculum resources. *Agora*, 52(3), 45–49. 10.3316/ielapa.069624171627356

Curtis, E., Jones, R., Tipene-Leach, D., Walker, C., Loring, B., Paine, S.-J., & Reid, P. (2019). Why Cultural Safety rather than cultural competency is required to achieve health equity: A literature review and recommended definition. *International Journal for Equity in Health*, 18(1), 174. 10.1186/s12939-019-1082-3

Delbridge, R., Garvey, L., Mackelprang, J. L., Cassar, N., Ward-Pahl, E., Egan, M., & Williams, A. (2021). Working at a cultural interface: Co-creating Aboriginal health curriculum for health professions. *Higher Education Research & Development*, 41(5), 1–16. 10.1080/07294360.2021.1927999

DeSouza, R. (2008). Wellness for all: The possibilities of Cultural Safety and cultural competence in New Zealand. *Journal of Research in Nursing: JRN*, 13(2), 125–135. 10.1177/1744987108088637

De Souza, R. (2018, December 4). *Is it enough? Why we need more than diversity in nursing – Australian College of Nursing*. Australian College of Nursing. https:// www.acn.edu.au/publications/the-hive-2018/is-it-enough-why-we-need-more-than-diversity-in-nursing

DeSouza, R., & Higgins, R. (2020). Cultural safety: An overview. In J. Lillie, K. Larsen, C. Kirkwood, & J.J. Brown (Eds.), *The relationship is the project: Working with communities*. (pp. 81–88). Australia: Brow Books.

Doran, F., Wrigley, B., & Others (2018). Cultural Safety and Implications for building staff capacity: Snapshot of Findings from a study with nurse academics. *Australian Nursing and Midwifery Journal*, 25(9), 22.

Drummond, A. (2020). Embodied Indigenous knowledges protecting and privileging Indigenous peoples' ways of knowing, being and doing in undergraduate nursing education. *The Australian Journal of Indigenous Education*, 49(2), 127–134. 10.1017/ jie.2020.16

Drummond, A., & Cox, L. (2016). Indigenous history, health, wellness and culture within nursing curriculum. *Australian Nursing & Midwifery Journal*, 23(8), 35.

Duffy, P., & Powers, B. (2018). Blind to what's in front of them: Theatre of the Oppressed and teacher reflexive practice, embodying culturally relevant pedagogy with pre-service teachers. *Youth Theatre Journal*, 32(1), 45–59. 10.1080/08929092. 2018.1445677

Forsyth, S. (2007). Telling stories: Nurses, politics and Aboriginal Australians, circa 1900–1980s. *Contemporary Nurse, 24*(1), 33–44. 10.5172/conu.2007.24.1.33

Harrowell, E., Davies, T., & Disney, T. (2018). Making space for failure in geographic research. *The Professional Geographer: The Journal of the Association of American Geographers, 70*(2), 230–238. 10.1080/00330124.2017.1347799

Hassouneh, D. (2006). Anti-Racist pedagogy: Challenges faced by faculty of color in predominantly white schools of nursing. *Journal of Nursing Education; Thorofare, 45*(7), 255–262.

Holmes, C., & Lindsay, D. (2018). "Do you want fries with that?": The McDonaldization of University education—Some critical reflections on nursing higher education. *SAGE Open, 8*(3), 2158244018787229. 10.1177/2158244018787229

Holmes, D., Roy, B., & Perron, A. (2008). The use of postcolonialism in the nursing domain: Colonial patronage, conversion, and resistance. *ANS. Advances in Nursing Science, 31*(1), 42–51. 10.1097/01.ANS.0000311528.73564.83

hooks, b. (1990). *Yearning.* Boston: South End Press.

Jakubowicz, A. (2002). White noise: Australia's struggle with multiculturalism. In C. Levine-Rasky (Ed.) *Working through Whiteness: International perspectives* (pp. 107–112). New York: State University of New York Press.

Jenkins, K., Kinsella, E. A., & DeLuca, S. (2021). Being and becoming a nurse: Toward an ontological and reflexive turn in first-year nursing education. *Nursing Inquiry, 28*(4), e12420. 10.1111/nin.12420

Kagan, P. N., Smith, M. C., & Chinn, P. L. (2014). *Philosophies and practices of emancipatory nursing: Social justice as praxis.* Routledge. https://market.android.com/details?id=book-OWMKBAAAQBAJ

Kauanui, J. K., & Wolfe, P. (2012). Settler colonialism then and now. A conversation between. *Politica & Società, 1*(2), 235–258. https://www.rivisteweb.it/doi/10.4476/37055

Kowal, E., Franklin, H., & Paradies, Y. (2013). Reflexive antiracism: A novel approach to diversity training. *Ethnicities, 13*(3), 316–337. 10.1177/1468796812472885.

McLaughlin, J. M., & Whatman, S. L. (2007). Embedding Indigenous perspectives in University teaching and learning: Lessons learnt and possibilities of reforming/decolonizing curriculum. In Proceedings *4th International Conference on Indigenous Education.* Vancouver, Canada: Asia/Pacific.

Middlewick, Y., Kettle, T. J., & Wilson, J. J. (2012). Curtains up! Using forum theatre to rehearse the art of communication in healthcare education. *Nurse Education in Practice, 12*(3), 139–142. 10.1016/j.nepr.2011.10.010

Mountz, A., Bonds, A., Mansfield, B., Loyd, J., Hyndman, J., Walton-Roberts, M., Basu, R., Whitson, R., Hawkins, R., Hamilton, T., & Others. (2015). For slow scholarship: A feminist politics of resistance through collective action in the neoliberal university. *ACME: An International E-Journal for Critical Geographies, 14*(4), 1235–1259. https://acme-journal.org/index.php/acme/article/download/1058/1141/0

Mukandi, B. (2019). Beyond Hermes: Metaphysics in a new key. *Utafiti, 14*(1), 145–161. 10.1163/26836408-14010008

Mukandi, B., & Bond, C. (2019). "good in the hood" or "burn it down"? Reconciling black presence in the academy. *Journal of Intercultural Studies, 40*(2), 254–268. 10.1080/07256868.2019.1577232

Nanni, G., & James, A. (2013). *Coranderrk: We will show the Country.* Canberra: Aboriginal Studies Press.

Nursing and Midwifery Board of Australia. (2018). Code of conduct for nurses. Retrieved January 30, 2022. https://www.nursingmidwiferyboard.gov.au/codes-guidelines-statements/professional-standards.aspx

Perron, A. (2013). Nursing as "disobedient" practice: Care of the nurse's self, parrhesia, and the dismantling of a baseless paradox. *Nursing Philosophy: An International Journal for Healthcare Professionals, 14*(3), 154–167. 10.1111/nup.12015

Puzan, E. (2003). The unbearable whiteness of being (in nursing). *Nursing Inquiry, 10*(3), 193–200. 10.1046/j.1440-1800.2003.00180.x

Ramsden, I. M. (n.d.). *Cultural Safety and Nursing Education in Aotearoa and Te Waipounamu.* https://www.croakey.org/wp-content/uploads/2017/08/RAMSDEN-I-Cultural-Safety_Full.pdf

Rieger, K. L., Chernomas, W. M., McMillan, D. E., Morin, F. L., & Demczuk, L. (2016). Effectiveness and experience of arts-based pedagogy among undergraduate nursing students: A mixed methods systematic review. *JBI Database of Systematic Reviews and Implementation Reports, 14*(11), 139–239. 10.11124/JBISRIR-2016-003188

Smith, L., Kashubeck-West, S., Payton, G., & Adams, E. (2017). White professors teaching about racism: Challenges and rewards. *The Counseling Psychologist, 45*(5), 651–668. 10.1177/0011000017717705

Tang Yan, C., Orlandimeje, R., Drucker, R., & Lang, (2021). Unsettling reflexivity and critical race pedagogy in social work education: Narratives from social work students. *Social Work in Education,* 1–24. 10.1080/02615479.2021.1924665

Thorne, S. (2017). Isn't it high time we talked openly about racism? *Nursing Inquiry, 24*(4). 10.1111/nin.12219

Tuck, E. (2009). Suspending damage: A letter to communities. *Harvard Educational Review, 79*(3), 409–427. 10.17763/haer.79.3.n0016675661t3n15

Valderama-Wallace, C. P., & Apesoa-Varano, E. C. (2020). "The Problem of the Color Line": Faculty approaches to teaching Social Justice in Baccalaureate Nursing Programs. *Nursing Inquiry, 27*(3), e12349. 10.1111/nin.12349

Van Bewer, V., Woodgate, R. L., Martin, D., & Deer, F. (2021a). An Indigenous and arts-influenced framework for anti-racist practice in nursing education. *Journal of Professional Nursing: Official Journal of the American Association of Colleges of Nursing, 37*(1), 65–72. 10.1016/j.profnurs.2020.11.002

Van Bewer, V., Woodgate, R. L., Martin, D., & Deer, F. (2021b). Exploring theatre of the oppressed and forum theatre as pedagogies in nursing education. *Nurse Education Today, 103,* 104940. 10.1016/j.nedt.2021.104940

Woodland, L., Blignault, I., O'Callaghan, C., & Harris-Roxas, B. (2021). A framework for preferred practices in conducting culturally competent health research in a multicultural society. *Health Research Policy and Systems / BioMed Central, 19*(1), 24. 10.1186/s12961-020-00657-y

10a Artificial Intelligence for Health and Care Is Not Inevitable: Introduction and Critical Vocabulary

Rae Walker

I can't remember the very first time I heard the term *artificial intelligence* (AI) but I think it was during middle school, perhaps from a battered copy of one of Isaac Asimov's futuristic novels I'd picked up at my town library's annual used book sale. In a 1942 short story titled *Runaround*, Asimov introduced what are now known as the "Three Laws of Robotics:"

> First Law: A robot may not injure a human being or, through inaction, allow a human being to come to harm.
>
> Second Law: A robot must obey the orders given it by human beings except where such orders would conflict with the First Law.
>
> Third Law: A robot must protect its own existence as long as such protection does not conflict with the First or Second Laws.

Though fictional in origin, principles undergirding Asimov's laws are now foundational to contemporary understandings of AI *ethics* (Salge, 2017). At the time, I didn't understand how AI worked, other than that it involved computers and some type of advanced robotics yet to be discovered. Whatever it was, it seemed mysterious, far off and futuristic: an alien technology more likely to be found on the set of the sci-fi series *Star Trek: The Next Generation* than in my living room or car. Fast-forward a few decades and now it seems like AI is everywhere, including within health systems.

Artificial intelligence is an intentionally fluid concept that evolves to contain the aims of whatever powers deploy it (Katz, 2020). McGrow defines AI as "the theory and development of computer systems able to complete tasks that typically require human intelligence, such as visual perception, speech recognition, decision-making, and/or language translation" (McGrow, 2019, p. 48). Table 10a.1 Glossary of Common Terms in Artificial Intelligence outlines just a few of the myriad concepts commonly associated with AI, from natural language processing to computer vision.

My professional introduction to AI didn't come until decades after I first stumbled across the writings of Asimov. I am a housed employed fat white

DOI: 10.4324/9781003245957-14

Table 10a.1 Glossary of Common Terms in Artificial Intelligence

Term	Definition
Algorithm	A process or set of rules designed to be followed when making calculations or problem-solving.
Big Data	A collection of data considered so large in volume and complexity that traditional data management tools cannot store or analyze it effectively.
Machine Learning-ready Dataset	Data organized and stored in such a way that it can readily be analyzed by machine learning algorithms.
Machine Learning	A branch of computer science intended to imitate how humans learn, through the application of statistical applications or algorithms to big data.
Natural Language Processing	A branch of computer science and AI focused on computers analyzing and responding to text and spoken words.
Computer Vision	A field of AI originally developed for military purposes and focused on enabling computers to analyze, categorize or interpret visual inputs such as digital images or videos.
Facial Recognition	Surveillant and easily weaponized technologies that deploy computer vision with the aim of correctly identifying and labeling human faces from visual inputs such as photographs and video.
Supervised Learning	Involves "teaching" a model (a set of algorithms) by feeding it labeled data. Labeled data are input data paired with their "correct" outputs, as determined by whatever humans previously labeled the data (a process rife with possibilities for error and bias).
Unsupervised Learning	Involves teaching a model to look for patterns in a dataset that has no labels, with minimal human supervision. Humans do not tell the model what it must "learn," allowing it to detect patterns and propose conclusions from unlabeled data. Lack of supervision contributes to potential the model may detect harmful patterns and amplify violent conclusions, as seen in 2016 with Microsoft's racist chatbot "Tay."

queer trans-non-disabled tenured academic settler nurse inventor working through a global pandemic on lands that were stolen from the Nipmuc Nation, many of whose members are still here. These positionalities mean I possess tremendous unearned power and privilege. And as a queer, trans, and non-binary person I also regularly witness ways in which my identities, body, and perspectives do not "fit" certain societal norms, institutions, architectures, and dominant data models—experiences that inform both my scholarship and activism. I rely on relationships with a number of accountability partners from whom I continue to learn and unlearn. Some I live near and see on a regular basis—though given the highly siloed and segregated nature of academe and society, I originally connected with many of them through digital platforms like Twitter. I currently use they/them pronouns in most professional and social settings, and my school-aged kids call me "mom." In the fall of 2015, I was a brand new assistant professor asked to help write a grant to sponsor the creation of a new interdisciplinary center that would combine nursing knowledge of symptom science with technologies developed by disciplines such as engineering and computer science to improve the health and well-being of persons managing chronic conditions. I was working on multiple studies addressing chronic fatigue at the time, one of many invisible symptoms notoriously ignored and under-treated in contemporary health care settings— a phenomenon we dubbed *medical gaslighting*, though we were likely not the first (Gance-Cleveland et al., 2020).

As we deliberated about the research questions we might answer in this grant proposal, a colleague from computer science, Deepak Ganesan, approached me with a new technology from his lab called iShadow. The iShadow was a set of computational eyeglasses invented by one of his doctoral students, Addison Mayberry. He wondered if his technology, an eye-tracker capable of continuously recording and characterizing rapid and minute movements of the eye, might be useful to our research. We hypothesized perhaps this sensor could quantitatively characterize changes in eye function associated with increased fatigue, putting empirical data and an actual number to a phenomenon otherwise imperceptible to anyone other than, perhaps, the fatigued individual. Early prototypes involved a plastic 3D-printed glasses frame, hooked up to a small circuit board glued to the side and small outward and inward-facing cameras, as presented by Dr. Mayberry at the 21st Annual International Conference on Mobile Computing and Networking in 2015, and shown in Figure 10a.1 Early prototype of iShadow computational eyeglasses (Mayberry et al., 2016).

At the time, the National Institute of Nursing Research (NINR) was actively encouraging nurse scientists to focus on developing *digital health* through use of "technologies that passively monitor biology, behavior, and context of use" like wearable sensors (NINR, n.d.). The innovation of this particular

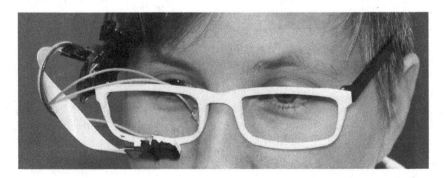

Figure 10a.1 Early Prototype of iShadow Computational Eyeglasses.

eyetracker was in its use of *machine learning*, a form of AI, to calculate the directionality of the wearer's gaze using less information, and more specifically, *fewer camera pixels*, than a typical research-grade eyetracker would require. It relied on a form of *computer vision* not unlike that used by *facial recognition software*. Reduced data burden meant increased energy efficiency requiring less battery power. Inventors of the iShadow hoped the eyetracker would eventually power itself entirely through wireless signals instead of relying on a bulky external battery pack (Mayberry et al., 2014). Freed of an external battery pack, this innovation would allow future generations of the glasses to render the small cameras and other hardware essentially invisible, allowing the user to appear like they were just wearing eyeglasses, rather than a high-tech surveillance apparatus.

In order to pitch this innovation to funders at the NIH, I had to teach myself about *machine learning* (ML)—or at very least, basic concepts underlying this area of computer science. I never learned about ML in nursing school, nor in any of the myriad graduate statistics courses I'd taken. I pulled research papers and read what I could online to catch up with the science. When it came to the actual grant submission, no one inquired about the ethical implications of this new surveillant tech beyond standard IRB compliance. We got the NIH center grant on our first try. Like so many other clinicians, researchers, and technologists associated with powerful institutions with federal funding, I was handed fire before I even knew what I was holding, or how to use it. And now that fire is everywhere.

AI is a powerful and transformative set of technologies (McGrow, 2019). These technologies may have the capacity to bring light to new and generative possibilities for the future of health and care. And like fire, AI can scale and burn, causing harm and destruction in ways that may be unpredictable and beyond its creators' control. While federal funders, industry groups, and professional conferences tout AI as imperative for the future of health and care (Ahuja, 2019; Cato et al., 2020), contemporary examples abound of harmful AI tech that amplifies coded bias within electronic health records (Obermeyer et al., 2019), fails to function properly on bodies that don't conform to the narrow norms of whiteness and cisheteropatriarchy (Benjamin, 2019), and punishes immigrants, Indigenous communities, and the poor (Eubanks, 2017). Such hard coding has already been skillfully demonstrated by scholars such as Safiya Noble, whose book *Algorithms of Oppression: How Search Engines Reinforce Racism* examines ways in which popular search algorithms like Google systematically reproduce data discrimination against people of color and especially, Black women (Noble, 2019). Mathematician Cathy O'Neil's *Weapons of Math Destruction: How Big Data Increases Inequality and Threatens Democracy* provides a similar critique, particularly, how mathematical models driving AI like search engines remain unregulated and uncontestable, by design, even when they're demonstrably causing harm (O'Neil, 2016). Many of the algorithms that animate AI in health care are proprietary and therefore black-boxed, making them hard to

spot-in-action and even more difficult to evaluate. This is particularly pernicious in praxes like nursing and medicine that often (and uncritically) rely
on such technologies in a compulsory fashion, like sensors and clinical
decision-making prompts embedded in electronic health records (Dillard-
Wright, 2019).

AI technologies and the datasets that drive them are products of human
choices and power arrangements that have real and lasting implications for
human and planetary health (Crawford, 2021). Scholars who've made it their
career's work to study the operation of these innovations, like Ruha Benjamin,
argue no technology is politically neutral as all design is, at its heart, a colonizing enterprise (Benjamin, 2019). Accepting this as true, we must conclude
that no AI, no matter how well-designed or deployed, is completely free of risk
for harm and abuse. The question for nurses and other healers is not, "How do
we design technology for good?" but rather, "What are the conditions that
need to be created for any technology we create to support health, healing, and
collective liberation?" This question informs the second part of this essay
titled Artificial Intelligence for Health and Care Is Not Inevitable: Part II
Ten Commitments to New Futures where I challenge dominant narratives of
AI as an imperative for health and care, and outline ten commitments to
more just and equitable futures. The following critical vocabulary provides an
introduction and foundations for that discussion.

Matrix of Domination

AI, like all technologies, exists, operates, and is produced under the matrix of
domination. The *matrix of domination* is a paradigm developed by sociologist
Patricia Hill Collins to describe the overall social organization within which
intersecting oppressions originate, develop, and are contained (Hill Collins,
1990). Hill Collins originally published these ideas in her landmark book, *Black
Feminist Thought: Knowledge, Consciousness, and the Politics of Empowerment*.
There are four levels of power within the matrix: structural, disciplinary, hegemonic, and interpersonal. At each level, intersecting oppressions (e.g.,
whiteness, settler colonialism, capitalism, cisheteropatriarchy) operate to
maintain a violent and unjust status quo wherein systems operate precisely as
designed: to maintain the power and unearned advantages of dominating groups
at the expense of all others.

Technochauvinism

Introduction of new technology is often treated synonymously with the concept
of "innovation" for positive change in the realm of health and care. The underlying assumption for this association is that new technology translates to
better outcomes. Computer scientist and journalism professor Meredith
Broussard coined a term for this logic: *technochauvinism* (Broussard, 2018).
"Technochauvinism is the assumption that computers are superior to people, or

that a technological solution is superior to any other" (Broussard, 2019). Such logic has also been identified as a common characteristic of institutionalized cultures of white supremacy that many of us existing within them have been socialized to accept as normal, even though such belief systems propagate violence and a sense of disconnection (Okun, 2021). In her book, *Race After Technology: Abolitionist Tools for the New Jim Code*, sociologist Ruha Benjamin names *technological benevolence* as similarly problematic (Benjamin, 2019). She provides example upon example of technological "fixes," pitched by well-intentioned people, that work to reinforce and extend racism and related structures of oppression Benjamin has dubbed, "New Jim Code Systems," a sort of 21st century white saviorism (Yerian, 2020).

Algorithmic Exceptionalism

Since its inception, AI has been associated with technological advancement, complexity, and more objective, data-driven decision-making (Katz, 2020). This expectation is reflected in common classification systems for AI in health care, outlined in Table 10a.2. Examples of AI for Health Care Classifications that can

Table 10a.2 Examples of AI for Health Care Classifications

Classification Systems	Categories and Definitions
Technology-Dependence Model Locsin, 2017	• **Completer:** A.I. technology as completer of human beings • **Tool:** A.I. technology as instruments and gadgets that facilitate human caring of persons • **Mimic:** A.I. that "mimics" human beings
Big Data Analytics McGrow, 2019	• **Clinical Analytics:** Focus on improving medical treatment insights and outcomes • **Operational Analytics:** Focus on improving systems efficiency and effectiveness, defined by some as medical claims fraud identification and revenue enhancement • **Behavioral Analytics:** Focus on examining "consumer behavior patterns" that inform healthcare delivery
AI as a 3-Dimensional Space Zheng, 2017	AI as 3 Dimensions: • **Strength:** the "intelligence level" of AI systems • **Extension:** scope of problems that can be solved • **Capacity:** the average solution quality
Netnographic taxonomy of A.I. for health care in media Erikkson and Saltzmann	Media depictions of AI in health care reflect it as: • **Droids:** Simple, box-like helpers • **Exoskeletons:** Designed to "strengthen weakness," either physical or cognitive, such as memory • **Humanoids:** Robots mimicking human behaviors that appear to have greater autonomy and "intelligence"

found at the end of this essay. The notion of *algorithmic exceptionalism*, a sort of magic, pervades discourse on AI, lending these technologies the air of superlative and mysterious power that transcends the capacities of mere mortals (Crawford, 2021). Gabriel Krieshok explains, "AI has a black box problem where we can't peer into the decision-making logic of the algorithm—and so how do we interpret the findings? Magical. Well, not magical *per se*, but we still tend to give the algorithm the benefit of the doubt, and it's almost as if the black box nature of the systems lend them even *more* credibility in the eyes of the lay person reading the interpretation" (Krieshok, 2020). Disturbingly, scientists from Harvard University and UC-Berkeley have already demonstrated this bias towards algorithmic judgment, called *algorithmic appreciation*, in a series of controlled experiments (Logg et al., 2019). Their research indicated humans, and especially lay persons, were more likely to rely on a judgment to make an important decision if they thought the information informing that decision came from a computer, as opposed to a human.

Abolition

Origins of AI are rooted in settler colonialism, militarism, and dominating aims of empire (Crawford, 2021; Katz, 2020). We cannot expect to disrupt such violent systems by relying on the same structures that brought us to our present moment. Creating new futures for health and care in an AI era will require *abolition* (Benjamin, 2019). Abolition is a mindset and a movement rooted in transformative justice. It is not a homogenous or hierarchical movement, but the work of many hands over generations. Foundations of abolition were built by Black and Indigenous organizers and activists, especially Black women and queer and trans people of color, laboring in varied and diverse contexts with equally varied and diverse strategy and tactics (Rothman, 2016). Abolition is not just about the destruction or dismantling of profoundly unjust systems, such as racist, ableist, and transmisic surveillance regimes and technologies like credit scores, facial recognition technologies, or predictive policing algorithms that punish, coerce, incarcerate and exterminate individuals and communities at the margins (Eubanks, 2017; Hamid, 2020). Abolition is also about creating the conditions to support human flourishing, without relying on carcerality, structural forms of oppression, or the violent systems that increase it (Kaba, 2021).

In her 2021 collection of essays, *We Do This 'Til We Free Us: Abolitionist Organizing and Transforming Justice*, organizer Mariame Kaba describes abolition as "a vision of a restructured society in a world where we have everything we need: food, shelter, education, health, art, beauty, clean water, and more things that are foundational to our personal and community safety" (2021, p. 2). Her essay, "So you're thinking about becoming an abolitionist," provides several suggestions for adopting an abolitionist mindset: First, that transforming society involves transforming ourselves, including unlearning internalized and interlocking logics of oppression such as white supremacy, misogyny, ableism, classism, homophobia, transphobia and racial capitalism; Second, that we must imagine and experiment with new collective structures that enable us to take more principled action, such as collective responsibility for resolving conflicts (she points to the successes of Brazil's Landless Workers Movement, which has sought to create governance structures that are less hierarchical and more transparent); Third, that we must simultaneously engage in strategies designed to reduce contact between people and the systems that harm them, such as the criminal legal system, from which we must divest; And fourth, that changing one aspect of this world, such as how we address harm, involves changing everything, as all oppressions are interconnected. Rather than beginning from the standpoint of "What do we have now and how can we make it better?," Kaba encourages us to ask, more expansively, "What can we imagine for ourselves and the world?" and to work, collectively, towards that vision (Kaba, 2021).

Communities of Practice

In the absence of obvious and accessible resources and clinical practices designed to disrupt and reimagine AI for health and care, nurses must build their own. This will require fostering new communities of practice around our shared commitments to new and different health and care in the age of AI wherein practitioners hold themselves and each other accountable. A *community of practice* can be defined by three shared characteristics: (a) common domain of interest; (b) persons who engage and communicate with each other; and (c) regular practice working with each other to identify and overcome challenges, learn together, and build specific skills (Wenger, 1998). Through *engagement*, the group fosters sustained intensity and *elations of mutuality* through group activities, community-building conversations, and the co-creation of meaningful artifacts (Wenger, 1998, p. 84). "*Imagination* is the act of thinking what could be and using this alternative vision to excite the members of the community" (Campbell & Lavallee, 2020, p. 413). When diverse perspectives are brought together, the group moves toward a unified purpose or *alignment*. Once formed, the community of practice shares a common repertoire of skills and a shared vocabulary that can be used as a foundation to welcome new members and sustain ongoing practice.

Numerous experts working with communities disproportionately harmed by historical and current forms of AI and big data have argued that unless the innovation ecosystems are profoundly disrupted and power redistributed within these systems, these technologies will only serve to reinforce and deepen existing forms of injustice (Benjamin, 2019; Crawford, 2021; Fischer, 2019; O'Neil, 2016; Zuckerman, 2021). Those of us in the clinical professions and academe are increasingly incentivized, if not compelled, by funders, professional organizations, industry, academic institutions, and our governments to engage, design, evaluate, deploy and exist within these data regimes and technologies (National Academies of Science, Engineering, and Medicine, 2021). In a health care landscape increasingly colonized by AI and big data, what are our commitments to each other and to new and more liberatory futures—as healers, and as human beings? In the next chapter, I outline ten commitments I consider fundamental for the co-creation of new and more liberatory futures. I offer these thoughts with humility— mindful I do not (cannot) speak *for* anyone but myself—reflexive about the hard-fought foundations laid by many generations of healers, scholars, organizers, artists, and activists upon which these ideas build—and with every expectation that they will continue to grow and evolve.

References

Ahuja, A. S. (2019). The impact of artificial intelligence in medicine on the future role of the physician. *PeerJ, 7*, e7702. 10.7717/peerj.7702

Benjamin, R. (2019). *Race after technology: Abolitionist tools for the new jim code.* Polity.

Broussard, M. (2018). *Artificial unintelligence: How computers misunderstand the world.* MIT Press.

Broussard, M. (2019, June 17). Letting go of technochauvinism. *Public Books.* https://www.publicbooks.org/letting-go-of-technochauvinism/

Campbell, A. C., & Lavallee, C. A. (2020). A community of practice for social justice: Examining the case of an international scholarship alumni association in Ghana. *Journal of Studies in International Education, 24*(4), 409–423. 10.1177/102831531 9842343

Cato, K. D., McGrow, K., & Rossetti, S. C. (2020). Transforming clinical data into wisdom: Artificial intelligence implications for nurse leaders. *Nursing Management, 51*(11), 24–30. 10.1097/01.NUMA.0000719396.83518.d6

Crawford, K. (2021). *Atlas of AI.* Yale University Press.

Dillard-Wright, J. (2019). Electronic health record as a panopticon: A disciplinary apparatus in nursing practice. *Nursing Philosophy, 20*(2), e12239. 10.1111/nup.12239

Eriksson, H., & Salzmann-Erikson, M. (2017). The digital generation and nursing robotics: A netnographic study about nursing care robots posted on social media. *Nursing Inquiry, 24*(2), e12165. 10.1111/nin.12165

Eubanks, V. (2017). *Automating inequality: How high-tech tools profile, police, and punish the poor.* St. Martin's Press.

Fischer, M. (2019). *Terrorizing gender: Transgender visibility and the surveillance practices of the U.S. security state.* University of Nebraska Press.

Gance-Cleveland, B., McDonald, C. C., & Walker, R. K. (2020). Use of theory to guide development and application of sensor technologies in Nursing. *Nursing Outlook, 68*(6), 698–710. 10.1016/j.outlook.2020.04.007

Hamid, S. T. (2020, August 21). *Community defense: Sarah T. Hamid on abolishing carceral technologies.* Logic Magazine. https://logicmag.io/care/community-defense-sarah-t-hamid-on-abolishing-carceral-technologies/

Hill Collins, P. (1990). *Black feminist thought: Knowledge, consciousness, and the politics of empowerment.* Hyman. https://www.amazon.com/Black-Feminist-Thought-Consciousness-Empowerment/dp/0415964725

Kaba, M. (2021). *We do this 'til we free us: Abolitionist organizing and transforming justice.* Haymarket Books.

Katz, Y. (2020). *Artificial whiteness: Politics and ideology in artificial intelligence.* Columbia University Press.

Krieshok, G. (2020, September 14). *Magical thinking of AI.* Gabriel Krieshok. https://gabrielkrieshok.com/blog/magical-thinking-of-ai/

Locsin, R. C. (2017). The Co-existence of technology and caring in the theory of technological competency as caring in nursing. *The Journal of Medical Investigation*, 64(1.2), 160–164. 10.2152/jmi.64.160

Logg, J. M., Minson, J. A., & Moore, D. A. (2019). Algorithm appreciation: People prefer algorithmic to human judgment. *Organizational Behavior and Human Decision Processes*, 151, 90–103. 10.1016/j.obhdp.2018.12.005

Mayberry, A., Hu, P., Marlin, B., Salthouse, C., & Ganesan, D. (2014). iShadow: Design of a wearable, real-time mobile gaze tracker. *MobiSys ...: The International Conference on Mobile Systems, Applications and Services. International Conference on Mobile Systems, Applications, and Services*, 2014, 82–94. 10.1145/2594368.2594388.

Mayberry, A., Tun, Y., Hu, P., Smith-Freedman, D., Marlin, B., Salthouse, C., & Ganesan, D. (2016). CIDER: Enabling robustness-power tradeoffs on a computational eyeglass. *Proceedings of the 21st Annual International Conference on Mobile Computing and Networking. Eye Tracking Research & Applications Symposium*, 313–314. 10.1145/28574 91.2884063.

McGrow, K. (2019). Artificial intelligence: Essentials for nursing. *Nursing*, 49(9), 46–49. 10.1097/01.NURSE.0000577716.57052.8d

National Academies of Science, Engineering, and Medicine. (2021). *The future of nursing 2020–2030: Charting a path to achieve health equity*. National Academies Press. https://nam.edu/publications/the-future-of-nursing-2020-2030/

NINR. (n.d.). *NINR areas of interest*. Retrieved April 19, 2022, from https://www.ninr. nih.gov/researchandfunding/desp/oep/fundingopportunities/sb-areas

Noble, S. U. (2019). *Algorithms of oppression: How search engines reinforce racism*. New York University Press.

Obermeyer, Z., Powers, B., Vogeli, C., & Mullainathan, S. (2019). Dissecting racial bias in an algorithm used to manage the health of populations. *Science*, 366(6464), 447–453. 10.1126/science.aax2342

Okun, T. (2021). *Progress is bigger & more*. White Supremacy Culture. https://www. whitesupremacyculture.info/progress--quantity.html

O'Neil, C. (2016). *Weapons of math destruction: How big data increases inequality and threatens democracy*. Broadway Books.

Rothman, A. (2016, April). *The truth about abolition*. The Atlantic. https://www. theatlantic.com/magazine/archive/2016/04/the-truth-about-abolition/471483/

Salge, C. (2017, July 11). *Asimov's laws won't stop robots from harming humans, so we've developed a better solution*. Scientific American. https://www.scientificamerican.com/ article/asimovs-laws-wont-stop-robots-from-harming-humans-so-weve-developed-a-better-solution/

Wenger, E. (1998). Communities of practice: Learning as a social system. *Systems Thinker*, 9(5), 2–3.

Yerian, N. (2020, February 4). Benevolence and solidarity in ruha benjamin's race after technology. *Digital Public History*. https://digitalpublichistory.wordpress.com/2020/02/ 04/benevolence-and-solidarity-in-ruha-benjamins-race-after-technology/

Zheng, N., Liu, Z., Ren, P., Ma, Y., Chen, S., Yu, S., Xue, J., Chen, B., & Wang, F. (2017). Hybrid-augmented intelligence: Collaboration and cognition. *Frontiers of Information Technology & Electronic Engineering*, 18(2), 153–179. 10.1631/FITEE. 1700053

Zuckerman, E. (2021). *Mistrust: Why losing faith in institutions provides the tools to transform them*. W. W. Norton & Company.

10b Artificial Intelligence for Health and Care Is Not Inevitable: Ten Commitments to New Futures

Rae Walker

No matter how compelling the narrative, predicted A.I. futures are not inevitable—they are products of power and human choices. The question is not, "How to do we create *AI for good?*" but "How will we create the conditions in which health, healing, and collective liberation are possible – not just for a select few for whom these technologies are designed and function, but for all and especially communities occupying the margins?". This essay outlines ten commitments for nurses and other healers confronted with increasing expansion of surveillance, big data, and AI for health and care. Drawing on intellectual labor, theory, and community-led frameworks from fields such as nursing, design justice, critical digital studies, sociology, data feminism, Black feminism, queer and gender studies, this chapter builds upon ideas and critical vocabulary laid out in Part I. All oppression is connected, therefore efforts to disrupt oppression must also be intersectional (UN Women, 2020). The ten commitments proposed here are interrelated and reciprocal, defying hierarchical classification. Figure 10b.1 titled Ten Commitments to New Futures depicts them arranged in the shape of a star surrounded by a circle, a *pentacle*. Pentacles are powerful symbols associated with stewardship of bodies, communities, the land, and other creatures that inhabit it (Snow, 2020). The pentacle reminds us that as nurses we must be good stewards. These commitments are promises we are making to each other, communities we accompany in care, and to all living beings on our planet.

Commitment #1: Recognize All AI Is Political and Subject to Forces Under the Matrix of Domination That Affect its Design, Impacts, and Evolution

The term *artificial intelligence* was coined by logician John McCarthy in 1956 to describe a meeting he convened with a group of male scholars around the concept of "intelligence" and specifically, intelligence involving machines (Crawford, 2021). The field locates its roots in the American industrial-military complex, and specifically, unrestricted funding provided to several of its early co-founders, including McCarthy, by the Pentagon's research agency, later renamed the Defense Advanced Research Projects Agency (DARPA).

DOI: 10.4324/9781003245957-15

178   *Rae Walker*

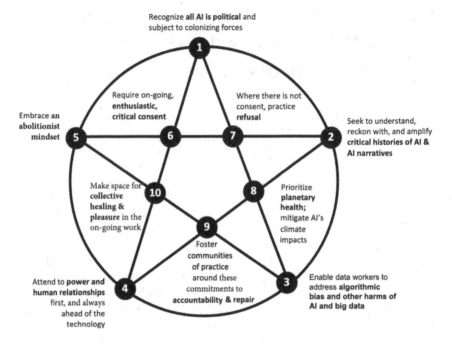

Figure 10b.1 Ten Commitments to New Futures.

> AI's subfields were from the start organized around a militaristic frame: vision research to detect "enemy" ships and spot resources of interest from satellite images, speech recognition for surveillance and voice-controlled aircraft control, robotics to develop autonomous weaponry, and so on.
>
> (Katz, 2020, p. 35)

A project of empire and capitalism, AI has also been described as a *technology of whiteness*, reinforcing patriarchy, heteronormativity, and systemic racism even as many of its creators' claim emancipatory aims (Katz, 2020).

In *Data Feminism*, Catherine D'Ignazio and Laura F. Klein describe how power unfolds in and around data under the *matrix of domination*, pointing to how demographics of the very fields that created specialties such as AI and data science fail to reflect society as whole (D'Ignazio & Klein, 2020). These fields are dominated by white cisgender highly educated men from the global north, replicating deep disparities along lines of race, gender, class, and citizenship. Pioneering algorithmic justice advocate and computer scientist Joy Buolamwini calls these fields the bastion of the "pale males" (Buolamwini, 2021). Unequal representation in these spaces creates what D'Ignazio and Klein refer to as a *privilege hazard*, where those afforded the most power over the creation of AI are also least well-equipped to recognize harms and oppressions in how it operates (2020). At the structural level, this also means that the politics, biases, and agendas of those at the top of the power hierarchy, and specifically, cis-gender non-disabled white settler men from the global North, may eventually "hard-code sexism, racism, and other forms of discrimination into the digital infrastructure of our societies" (D'Ignazio & Klein, 2020, p. 29).

This kind of hard-coded white cishetereopatriarchy is apparent in the collusion of AI and apparatuses of the state that weaponize welfare institutions as carceral interventions (Benjamin, 2019; Eubanks, 2017; Ford School, 2022; Haymarket Books, 2022). Historian of tech Melvin Kranzberg's words are echoed in the #TechIsNotNeutral hashtag of recent campaigns against the racist hyper-surveillance of Black communities borne out of partnerships between police departments and ICE and big tech companies like Microsoft, Google, NextDoor, and Amazon (Becker, 2021; Dickey, 2020). If we are to disrupt continuation and amplification of coded bias and oppressions into the future, we must acknowledge their presence and violent impacts now.

Commitment #2: Seek to Understand, Reckon with, and Amplify Critical History and Narratives about AI and Big Data

Popular narratives surrounding AI, particularly within academic medicine and the health care industry, lean heavily into a *technosolutionism* rooted in *technochauvinism* and belief in *technological benevolence* (Benjamin, 2019; Broussard, 2018). For evidence of this, we need look no further than the introduction of Boston Dynamics' AI-powered robotic "dog" (called Spot) into COVID triage tents of a large U.S.-based health system during the initial surges of the COVID-19 pandemic (Statt, 2020). The robot was originally developed by a military contractor with funding from DARPA. Prior to the pandemic, reporters had described the purpose of earlier prototypes in use by U.S. Marines as a way to search for enemies before entering a building (Roston, 2015). Some AI taxonomies would label Spot a humanoid robot (Eriksson & Salzmann-Erikson, 2017). Equipped with a tablet screen for a "head" and bedecked in video cameras with sensors designed to pick up on physiological parameters such as temperature and heart rate, the robots were presented as an innovative technological solution to an under-staffing crisis (Statt, 2020). Initial experiments involved only "healthy volunteers" and were intended to establish proof of concept the robot could serve as an effective alternative to hiring additional nursing staff. However, the robot was never formally deployed for this purpose (Etherington, 2020; Statt, 2020). The Spot robot has been reported to retail at $74,500 to $150,000 per unit (Stieg, 2020; Gault, 2022). For comparison, the median salary for a registered nurse in the United States in 2021 was $77,600. Certified medical technicians (frequently the ones to actually collect vital signs) earned an average of just $35,660. At these salaries, a hospital could hire a full-time registered nurse plus *two* certified medical assistants for one year for roughly the same cost as a single robot (*Average Registered Nurse Salary by State*, 2022).

In the wake of the COVID triage pilot, scientists and the company that created the Spot robots received positive media attention and plentiful data upon which to base future experiments and entrepreneurial efforts, even as the human nurses and other laborers at the hospital received no relief (Statt, 2020). A few months later, in November 2020, the same health system told nurses living with COVID+ household members such as a sick children they would need to show up to work, no matter what, even though no staff shortages were reported (Coupal, 2020). Conditions were even worse elsewhere. At many hospitals across the country, clinicians who'd responded to initial incentives such as hazard pay, overtime wages, and the opportunity to pitch in during initial COVID surges found themselves furloughed or fired as health systems scrambled to protect their profit margins. Hospitalized patients reported the disastrous impacts of their isolation from both loved ones and direct contact with clinical staff (Hwang et al., 2020). Cases in which the need for human connection was met through technology often involved relatively simple tablet devices and smartphones that did not require an entire robot dog attached. Since that time, Boston Dynamics has pivoted from primarily supplying defense requisitions to more commercial and warehouse operations like Amazon, searching for additional use cases for this military-grade, surveillant technology (Hadwick, 2021). One article describes deployment of Spot by Honolulu's police department to surveil unhoused community members as outsourcing "human interaction" to a \$150 K machine to do "the noble work of an \$11 thermometer" (Gault, 2022). More recent reports also show similar robot dogs mounted with automatic weapons (Vincent, 2021). Others have been deployed at the U.S. southern border as a "force multiplier" for Customs and Border Patrol (US Department of Homeland Security, 2022). Every bit of data collected by these robots potentially helps train the algorithms that power such machines. This case illustrates how all data, including data collected in humanitarian trials of robots-as-COVID-relief-workers, has the potential to be weaponized by the carceral state.

Commitment #3: Enable Data Workers, Including Nurses, to Address Algorithmic Bias and Other Harms of AI and Big Data

New algorithms are often introduced into health care systems behind the scenes. While these algorithms may have serious and even deadly repercussions, such negative impacts are frequently obscured from view due to siloing of data within systems and the appearance of seemingly objective, data-driven performance (Igoe, 2021). A recent report by researchers at the University of Chicago concluded commercial algorithms already widely integrated across health systems, such as Optum's algorithm for allocating additional resources and supportive care following hospitalization based on EHR data, are rife with *algorithmic bias* (Obermeyer et al., 2019). In their *Algorithmic Bias Playbook*, Obermeyer and colleagues recommend organizations using these technologies conduct their own algorithmic bias audits, beginning with *inventorying* all the algorithms being used or developed by the organization; *screening* each algorithm for bias relative to its ideal target outcomes; removing or *retraining* problematic algorithms to improve them; and finally developing accountability systems and structures to *prevent* introduction of biased algorithms in the future (Obermeyer et al., 2021). This is no small feat, and certainly not labor individual nurses should expect to take on themselves. It requires infrastructure and *collective action*, including collaboration and commitment from administrators, technologists, data scientists, patients, and other communities impacted by algorithmic bias.

Nurses generate tremendous amounts of data about the persons we accompany in care, which are then immortalized via platforms like insurance databases and electronic health records (EHR). By sheer volume of the global workforce (>27 million), nurses represent one of the largest contingents of data workers in the world (WHO, 2020). But this is not necessarily how we identify ourselves. Nor have nurses been trained to recognize and grapple with wider implications of the data we generate beyond attending to immediate patient outcomes and issues of compliance, such as when an EHR flags a missing field or medication. Curricula for nursing and other clinical professions have historically avoided issues of empire, power, and politics, including political economies surrounding data practices and technology (Barton et al., 2020). Although fields such as *AI ethics* and *accountable AI* are burgeoning, curricula for the clinical professions have yet to integrate such knowledge into prelicensure training or continuing education. This must change.

Entire social movements and fields, such as critical race and digital studies, have emerged to address not just the **how** of AI technologies, but the **why**, including the debate over whether some of these technologies *should* exist in the first place (Lopez & Land, 2019). Yet this scholarship is completely absent from this latest guidance from organizations like the AACN on nursing's curriculum (AACN, 2021). Though the recently revised *Essentials for Nursing Practice* make brief mention of ethics and compliance, none of the newly proposed competencies specifically address nurses' role in critically analyzing the evolution and operation of power in the domain of AI and big data (Walker et al., 2020, December 30). This too must change if nurses are to be effective advocates for institutional and structural transformation.

Even once nurses are equipped to recognize ethical dilemmas and harm associated with AI or big data that drive it, they likely still lack the time, resources, or authority necessary to enact meaningful changes in their workplaces, communities, regulatory structures, and governments. Part of the work of creating the conditions for a more liberatory AI, if such a thing can exist, involves improving regulatory mechanisms and accountability structures such as patient and community governance over tech industries and health systems (D4BL, n.d.). Expanded legal protections such as whistleblower laws and dedicated pro bono and legal aid funds are needed for both nurses and the public. Surveillant consumer technologies associated with the *internet of things,* like Amazon's Echo, and other forms of *ambient intelligence* designed to capture and interpret data from care environments, are increasingly present both in homes and hospital rooms (Schuster-Bruce, 2021). Accountability systems like consent forms and AHA's *Patient's Bill of Rights* must be updated to reflect threats posed by expanding surveillance and the commodification of data, including the right to privacy, the right to protection from harmful algorithms, the right to one's own data, and the right to receive clear and transparent information about when and how AI technologies have been applied to care, clinical decision-making, or resource allocation (Flynn, 2020).

We must also prepare those who regularly generate and access data to incorporate ethical approaches to this work beyond strictly legalistic frameworks that center on the rights of living individuals. Electronic health records are a type of digital archive. In an essay for *Uncertain Archives: Critical Keywords for Big Data*, Daniela Agostinho suggests digital archivists adopt a new *critical ethics of care*: "Rather than conceiving of care as an exclusively positive and redressing affect immune to power differentials – such critiques point to how care already circulates within "non-innocent histories," given the centrality of care to operations of colonialism, empire, and capital" (Agostinho, 2021, p. 81). It is not enough for nurses to be caring in our approaches to data management. We must be reflexive about whose experiences, skills, labor, and knowledge have shaped these digital infrastructures, policies—like HIPAA—that govern them, and whose lives are valued in such environments.

Commitment #4: Attend to Power and Human Relationships First, and Always Before the Technology

New technologies are often used to obscure power relations among human actors, serving to (falsely) position the technology as apolitical and "objective." AI technologies and associated data practices can never be allowed to take precedence over attending to inequities and abuses of power within human networks, nor to further dehumanize or *other* persons already marginalized by extant systems. MIT Media Lab researcher Sasha Costanza-Chock opens the book *Design Justice: Community-led Practices to Build the Worlds We Need* with a poignant illustration of just how such dehumanization takes place within a technosolutionist surveillance state. In the chapter "#TravelingWhileTrans, Design Justice, and Escape from the Matrix of Domination," Costanza-Chock describes how TSA's millimeter wave scanners, which use AI to generate a rough image of a person's body and possible "anomalies," requires agents to code the individual being scanned as a man or woman before the algorithm is applied (Costanza-Chock, 2020). No matter what option the TSA agent chooses, persons whose identities, bodies, and outward appearances do not conform to a narrow and cisheteropatriarchal gender binary (particularly trans, non-binary, gender non-conforming, and intersex persons) inevitably receive extra and often invasive, humiliating body searches when passing through these airport security checkpoints. This is not strictly a problem with agents making incorrect decisions in a world where they've been given limited options, but rather, a problem with power, and ways in which technology is wielded to reinforce both the gender binary and white cisheteropatriarchal supremacy in the name of public safety (Fischer, 2019). Although TSA scanners are not typically considered health technologies, they are by no means atypical when it comes to the long history of assessment of the human body. Indeed, many of the foundational physical assessment skills and tools now used to generate data in health systems were founded on equally problematic foundations that encode gender essentialism (for example, many breast cancer screening tools that assume gender is not only static and assigned at birth but that respondents are 100% cisgender and female), biological racism (such as "race corrections" for lung volume or eGFR), and ableism (exam tables inaccessible to some chair users) into the very fabric of health care's data systems and technologies (Benjamin, 2019; Hogarth, 2017; Goldberg et al., 2022; Morris et al., 2017).

Attending to power and human relationships first also means making transparent the myriad ways in which invisible human labor props up AI systems. In *Data Feminism*, authors Catherine D'Ignazio and Lauren Klein devote an entire chapter to "making labor visible" (2020). They highlight recent scholarship by technology researcher Kate Crawford and design scholar Vladan Joler, who mapped the human inputs required to generate and operate a single Amazon Echo—an increasingly common household technology that relies on *natural language processing* to respond to verbal commands from a user (Crawford & Joler, 2018). These inputs included mineral extraction to produce the electronic components (sometimes requiring child labor and further pollution of the environment), refining, assembling, distributing, and transporting the components both virtually and physically via Amazon's "fractal chains of production and exploitation" (Crawford, 2021). Their map includes invisible inputs such as the labor of academics and engineers, unpaid or low-wage labor from students and crowd workers labeling training data via services like Amazon's Mechanical Turk, and unrecognized labor such as completion of ReCaptchas (critical data labeling). They conclude, "At every level of contemporary technology is deeply rooted in and running on the exploitation of human bodies" (Crawford & Joler, 2018). Their visualization and essay are available at: https://anatomyof.ai/.

AI-washing is not limited to new start-up ventures. Data and Society's recent expose on *repair work* associated with implementation of AI in hospital settings highlights widespread potential for AI-washing in health care as well. Their in-depth reporting on impacts of Duke's Sepsis Watch protocol, designed to detect and intervene on hospitalized patients at high risk of developing sepsis concludes, "integration of an AI system creates breakages in social structures that must be repaired in order for the technology to work as intended" (Elish & Watkins, 2020). Rapid Response Nurses at the hospital took on the bulk of this hidden and undervalued repair work after the sepsis algorithm was implemented in the EHR. Nurses mediated professional hierarchies and performed emotional labor to strategically communicate patients' risk scores to doctors (Elish & Watkins, 2020). Multiple automated alerts, most of which were false positives, sent nurses scurrying to ensure the *human labor* of implementing sepsis protocols occurred even though it caused sudden and unpredictable disruptions to their workflows and impaired their capacity to attend to other patients' urgent needs. Since then, newly published research indicates proprietary sepsis detection algorithms introduced to EHR software like Epic may do little to *actually* improve patient outcomes. One report concluded the company's algorithm failed to identify two-thirds of the roughly 2,500 sepsis cases (Simonite, 2021). Had innovators begun with an equity-centered design approach that focused first on power and human relationships: engaging all parties impacted these systems (including patient advocates, nurses, unit clerks, and other staff) to define the *actual design challenge* requiring intervention, they might have identified a different problem with a better solution and improved outcomes for all (Creative Reaction Lab, 2019). Instead, siloed algorithmic innovators often receive acclaim, and industry reaps profits of its proprietary tech, while patients and health care workers especially nurses shoulder the consequences. Technologists and health systems must do better.

Commitment #5: Embrace an Abolitionist Mindset and Principles That Center the Priorities and Expertise of Persons Occupying the Margins, Recognizing Communities' Strengths, and Lifting up Those Already Doing the Work

Nurses and other healers could take a page from communities already engaged in such projects grounded first and foremost in re-imagining relationships with regards to people and power. An abolitionist mindset for dismantling that which is not serving us or our communities and co-creating new forms of AI that do also requires *design justice*. Design justice is a network of practitioners and a dynamic, living set of principles that originated out of a workshop planned by Una Lee, Jenny Lee, and Melissa Moore and presented by Una Lee and Wesley Taylor at the Allied Media Projects conference in 2015 (Costanza-Chock, 2020). Design justice work is guided by the core beliefs that "those directly affected by the issues a project aims to address must be at the center of the design process, and second, that absolutely anyone can participate meaningfully in design" (Costanza-Chock, 2020, p. 7). This entails building community accountability through approaches such as: centering community members as experts in the nature and definition of the AI design challenge, especially those who are regularly marginalized within or erased from design efforts; capacity-building through education and other efforts focused on equipping co-designers with the knowledge and tools necessary to co-create their own solutions; specifying clear mechanisms for community accountability from the inception of new projects; and investment in continued maintenance and improvement of projects beyond the innovation stage. Design justice encourages co-designers to address common pitfalls of institutionalized cultures of innovation like the Silicon Valley motto "move fast and break things," by avoiding the temptation to simply "parachute" nurse informaticists and other technologists into organizations and community settings where they have no prior history of relationship-building or local knowledge (Costanza-Chock, 2020).

Commitment #6: Require Ongoing, Enthusiastic, Critical Consent

Definitions of consent abound and vary dramatically in the digital and algorithmic space. Most of us are now accustomed to the long fine print in "terms of use" that accompany new downloads and digital platforms. In health care and research circles, we often discuss the concept of *informed consent*. What constitutes informed consent is usually determined at the level of the institution, such as by the members of an institutional review board. This type of consent is less about morals or ethical practice, and more about compliance with a legal requirement (Bazzano et al., 2021). With few exceptions, such as examples derived from Black midwifery-grounded models of reproductive health or trans-led approaches to more inclusive, gender-affirming care, the culture of health care and innovation has not cultivated a culture around consent that goes anywhere beyond the bare minimum level of compliance, and even then, it often fails (Rabelais, 2020; Suarez, 2020). In some cases, even compliance with legal standards has done violence to communities, such as the situation of some Native nations whose sovereignty has been bypassed by the NIH's large-scale data repositories (Hansen & Keeler, 2018). If we are serious about cultivating more liberatory futures as they relate to AI and data practices, we must also re-imagine consent in the digital space. Not as a static, one-and-done sort of proposition involving long paper forms and legal-ese, but consent as a dynamic relationship between the person(s) about whom data are being generated and/or who are being impacted by products of AI and data science, and those collecting the data and/or developing the technologies and algorithms. Consent that is not only "informed," but affirmative, enthusiastic, ongoing, and given from a positionality of power (And Also Too, 2022).

This is a space wherein folks *on the margins*, such as many professional sex workers, and queer and feminist practitioners of bondage, discipline, sadism, and masochism [BDSM] or polyamory, could teach clinicians, data scientists, and technologists less familiar with consent practices beyond individualistic and transactional legal frameworks. Professional sex worker Chanelle Gallant, a long-time organizer and co-director of the Migrant Sex Worker Project in Toronto, Canada, explains:

> *I believe this is the most valuable lesson of sex workers to consent culture: the knowledge that consent is about power. Less power means less ability to establish meaningful consent. So if a sex worker is selling sex in an environment where they have a lot of power ... they can better negotiate for safer sex, they can better protect their boundaries, they can be really clear about what they want, what they don't want, at what time, and when and with whom. If a sex worker has less power, then they have less control and there is less real consent in the sexual interaction.*
> (Gallant, 2016)

In *Queer BDSM Intimacies: Critical Consent and Pushing the Boundaries,* German queer studies scholar Robin Bauer describes negotiation of relationships and power among self-described "dyke" and queer practitioners of BDSM (Bauer, 2014). This group, while not a monolith, provides a contrast to the hetero-normative *ideal of harmonic sex* wherein all couples are assumed to be egalitarian and therefore neutral, without power dynamics requiring mitigation or nego-tiation. This assumption is of course, a myth. But it comes eerily close to similar assumptions underlying many contemporary approaches to consent practices in health care and tech sectors, including, the collection of big data. Queer BDSM practitioners, by existing outside of these normative assumptions, throw them on their head, providing a model for consent practices in contexts where the default is never egalitarian or neutral. Bauer concludes:

> *The dyke + queer BDSM community developed technologies of negotiating critical and affective (rather than liberal and rational-choice) consent that offered a promising tool to invent new power-sensitive ways of dealing with difference and social hierarchy. Starting from an acknowledgment of interdependence rather than personal autonomy, they replaced the illusion of equality with the criterion of negotiating agency, which enabled individuals to state their desires and set limits in concrete, contained situations. The notion of agentic feminism that prevailed in the community entailed claiming one's own agency both to empower oneself and to interrogate one's own position of power critically.*
>
> (Bauer, 2014, p. 252)

How will we, as nurses and healers, create the conditions wherein individuals and communities impacted by AI and big data are able to engage in critical consent from a positionality of greater agency and power? We are far from that now. The ethics and accountability structures that currently exist in health care are not only inadequate for this task but also mired in the most basic moral debates regarding whether patients should even be informed AI has impacted their care in the first place (Darrell M. West & Allen, 2020). A recent legal brief in The Georgetown Law journal summarizes current legal controversies in the realm of patient consent related to the use of AI and machine learning (ML) technologies:

> First, when, if ever, under the law of informed consent do physicians need to tell patients that AI/ML was involved in helping to guide the treatment decision the physician ultimately adopted? Second, conditional on be-lieving such disclosure is sometimes appropriate, how much detail must they share about the AI/ML recommendation and the AI/ML system itself?
>
> (Cohen, 2020)

The world of health care compliance is still grappling with questions as basic as whether or not patients should be made aware of the degree to which algorithms and AI technologies have impacted their care and possible recommendations for treatment decision-making.

But here is where it gets tricky: whether the use of AI/ML to help direct their care matters to patients depends in part on (a) how commonly it is used and (b) how much patients know about how commonly it is used, which is itself at least somewhat related to (c) whether we require disclosure about the use of AI/ML today.

(Cohen, 2020)

If we are to co-create praxis that is truly emancipatory in the context of AI for health and care, nurses will need a new ethics of *critical consent*.

Commitment #7: Where There Is Not Consent, Practice a Feminist Politics of Refusal

There are many examples of refusal at work, particularly among communities marginalized under the matrix of domination. Native and Indigenous peoples have been forced to struggle against settler states, including Federal agencies such as the National Institutes of Health (NIH), for sovereignty over their own data and stories. For example, the National Congress for American Indians (NCAI), which represents the majority of 573 tribes in the United States, condemned the failure of researchers for the NIH-sponsored *All of Us* precision health study, a 1 million person+ longitudinal cohort study involving sequencing and archiving participants' genomes, to engage in good faith discussions with leaders of sovereign tribes before launching. Although the *All of Us* program has a Tribal Collaboration Working Group, there had been no tribal consultations that satisfy treaty or other requirements nine months into the program (The Tribal Collaboration Working Group Report, 2018). These data are sensitive and could have ramifications beyond just those for individual participants. Some Indigenous leaders called this effort to hoover up as much genomic and health data as possible on such a large group anew form of *biocolonialism* (Hansen & Keeler, 2018). Immediately following the research program's launch, the NCAI tweeted, "All of Us Research Program recruitment launch is a reminder that NIH and this program must consult and partner with tribes on how to best protect American Indian/Alaska Native (AI/AN) data and tribal sovereignty in research" (NCAI Policy Research, 2018). NIH responded with a press release in March 2021, that affirmed their "baseline commitments" to certain safety protocols for data collected from AI/AN participants, such as holding release of those data for 6 months to allow participants to consult with tribal leaders about their participation in the study (*NIH to Enhance Tribal Engagement Efforts for Precision Medicine Research*, 2021). Prior to engaging with these tribal communities, researchers at the NIH had already decided what types of data would be collected and how those categories would be defined. Even with certain "safety" agreements in place, tribal communities remain at the mercy of the research questions, frameworks and measures selected *a priori* by settler scientists. Social scientists Eve Tuck and K. Wayne Yang (2014) name and push back against this type of *settler gaze* in their pivotal essay, "R-Words: Refusing Research."

> Settler colonial knowledge is premised on frontiers; conquest, then, is an exercise of the felt entitlement to transgress these limits. Refusal, and stances of refusal in research, are attempts to place limits on conquest and the colonization of knowledge by marking what is off limits, what is not up for grabs or discussion, what is sacred, and what can't be known.
>
> (Tuck & Yang, 2014, p. 225)

Commitment #8: Attend to Planetary Health Implications of AI and Associated Extractive Economies

Artificial intelligence and big data have important implications for planetary health. Though some of these impacts may be positive, many exacerbate an already worsening climate emergency. Some researchers hypothesize applications of AI to the energy sector may result in greater efficiencies and reductions in greenhouse gas emissions (GHG) (Dutta, 2021). According to some models, AI is estimated to assist organizations in industries to fulfill up to 45% of the Paris Agreement targets by 2030 (Capgemini Research Institute, 2020). However, the use of AI to solve these sticky climate challenges also involves costs with non-trivial impacts on the environment. AI technologies require large amounts of energy and planetary resources to be produced. Precious minerals, such as lithium, are essential components of technologies like the batteries that power many robotic and automated systems, wearable sensors, "smart" devices like cell phones, computers, and electric vehicles. In *Atlas of AI*, computer scientist Kate Crawford opens the book with an excruciating tale about lithium mining and its poisonous consequences for communities and wildlife that once occupied what are now ghost towns scattered across the western United States (Crawford, 2021). In many cases, extraction of these minerals is conducted by large multi-billion dollar corporations on Indigenous and Native lands, contributing to environmental racism by draining and poisoning those ecosystems. Once built, these technologies also require copious amounts of energy to operate.

Researchers at the University of Massachusetts Amherst performed a life cycle assessment for training several common large AI models. They found that the process can emit more than 626,000 pounds of carbon dioxide equivalent—nearly five times the lifetime emissions of the average American car, including manufacture of the car itself (Hao, 2019). The study, by researchers Emma Strubell, Ananya Ganesh, and Andrew McCallum, specifically studied energy required to train model used to support natural language processing (NLP), a technology critical to the function of voice-activated applications like auto-scribes, Siri, and Cortana (Strubell et al., 2020). To date, nursing discourse on AI and big data has largely ignored climate implications of these technologies, even as they deploy climate-related metaphors. For example, a recent article on nursing leadership and data mining warns:

Today's nursing executives and managers are inundated by a *tsunami of data* from a variety of sources, including inpatient and ambulatory electronic health records (EHRs), finance and accounting data, claims data, human resources reports, demographic data, national and internal benchmarking data, research data, quality improvement and process improvement project outcomes data, and satisfaction reports for patients, physicians, and employees.

(Clancy & Gellinas, 2016)

Tsunami is used here as a metaphor for an overwhelming wave of data. *Actual* tsunamis are series of potentially catastrophic waves caused by earthquakes or undersea volcanic eruptions (NOAA, 2018). Human activity, such as commercial development of shorelines, compounds their devastating effects even as tsunamis are frequently described as natural phenomena. By referring to a *data tsunami*, nurse authors confer a sense of overwhelming force while simultaneously dodging complicity or control, as if data tsunamis were as inevitable as massive earthquakes or volcanic eruptions. Meanwhile, big data-driven AI and related technologies like blockchain, built and maintained by fellow humans, have been implicated in exacerbating global climate change thereby increasing the likelihood and human devastation of literal tsunamis around the planet (Browne, 2021; Strubell et al., 2020; Tully, 2021).

Organizations such as the Alliance of Nurses for Healthy Environments (ANHE) have committed to the development of curricula and action strategies nurses can use to disrupt unnecessary waste and other harmful practices, and to advocate for regulation and greater accountability of industries and governments (Anderko et al., 2016). Though not yet specifically named in any nursing organization's public commitments to address the climate emergency (Walker et al., 2020), going forward our efforts to protect planetary health must address technology waste and other ongoing planetary harms resulting from the maintenance of AI-powered systems and associated extractive economies. In pursuing these efforts, nurses should center the leadership of groups disproportionately impacted by the effects of a changing climate, such as disabled, queer, and trans people of color, and Indigenous and Native communities with generations of experience innovating in the face of adversity and stewarding the land (Sanderson et al., 2020).

Commitment #9: Foster Communities of Practice Surrounding These Commitments to New Futures, Accountability, and Repair

When establishing new communities of practice around responses to AI and big data, nurses should seek to support, amplify, learn from, and build upon the activism and intellectual labor of community-led organizations already doing the work (Costanza-Chock, 2020). My own introduction to the concept of *algorithmic accountability* came in 2019 while standing in my kitchen preparing dinner for my children and listening to a livestream of the 2nd annual Data for

Black Lives (D4BL) conference. The in-person event was at capacity, but the organization had made a commitment to making their work accessible to a wide audience including those of us who ultimately tuned in via YouTube. Data for Black Lives was established by data scientist and entrepreneur Yeshimabeit Milner for the purpose of using data science to create concrete and measurable change in the lives of Black people (D4BL, n.d.). The organization acknowledges that "tools like statistical modeling, data visualization, and crowdsourcing, in the right hands, are powerful instruments for fighting bias, building progressive movements, and promoting civic engagement," however, "history tells a different story, one in which data is too often wielded as an instrument of oppression, reinforcing inequality and perpetuating injustice" (D4BL, n.d.). One of their most recent campaigns, *Abolish Big Data* (hashtag #NoMoreData Weapons), is a call to action to reject the concentration of big data in the hands of a few, and to challenge the structures that allow data to be used as a weapon of political influence. Milner explains, "To abolish Big Data means to put data back in the hands of people who need it the most" (Milner, 2021).

Working alongside organizations like D4BL, the Algorithmic Justice League (AJL) was founded by computer scientist and self-proclaimed "poet of code" Joy Buolamwini. The algorithmic justice movement caught fire after Dr. Buolamwini gave a ground-breaking TED talk on algorithmic bias in 2017 that has since garnered more than one million views (Buolamwini, 2021). In her talk, Dr. Buolamwini demonstrated how facial recognition software commonly found across a wide range of computer applications and technologies routinely misclassified or failed to recognize faces, including her own, in ways that were systematically biased because "people who coded the algorithm hadn't taught it to identify a broad range of skin tones and facial structures" (Buolamwini, 2016). She called this bias the *coded gaze*. Since its founding in 2017, the Algorithmic Justice League has successfully fought for new laws in towns and cities banning use of facial recognition technologies in public spaces. They provide algorithmic auditing services, datasets, and expertise to guide policymakers and industry around more accountable use and regulation of AI.

The Our Data Bodies (ODB) Project was originally formed in 2015, predating both Data for Black Lives and the Algorithmic Justice League. Based in marginalized neighborhoods in Charlotte, North Carolina, Detroit, Michigan, and Los Angeles, California, the ODB project critically examines digital data collection and human rights, working with local communities, community organizations, and social support networks to show how different data systems impact re-entry, fair housing, public assistance, and community development (Our Data Bodies, n.d.). Through support of the Digital Trust Foundation, Our Data Bodies collaborated with co-creators from their local neighborhoods to develop the *Digital Defense Playbook*, an open-access workbook available in both English and Spanish that contains group-based education activities focused on data, surveillance, and community safety to co-create and share knowledge, analyses, and tools for data justice and data access for equity (Lewis et al., 2018). In the *Digital Defense Playbook*, one user writes, the implications of data are not imagined and predicted as they are in data science, but instead, embodied, experienced and felt. In the wrong hands, data has the power to dismantle, dividuate, and dissect. This is quite the antithesis to how data are materialised in data science – yet an important way forward if we want the more negative aspects of datafication to change.

(Pangrazio, 2020)

The workbook was designed to support "intersectional fights for racial justice LGBQ+ liberation, feminism, immigrant rights, economic justice, and other freedom struggles, to help us understand and address the impact of data-based technologies on our social justice work" (Lewis et al., 2018). Such tools are ready resources for nurses seeking to establish common vocabularies and *embodied* understandings around how data and data-driven technologies, such as AI, impact their health and the health of their communities, and how to fight back.

   In addition to partnering with movement leaders to foster new and expanded communities of practice, nurses can also draw upon existing community accountability practices. These have been informed by frameworks such as ending sexual violence, trauma-informed practice, harm reduction, healing justice, PIC abolition, and transformative justice (Kaba & Hassan, 2019). Many grew out of the labor of Black women and other women of color, Indigenous and disabled communities, queer and trans people of color, and other marginalized and stigmatized groups such as professional sex workers. Harm reduction is "a philosophy of living, surviving and resisting oppression and violence that centers self-determination and non-condemning access to an array of options" (Kaba & Hassan, 2019, p. 7).

Community accountability (CA) strategies aim at preventing, intervening in, responding to and healing from violence through strengthening relationships and communities, emphasizing mutual responsibility for addressing the conditions that allow violence to take place, and holding people accountable for violence and harm.

(The Audre Lorde Project, 2010)

This approach is especially important when community members—whether they are nurses or the persons nurses accompany in care—cannot rely on state systems or other institutions for safety. Mariame Kaba and Shira Hassan's working for community accountability facilitators, *Fumbling Towards Repair*, outlines 10 critical questions for any CA process. These include, "Where is the harm and where is the potential healing?"; "What change are you hoping for?"; and "How can I/we make this better?" (Kaba & Hassan, 2019, p. 33). These questions are intended to facilitate a process wherein community members show up for each other and especially those who've experienced harm, hold themselves and each other accountable, and work—where possible—toward *repair*.

Commitment 10. Make Space for Collective Healing and Pleasure in the Work

Disruption and transformation are not easy. It is work. It can be exhausting, even violent. Layered onto this is the trauma of an ongoing pandemic that has done untold damage to the health care workforce, to students, and to patients and communities, especially those already occupying the margins. Corporations, governments, health care industries, and other powerful entities deeply invested in maintaining the power status quo will (and have) quash disruption to hegemony. In January 2021, Google summarily fired AI ethics researcher Timnit Gebru along with one of her chief collaborators, AI scientist Margaret Mitchell. Their infraction? Internally circulating scholarly work demonstrating significant harms of some of the AI models the company relies on to sustain its search engines (Schiffer, 2021). Gebru, a well-respected scientist in AI circles, spoke out when the company claimed she had voluntarily resigned. She referred to this characterization of her firing as having been "resignated" (Axon, 2021). The hashtag #IStandWithTimnit made the rounds on social media alongside an outpouring of support from fellow advocates and AI researchers. The company denied it did anything wrong, or that the implications of Gebru's research influenced its decision to fire the Ethiopian-born computer scientist of Eritrean descent (Wakabayashi, 2021). Though some legal aspects remain pending, Gebru, Mitchell, and their collaborators have publicly documented an audit trail of internal emails and other documentation from Google executives capturing a systemic campaign of threats, intimidation, and gaslighting (Mitchell, 2022; Schiffer, 2021).

Gebru sought to disrupt and transform a very powerful corporate system from within. Despite some early wins and exquisite scholarship, her AI ethics research team was ultimately met with stonewalling, dismissal, and legal and financial consequences. Google immediately rushed to fill the void by launching an elaborate media campaign about how their new AI ethics division would be even bigger and better than the last (Ghaffary, 2021). The incident threw into sharp relief other *AI for good* efforts funded by large corporate sponsors, like Google, many of which now underwrite AI curricula at many institutions of higher education and sponsorships for health innovation events like *nurse hackathons*. The case of Timnit Gebru's firing forces us to ask, to what extent do these industry investments represent authentic efforts to promote a more just and verdant future—and to what degree do they co-opt public goodwill and trust in nurses to *nurse-wash* less savory realities about these industries and their impacts? If our success as healers means abolishing and transforming the violence of industries and structures invested in oppression, will industries invested in the status quo allow us to succeed in these efforts? Or are these industry partners invested in allowing only for the *optics of success* wherein only very small, incremental changes that can be advertised as proof of good faith are allowed?

If we are to not only survive but thrive in an AI era, nurses and other actors engaged in resistance, abolition, and rewriting the future of power in these ecosystems need community spaces where we can experience true solidarity, pleasure, and radical joy in our work, relationships, and bodies. Co-creation of such spaces requires intention, relationship-building, and trust. In her collection of essays, *Pleasure Activism: The Politics of Feeling Good,* adrienne maree brown writes about the healing power of collective engagement in *generative somatics,* a set of practices focused on transformative embodiment, acknowledging both pleasure and pain, and "how each of us has the power to help each other feel more, heal, and move toward our longing for liberation and justice together" (brown, 2019, p. 275). We cannot rely on legacy nursing professional associations to hold space for such critical yet intimate forms of engagement. While nursing has multiple professional groups focused on big data and AI, like the American Nursing Informatics Association (ANIA) and the American Academy of Nursing (AAN), such organizations retain highly hierarchical leadership structures wherein the membership largely reflects well-resourced, highly educated, and mainly white professionals focused on academic and scholarly discourse and advancement of the discipline. These are not safe spaces for radical praxis, particularly when it is coming from folks on the margins. If we cannot locate safe and generative spaces for community accountability and generative somatics within our discipline's professional associations, nurses may need to create new networks. Once again, we can look to the examples from leaders already doing the work, like Timnit Gebru. Gebru neither gave up nor ran back to the oppressive industry spaces that continued to fight her very success. On December 2, 2021, she circulated a press release announcing the launch of her latest endeavor: the Distributed AI Research Institute (DAIR).

DAIR's values are outlined on the landing page of their new website: Community, not exploitation; comprehensive, principled processes; proactive, pragmatic research; and healthy, thriving researchers. Under the latter they explain,

> we understand that the current environments in which we conduct this work do not prioritize our well-being. We value the commitments required to produce strong research and are committed to being a place where researchers do not have to choose between their work and their health.
>
> (DAIR Institute, 2021)

Nursing as a discipline, either on its own or in partnership with other disciplines and stakeholders, has yet to launch its own version of DAIR. But if we are to be successful in sustaining the creative efforts and resistance that will be required to co-create new and more liberatory futures, we will need to create refuges where this work can happen in partnership with community members who see and acknowledge our humanity, value our pleasure and collective well-being, and help us to locate the joy in this work.

Final Thoughts

Claims surrounding benefits of AI for health care are extensive and ever-expanding. AI for health care has been described in the nursing literature as an imperative for improvement of patient safety and health care quality, and especially central to the provision of *evidence-based, personalized* and *precision care* (Geum Hee Jeong, 2020; Ronquillo et al., 2021; Santoni de Sio & van Wynsberghe, 2016; Schleder Gonçalves et al., 2020). The fact some forms of AI sensing, such as wall-mounted sensors, can allow clinicians and administrators to "passively" surveil patients, bypassing the need for cooperation or consent from the persons being monitored, has been touted as a significant advantage of this technology (Barrera et al., 2020). Over and over in the literature, AI is proposed as the answer to sticky behavioral challenges, mental health, and poorly managed symptoms (Barrera et al., 2020).

When we examine where these narratives about the revolutionary benefits of AI for health care originate from, we see this varies widely. Claims in the peer-reviewed literature largely stem from engineers and academics, many who do not have a clinical background or who are no longer active in direct care roles. Quite a few philosophers have added to the discourse (Santoni de Sio & van Wynsberghe, 2016). Some claims stem from technologists, particularly engineers and computer scientists (Gholami et al., 2018; Zheng et al., 2017). There is also industry, particularly the giants of Silicon Valley championing the AI for good movements such as Amazon, Apple, Facebook, Google, and Microsoft (Benjamin, 2019). When we ask whose voices are absent from this discourse, we see a different picture. Notably, we observe comparatively little representation from folks outside of academe and the health care industry, such as patients, caregivers, and communities directly impacted by these technologies (Eubanks, 2017; McGrow, 2019; Ronquillo et al., 2021). Even the recent AI for health care think tank convened by the Nursing and Artificial Intelligence Leadership Collaborative (NAIL), titled "Artificial intelligence in nursing: social, ethical and legal implications," while inclusive of multidisciplinary perspectives, lacked any obvious representation from patients, caregivers, or community organizers (Ronquillo et al., 2021).

Much of the Federally funded health research involving AI and big data, such as the NIH's *All of Us* project, remains deeply entrenched in forms of positivistic empiricism, biological determinism, and deficit models of health borne out of sociopolitical realities, and especially, the historical and current dominance of white westernized biomedicine as the defining framework for what is considered health and care (Rabelais & Walker, 2021). The majority of machine learning-ready datasets for these projects are derived from Federal databases like the U.S. Census, electronic health records of large health systems, and private insurance companies with access to large swathes of patient data (Scudellari, 2021). Such archives tend to contain variables characterized as intrinsic to *individuals*, like physiological parameters and pathological diagnoses, while failing to capture historical, relational, institutional, or environmental factors that might better explain health not only as it manifests for a single person, but within and across social networks and communities over time (Dillard-Wright, 2019). *These are not data for liberation.* Data platforms such as electronic health records were designed to maintain a system of surveillance, legal compliance, billing, and payment wherein the ways in which health and care are defined, and what forms of these are accessible and valued, are defined by white settler-dominated bio-medical institutions, regulatory agencies, and especially industries like insurance and pharmaceuticals that profit from present power arrangements (Evans, 2016). Creating new futures in an era of AI and big data entails co-constructing new narratives about what constitute data for health and liberation, how they are analyzed and managed, and who is an expert or data scientist (Thylstrup et al., 2021).

AI for health and care is not intrinsically bad or good, nor are predicted futures a foregone conclusion. Timnit Gebru writes,

> We believe that artificial intelligence can be a productive, inclusive technology that benefits our communities, rather than work against them. However, we also believe that AI is not always the solution and should not be treated as an inevitability. Our goal is to be proactive about this technology and identify ways to use it to people's benefit where possible, caution against potential harms and block it when it creates more harm than good.
>
> (DAIR Institute, 2021)

Manifesting emancipatory nursing futures in an AI era requires continuously recommitting to each other, our communities, and the planet. Though the work can seem daunting, nurses have an exciting opportunity to build new shared vocabularies, communities of practice, frameworks for codesign, and negotiating power and consent around AI, including what constitutes data for health and liberation. Glitch feminist Legacy Russell asks, "Can a break be a form of building something new? Can our breaking shit be a correction, too?" (Russell, 2020). In our collective endeavors to create the circumstances in which liberation is possible, nurses must be prepared to break a lot of shit along the way.

References

AACN. (2021). *The New AACN Essentials.* https://www.aacnnursing.org/AACN-Essentials

Agostinho, D. (2021). Care. In *Uncertain archives: Critical keywords for big data.* The MIT Press.

And Also Too. (2022). *The Consentful Tech Project.* https://www.consentfultech.io/

Anderko, L., Schenk, E., Huffling, K., & Chalupka, S. (2016). *Climate change, health, and nursing: A call to action.* https://envirn.org/climate-change-health-and-nursing/

Average Registered Nurse Salary by State (2022). (2021, December 13). Incredible Health. https://www.incrediblehealth.com/blog/the-highest-paying-states-for-nurses/

Axon, S. (2021, May 3). Yet another Google AI leader has defected to Apple. *Ars Technica.* https://arstechnica.com/gadgets/2021/05/apple-hires-yet-another-ex-google-ai-leader/

Barrera, A., Gee, C., Wood, A., Gibson, O., Bayley, D., & Geddes, J. (2020). Introducing artificial intelligence in acute psychiatric inpatient care: Qualitative study of its use to conduct nursing observations. *Evidence Based Mental Health, 23*(1), 34–38. 10.1136/ebmental-2019-300136

Barton, A. J., Brandt, B., Dieter, C. J., & Williams, S. D. (2020). *Social Determinants of Health: Nursing, Health Professions and Interprofessional Education at a Crossroads.* 32.

Bauer, R. (2014). *Queer BDSM intimacies: Critical consent and pushing boundaries.* Palgrave Macmillan.

Bazzano, L. A., Durant, J., & Brantley, P. R. (2021). A modern history of informed consent and the role of key information. *The Ochsner Journal, 21*(1), 81–85. 10.31486/toj.19.0105

Becker, C. R. (2021, July 10). *The first law of technology.* Medium. https://uxdesign.cc/the-first-law-of-technology-41de427c4ee4

Benjamin, R. (2019). *Race after technology: Abolitionist tools for the new jim code.* Polity.

brown, adrienne maree. (2019). *Pleasure activism: The politics of feeling good.* AK Press.

Browne, R. (2021, February 5). *Bitcoin's wild ride renews worries about its massive carbon footprint.* CNBC. https://www.cnbc.com/2021/02/05/bitcoin-btc-surge-renews-worries-about-its-massive-carbon-footprint.html

Broussard, M. (2018). *Artificial unintelligence: How computers misunderstand the world.* MIT Press.

Buolamwini, J. (2016, November). *How I'm fighting bias in algorithms.* https://www.ted.com/talks/joy_buolamwini_how_i_m_fighting_bias_in_algorithms

Buolamwini, J. (2021, February 26). *Joy buolamwini: How do biased algorithms damage marginalized communities?* NPR.Org. https://www.npr.org/2021/02/26/971506520/joy-buolamwini-how-do-biased-algorithms-damage-marginalized-communities

Capgemini Research Institute. (2020). Climate AI: How artificial intelligence can power your climate action strategy. *Capgemini US.* https://www.capgemini.com/us-en/research/climate-ai/

Clancy, T. R., & Gellinas, L. (2016). Knowledge discovery and data mining: Implications for nurse leaders. *JONA: The Journal of Nursing Administration, 46*(9), 422–424. 10.1097/NNA.0000000000000369

Cohen, I. G. (2020). Informed consent and medical artificial intelligence: What to tell the patient? *SSRN Electronic Journal.* 10.2139/ssrn.3529576

Collins, S., Couture, B., Kang, M. J., Dykes, P., Schnock, K., Knaplund, C., Chang, F., & Cato, K. (2018). Quantifying and visualizing nursing flowsheet documentation burden in acute and critical care. *AMIA Annual Symposium Proceedings, 2018,* 348–357.

Costanza-Chock, S. (2020). *Design justice: Community-led practices to build the worlds we need.* The MIT Press.

Coupal, B. (2020, November 24). *Union: Brigham and Women's Hospital telling nurses living with coronavirus-positive relatives to report to work.* https://whdh.com/news/union-brigham-and-womens-hospital-telling-nurses-living-with-coronavirus-positive-relatives-to-report-to-work/

Crawford, K. (2021). *Atlas of AI.* Yale University Press.

Crawford, K., & Joler, V. (2018, September 7). *Anatomy of an AI System.* AI Now Institute and Share Lab. http://www.anatomyof.ai

Creative Reaction Lab. (2019). *Field guide: Equity-centered community design.* Creative Reaction Lab. https://www.creativereactionlab.com/shop/p/field-guide-equity-centered-community-design

D4BL. (n.d.). *Data for Black Lives.* Retrieved January 15, 2022, from https://d4bl.typeform.com/to/wg6agF

DAIR Institute. (2021, December 2). *The DAIR institute.* https://www.dair-institute.org/press-release

West, D.M., & Allen, J. R. (2020). *Turning point: Policymaking in the era of artificial intelligence.* Brookings Institution Press.

Dickey, M. R. (2020, August 20). Tech is not neutral campaign urges companies to stop working with law enforcement agencies | TechCrunch. *TechCrunch+.* https://techcrunch.com/2020/08/20/tech-is-not-neutral-campaign-urges-companies-to-stop-working-with-law-enforcement-agencies/

D'Ignazio, C., & Klein, L. F. (2020). *Data feminism.* The MIT Press.

Dillard-Wright, J. (2019). Electronic health record as a panopticon: A disciplinary apparatus in nursing practice. *Nursing Philosophy, 20*(2), e12239. 10.1111/nup.12239

Dutta, A. (2021, September 23). *Council post: How cloud migration and AI can help reduce carbon footprint.* Forbes. https://www.forbes.com/sites/forbestechcouncil/2021/09/23/how-cloud-migration-and-ai-can-help-reduce-carbon-footprint/

Elish, M. C. , & Watkins, E. A. (2020). Repairing innovation: A study of integrating AI in clinical care. Data & Society.

Eriksson, H., & Salzmann-Erikson, M. (2017). The digital generation and nursing robotics: A netnographic study about nursing care robots posted on social media. *Nursing Inquiry, 24*(2), e12165. 10.1111/nin.12165

Etherington, D. (2020, August 19). MIT and Boston Dynamics team up on 'Dr. Spot,' a robot for remote COVID-19 vital sign measurement. *TechCrunch.* https://social.techcrunch.com/2020/08/19/mit-and-boston-dynamics-team-up-on-dr-spot-a-robot-for-remote-covid-19-vital-sign-measurement/

Eubanks, V. (2017). *Automating inequality: How high-tech tools profile, police, and punish the poor.* St. Martin's Press.

Evans, R. S. (2016). Electronic health records: Then, now, and in the future. *Yearbook of Medical Informatics, 25*(S 01), S48–S61. 10.15265/IYS-2016-s006

Fischer, M. (2019). *Terrorizing gender: Transgender visibility and the surveillance practices of the U.S. security state.* University of Nebraska Press.

Flynn, L. (2020, February 18). *When AI is watching patient care: Ethics to consider.* Bill of Health. https://blog.petrieflom.law.harvard.edu/2020/02/18/when-ai-is-watching-patient-care-ethics-to-consider/

Ford School. (2022, April 5). *Master Class in Activism: Dorothy Roberts, "Torn Apart".* https://www.youtube.com/watch?v=tXLehaRaVMw

Gallant, C. (2016, August 19). Sex workers are experts at sexual consent. *Femifesto.* http://www.femifesto.ca/sex-workers-are-experts-at-sexual-consent/

Gault, M. (2022, January 26). Police outsourcing human interaction with homeless people to Boston dynamics' robot dog. *Vice.* https://www.vice.com/en/article/v7dz7b/police-outsourcing-human-interaction-with-homeless-people-to-boston-dynamics-robot-dog

Geum Hee Jeong. (2020). Artificial intelligence, machine learning, and deep learning in women's health nursing. *Korean Journal of Women Health Nursing, 26*(1), 5–9. 10.4069/kjwhn.2020.03.11

Ghaffary, S. (2021, June 2). *Google says it's committed to ethical AI research. Its ethical AI team isn't so sure.* Vox. https://www.vox.com/recode/22465301/google-ethical-ai-timnit-gebru-research-alex-hanna-jeff-dean-marian-croak

Gholami, B., Haddad, W. M., & Bailey, J. M. (2018). AI in the ICU: In the intensive care unit, artificial intelligence can keep watch. *IEEE Spectrum, 55*(10), 31–35. 10.1109/MSPEC.2018.8482421

Goldberg, J. E., Moy, L., & Rosenkrantz, A. B. (2022). Assessing transgender patient care and gender inclusivity of breast imaging facilities across the United States. *Journal of the American College of Radiology.* https://edhub.ama-assn.org/jacr/module/2792678

Hadwick, A. (2021, May 20). From DARPA to distribution centre: How Boston Dynamics went from military to warehouse operations. *Reuters News.* https://www.reutersevents.com/supplychain/technology/darpa-distribution-centre-how-boston-dynamics-went-military-warehouse-operations

Hansen, T., & Keeler, J. (2018, December 21). *The NIH is bypassing tribal sovereignty to harvest genetic data from native Americans.* https://www.vice.com/en/article/8xp33a/the-nih-is-bypassing-tribal-sovereignty-to-harvest-genetic-data-from-native-americans

Hao, K. (2019, June 6). *Training a single AI model can emit as much carbon as five cars in their lifetimes.* MIT Technology Review. https://www.technologyreview.com/2019/06/06/239031/training-a-single-ai-model-can-emit-as-much-carbon-as-five-cars-in-their-lifetimes/

Haymarket Books. (2022, January 18). *Understanding E-Carceration: A Book Launch.* https://www.youtube.com/watch?v=fc2JaRJWcFM

Hogarth, R. A. (2017). *Medicalizing Blackness: making racial difference in the Atlantic world,* 1780–1840. UNC Press Books.

Hwang, T.-J., Rabheru, K., Peisah, C., Reichman, W., & Ikeda, M. (2020). Loneliness and social isolation during the COVID-19 pandemic. *International Psychogeriatrics,* 1–4. 10.1017/S1041610220000988

Igoe, K. (2021, March 12). *Algorithmic bias in health care exacerbates social inequities—How to prevent it.* Harvard T.H. Chan School of Public Health. https://www.hsph.harvard.edu/ecpe/how-to-prevent-algorithmic-bias-in-health-care/

Kaba, M., & Hassan, S. (2019). *Fumbling toward repair: A workbook for community accountability facilitators.* The NIA Project and Just Practice.

Katz, Y. (2020). *Artificial whiteness: Politics and ideology in artificial intelligence.* Columbia University Press.

Lewis, T., Gangadharan, S., Saba, M., & Petty, T. (2018). *Digital defense playbook: Community power tools for reclaiming data.* Our Data Bodies.

Lopez, L. K., & Land, J. (2019, April 18). *Critical race & digital studies syllabus.* Center for Critical Race and Digital Studies. https://criticalracedigitalstudies.com/syllabus/

McGrow, K. (2019). Artificial intelligence: Essentials for nursing. *Nursing, 49*(9), 46–49. 10.1097/01.NURSE.0000577716.57052.8d

Milner, Y. (2021, March 4). *Databite No. 129: Abolish big data.* Data & Society. https://datasociety.net/library/abolish-big-data/

Mitchell, M. (2022, January 13). 1 yr ago today, Google leaders still didn't seem to see what the big deal was abt what they did firing @timnitGebru + pretending it was a resignation. I participated in hours of questioning. I was warned I would be fired and smeared. I was a zombie from lack of sleep. [Tweet]. *@mmitchell_ai.* https://twitter.com/mmitchell_ai/status/1481667415410806785

Morris, M. A., Maragh-Bass, A. C., Griffin, J. M., Finney Rutten, L. J., Lagu, T., & Phelan, S. (2017). Use of accessible examination tables in the primary care setting: A survey of physical evaluations and patient attitudes. *Journal of General Internal Medicine, 32*(12), 1342–1348. 10.1007/s11606-017-4155-2

NCAI Policy Research. (2018, May 7). Tweet [Tweet]. @NCAIPRC https://twitter.com/NCAIPRC/status/993569695704985601

NIH to enhance tribal engagement efforts for precision medicine research. (2021, March 25). National Institutes of Health (NIH)—All of Us. https://allofus.nih.gov/news-events-and-media/announcements/nih-enhance-tribal-engagement-efforts-precision-medicine-research

NOAA. (2018). Tsunamis. Retrieved on July 23, 2022. http://www.noaa.gov/education/resource-collections/ocean-coasts/tsunamis

Obermeyer, Z., Nissan, R., Stern, M., Eaneff, S., Bembeneck, E. J., & Mullainathan, S. (2021). *Algorithmic bias playbook.* Center for Applied AI at Chicago Booth.

Obermeyer, Z., Powers, B., Vogeli, C., & Mullainathan, S. (2019). Dissecting racial bias in an algorithm used to manage the health of populations. *Science, 366*(6464), 447–453. 10.1126/science.aax2342

Our Data Bodies. (n.d.). *About Us.* Retrieved January 15, 2022, from https://www.odbproject.org/about-us-2/

Pangrazio, L. (2020, July 29). Materialising the implications of data: The digital defense playbook. *New Ways of Understanding Digital Data.* https://materialising-data.org/2020/07/29/materialising-the-implication-of-data-the-digital-defense-playbook/

Rabelais, E. (2020). Missing ethical discussions in gender care for transgender and non-binary people: Secondary sex characteristics. *Journal of Midwifery & Women's Health, 65*(6), 741–744. 10.1111/jmwh.13166

Rabelais, E., & Walker, R. K. (2021). Ethics, health disparities, and discourses in oncology nursing's research: If we know the problems, why are we asking the wrong questions? *Journal of Clinical Nursing, 30*(5–6), 892–899. 10.1111/jocn.15569

Ronquillo, C. E., Peltonen, L.-M., Pruinelli, L., Chu, C. H., Bakken, S., Beduschi, A., Cato, K., Hardiker, N., Junger, A., Michalowski, M., Nyrup, R., Rahimi, S., Reed, D. N., Salakoski, T., Salanterä, S., Walton, N., Weber, P., Wiegand, T., & Topaz, M. (2021). Artificial intelligence in nursing: Priorities and opportunities from an international invitational think-tank of the nursing and artificial intelligence leadership collaborative. *Journal of Advanced Nursing, 77*(9), 3707–3717. 10.1111/jan.14855

Roston, B. A. (2015, September 21). *Boston dynamics' spot robo-dog being tested by marines.* SlashGear. https://www.slashgear.com/boston-dynamics-spot-robo-dog-being-tested-by-marines-21405681/

Russell, L. (2020). *Glitch feminism: A manifesto.* Verso.

Sanderson, D., Mirza, N., Polacca, M., Kennedy, A., & Bourque-Bearskin, R. L. (2020). Nursing, indigenous health, water, and climate change. *Witness: The Canadian Journal of Critical Nursing Discourse, 2*(1), 66–83. 10.25071/2291-5796.55

Santoni de Sio, F., & van Wynsberghe, A. (2016). When should we use care robots? The nature-of-activities approach. *Science and Engineering Ethics, 22*(6), 1745–1760. 10.1007/s11948-015-9715-4

Schiffer, Z. (2021, March 5). *Timnit gebru was fired from Google—Then the harassers arrived.* The Verge. https://www.theverge.com/22309962/timnit-gebru-google-harassment-campaign-jeff-dean

Schleder Gonçalves, L., de Medeiros Amaro, M. L., Miranda Romero, A., de, L., Schamne, F. K., Fressatto, J. L., & Wrobel Bezerra, C. (2020). Implementation of an Artificial Intelligence Algorithm for sepsis detection. *Revista Brasileira de Enfermagem*, 73(3), 1–5. 10.1590/0034-7167-2018-0421

Schuster-Bruce, C. (2021, October 26). Amazon is putting Alexa next to hospital beds throughout the US. It says it will boost productivity because staff can go into patients' rooms less. *Business Insider*. https://www.businessinsider.com/amazon-alexa-hospitals-echo-next-to-us-hospital-bed-2021-10

Scudellari, M. (2021, March 29). *Machine learning faces a reckoning in health research*. IEEE Spectrum. https://spectrum.ieee.org/machine-learning-faces-a-reckoning-in-health-research

Simonite, T. (2021). Algorithim predicts deadly infections often flawed. Wired [blog]. https://www.wired.com/story/algorithm-predicts-deadly-infections-often-flawed/

Snow, C. (2020). *Queering your craft: Witchcraft from the margins*. Weiser Books.

Statt, N. (2020, April 23). *Boston dynamics' spot robot is helping hospitals remotely treat coronavirus patients*. The Verge. https://www.theverge.com/2020/4/23/21231855/boston-dynamics-spot-robot-covid-19-coronavirus-telemedicine

Stieg, C. (2020). This $75,000 Boston Dynamics robot 'dog' is for sale—take a look. CNBC. https://www.cnbc.com/2020/06/22/75000-boston-dynamics-robot-dog-for-sale-take-a-look.html

Strubell, E., Ganesh, A., & McCallum, A. (2020). Energy and policy considerations for modern deep learning research. *Proceedings of the AAAI Conference on Artificial Intelligence*, 34(09), 13693–13696. 10.1609/aaai.v34i09.7123

Suarez, A. (2020). Black midwifery in the United States: Past, present, and future. *Sociology Compass*, 14(11), e12829. 10.1111/soc4.12829

The Audre Lorde Project. (2010, August 9). *Community Accountability and Transformative Justice Groups Connect with S.O.S./ALP, YWEP, Creative Interventions, and the Revolution Starts at Home Collective*. The Audre Lorde Project. https://alp.org/community-accountability-and-transformative-justice-groups-connect-sosalp-ywep-creative-intervention

The Tribal Collaboration Working Group Report. (2018). *Considerations for Meaningful Collaboration with Tribal Populations*. 22.

Thylstrup, N. B., Agostinho, D., Ring, A., D'Ignazio, C., & Veel, K. (2021). *Uncertain archives: Critical Keywords for Big Data*. The MIT Press.

Tuck, E., & Yang, K. W. (2014). R-Words: Refusing research. In *Humanizing research: Decolonizing qualitative inquiry with youth and communities*. Routledge.

Tully, S. (2021, October 26). Every Bitcoin transaction consumes over $100 in electricity | Fortune. *Forbes*. https://fortune.com/2021/10/26/bitcoin-electricity-consumption-carbon-footprin/

UN Women. (2020, July 1). Intersectional feminism: What it means and why it matters right now. *Medium*. https://un-women.medium.com/intersectional-feminism-what-it-means-and-why-it-matters-right-now-7743bfa16757

US Department of Homeland Security. (2022, February 15). *Feature Article: Robot Dogs Take Another Step Towards Deployment | Homeland Security*. https://www.dhs.gov/science-and-technology/news/2022/02/01/feature-article-robot-dogs-take-another-step-towards-deployment

Vincent, J. (2021, October 14). *They're putting guns on robot dogs now*. The Verge. https://www.theverge.com/2021/10/14/22726111/robot-dogs-with-guns-sword-international-ghost-robotics

Wakabayashi, D. (2021, December 9). Google chief apologizes for A.I. researcher's dismissal. *The New York Times.* https://www.nytimes.com/2020/12/09/technology/timnit-gebru-google-pichai.html

Walker, R.K., Dillard-Wright, J., Rabelais, E., Valdez, A., Cogan, R., Glickstein, B. & Valderama-Wallace, C. (2020, December 30). AACN essentials national faculty meeting feedback. *Nursing Mutual Aid.* Retrieved April 20, 2022, from https://drive.google.com/file/d/1xCIl7jaMNUci4nr8QNolK-loWhOWIJWG/view?usp=sharing&usp=embed_facebook

Walker, R. K., Pereira-Morales, S., Kerr, R., & Schenk, E. (2020). Climate change should be on every nursing research agenda. *Oncology Nursing Forum, 47*(2), 135–144. 10.1188/20.ONF.135-144

WHO. (2020, April 6). State of the world's nursing 2020: Investing in education, jobs and leadership. https://www.who.int/publications-detail-redirect/9789240003279

Zheng, N., Liu, Z., Ren, P., Ma, Y., Chen, S., Yu, S., Xue, J., Chen, B., & Wang, F. (2017). Hybrid-augmented intelligence: Collaboration and cognition. *Frontiers of Information Technology & Electronic Engineering, 18*(2), 153–179. 10.1631/FITEE.1700053

Part IV

Getting There: Speculative Paths for the Present/Future

In the fourth part of this compendium, we invited authors to describe the potentiality that nursing holds in developing equitable futures for nursing students and the folks we accompany in care. These futures cross the disciplinary spectrum and include nursing education, practice, and research. Bursting forth from this speculative vision, collectively the authors highlight the possibility of antiracist teaching practices, abolition, planetary care, and democratic knowledge generation. The authors' visions embrace the generative potential of a radical future that is collaborative, communal, and just. Their words remind us of other liberatory calls to action, such as the Mental Health First initiative of the AntiPolice Terror Project in the Bay Area; New York City's the People's Forum, an incubator for transversal solidarity; and William Barber III's Poor People's Campaign.

In Chapter 11, *Horizons: Shifting the Gaze and Topography of Nursing Education*, authors DaJane Gresham-Ryder, Venika Marwaha, and Clarie Valderama-Wallace deeply interrogate the racist origins of nursing education and its perpetuation in the present. The authors critique the current narratives surrounding professionalism, accreditation standards, calls for diversity in nursing education, and future visions upheld by the neoliberal empire. Here, they argue that the current systems and structures that are in place are unable to bring about equity and "fall short of the possibility for freedom." Amid these faults, the authors excavate the oppressive practices of standardized testing in nursing and its marginalizing impact on students from historically-underserved backgrounds. From these roots of these injustices, Gresham-Ryder, Venika, and Valderama-Wallace endeavor to develop and build anti-racist admission practices and pedagogies grounded in justice through systems of faculty and institutional accountability.

In Chapter 12, *Open Nursing Science: Using Citizen Science to Break Nursing Knowledge Wide-open*, author Patrick McMurray envisions a future for nursing knowledge development that is unbolted, accessible, fluid, and democratizing in its approach. In an attempt to redefine what counts as research in nursing, McMurray explores the potentiality of citizen science as a mode of inquiry to unmoor the current epistemological practices of the discipline and to make them accessible to the folks we accompany and to all nurses regardless of

DOI: 10.4324/9781003245957-16

formal academic training. The author begins by describing the history and basic principles of citizen science as a mechanism to engage the public in a partnership of inquiry. From this starting point, the author makes the case for citizen science to dismantle the hegemonic hierarchy and boundaries of what counts as nursing knowledge. As McMurray states, "in nursing, the academy jealously guards who gets to be viewed as a scholar, scientist, theorist, leader, innovator, and change-maker." Citizen science disassembles these boundaries, inviting others in. McMurray notes that nursing has a stark history of "researching at people" rather than being equal partners in knowledge-making practices, issuing a call "for nurses (and others) to be part of doing science out loud and in the open."

In Chapter 13, *Metamorphosing Nursing Education for a Dying Planet*, author Brandon Blaine Brown envisions a future for nursing in which the environs of care are expanded to include nonhumans, plants, animals, and the Earth itself. Brown begins by describing the current epoch of time known as the Anthropocene and its impact upon the Earth and all of its denizens, living, nonliving, and dead. The author then focuses on nursing education's failure to address climate change and its driving force of capitalism. Brown elucidates that reasons for nursing education's negligence in addressing environmental degradation stem from the construction of the discipline caught in the throes of humanism and its operation within the commodified territories of higher education and healthcare. The author ends with a call for the academy to transform its pedagogical practices and transmission of knowledge towards an ecological and relational approach that emphasizes rhizomatic learning and making kin with the earth.

In Chapter 14, *#AbolishNursing: An Ethics for Creating Safer Realities*, author Em Rabelais proposes a liberatory future through the abolishment of nursing practice and education in its current form. The chapter is divided into two sections. In the first section, Rabelais begins by describing the harms that have been done and continue to be reproduced in the field through whiteness, ableism, and transmisia. The author deeply chronicles the impact of poor nursing care that has been perpetrated upon the trans community and other historically underserved groups. Rabelais goes on to illustrate that the "exercise of nursing itself is an exercise of white supremacy." The author offers a call for abolitionist frameworks that emphasize "we can only do this together, not alone" and that "abolition is a community event" summoning nurse educators and nurses to believe their patients and students. As Rabelais eloquently proclaims, "when we do not believe our students, we are actively teaching them not to believe their patients." Moving forward, in the second section of the chapter, the author outlines how we get to a liberatory future through the destruction and creation of something else that is not oppressive. Rabelais describes that this liberatory future will only be achieved when those who are currently in leadership step down and cede control to Black and Brown, transgender, disabled, and non-Christian communities.

As illustrated by the aforementioned brief overview of each chapter, we are inspired. Each of the author's speculative visions makes clear that there is a bountiful groundswell of liberatory futures and dreamers within the discipline. Each of their works offers us new ways of thinking about nursing that break apart the boundaries, limitations, and the confining ethos of the present, offering us paths forward for a more just present-future.

11 Horizons: Shifting the Gaze and Topography of Nursing Education

DaJanae Gresham-Ryder, Venika Marwaha, and Claire Valderama-Wallace

Authors' Positionalities

DaJanae Gresham-Ryder: As an African American nurse born and raised in Stockton, California, it has helped mold my perspective on healthcare disparities and the long-haul disadvantages the Brown and Black community have suffered for decades. The lack of healthcare resources in the African-American community has caused my ancestors to be maternally ignored and experimental subjects, resulting in a lack of trust in the healthcare system. The outlook of a human of color is optimistic, visionary, and cultivated; the future will partake in a direction that will guide equitable healthcare for all.

Venika Marwaha: I was born in Oakland, California to parents who emigrated from India. Having worked in hospitals through rotations as a previous nursing student, and in the community setting as a nursing assistant and mental health rehabilitation worker, I've seen disparities in the quality of care. Currently, I see a system focused on treating diagnoses and I envision a healthcare system with a more proactive desire to care for the needs of the community and healing.

Claire Valderama-Wallace: As a Filipino woman born and raised in the United States, I am particularly mindful of how colonialism and American imperialism created the conditions that brought my family to unceded Ohlone territory and continue to shape our lives. A vision for internationalist, anticolonial, and anti-imperialist futures shapes my every day.

Purpose

Systems built upon the violent pillars of white supremacy, colonialism, and imperialism thrive in the silencing of liberatory ways of thinking, living, learning, healing, communicating, and loving. These same pillars have created the landscape of nursing education, fraught with the perpetuation of unjust power dynamics as well as resistance. What Mariame Kaba (2021) said, "There is no road map for justice, because under this system we have never seen it. But the current system has been thoroughly mapped, and it has already failed." (p. 70) While Kaba described the prison industrial complex, this statement also applies to health professions education. Despite the increase in diversity, equity,

DOI: 10.4324/9781003245957-17

and inclusion (DEI) statements by nursing organizations (Knopf et al., 2021) and the formation of DEI committees, material shifts in the distribution of power remain elusive. The same people, formations, and policies which have invested in and benefit from racism, ableism, patriarchy, and transmisia in nursing remain deeply entrenched and are among those seeking to remain relevant (McFarling, 2021). For nursing to live up to the promise and claim of social justice (American Nurses Association, 2015), systematic disruption, transformation, and sustained non-transactional partnerships are necessary. The purpose of this chapter is to map this landscape, consider recent efforts, and envision steps to uproot contradictions.

Conceptual Framework

Critical Race Theory (CRT) and Critical Latin Epidemiology are the frameworks guiding our work, propelling us toward liberatory epistemologies where dismantling systems of oppression and epistemicide are centered. Futures of nursing education where health equity is paramount requires fluency about systems of oppression, the social and political construction of race, and the need for counternarratives and structural change (Bell, 1975; Ladson-Billings & Tate, 2016). We also draw inspiration from Breilh's theory of Critical Latin Epidemiology, which centers social determination of health, collective health, and the undoing of colonialism's biomedical tenets of individualism, linear causation, and risk factors (Breilh, 2021). Transforming nursing education requires intentional divestment from the biomedical model, which will not be possible through a patchwork of incremental changes in curricula, haphazard diversity initiatives, reform of accreditation standards, and ongoing reliance on testing industries.

The Topography of Nursing Education

Myths of Nursing Education and the Profession

Nursing is a remarkable profession created to care for patients holistically (Practicalnursing.org Staff Writers, 2021). Myths, however, have created misconceptions that continue to impact the workforce. Debunking myths in nursing is essential to uprooting the impact of systems of oppression. For example, the work of historians has unveiled that Florence Nightingale was not the only influential nurse in history (Smith, 2021). Another common myth is that the nursing profession is built around inclusion and diversity. The tragic deaths of George Floyd and multiple African-Americans have revealed what it means to be a person of color in the United States. Nursing is not immune from systemic racism. In reality, racism is still alive in the nursing profession, and this crisis must be acknowledged by those who pretend all nurses are equal.

Nursing education does not systematically combat racism. Nursing programs were established to produce competent nurses, but notions of competency have

Table 11.1 Myths That Serve as Vehicles of Oppression in Nursing

1 Nurses are not capable of and do not perpetuate racism.
2 Nurses with BSNs are more competent than LVNs and nurses with an ADN.
3 Ethnic studies, social sciences, the arts and humanities are not essential.
4 Nursing students have neither power nor voice.
5 Diversity, equity, and inclusion statements from nursing institutions without material and epistemic changes will bring about health equity.
6 Gatekeeping through accreditation and licensure examination ensures safe care.
7 When students ask faculty for clarification, it's to earn more points and challenge authority.
8 Cultural competency is still relevant, necessary, and causes no harm.
9 Only nurses should be faculty in nursing programs.
10 Emphasizing niceness and civility does not silence nor harm.
11 Educators who have been nurses for decades do not teach incorrect concepts and content.
12 Medical missions to areas of concentrated poverty, on Turtle Island and around the world, do not warrant an examination of power dynamics and whiteness.
13 Nurses currently in leadership are the best positioned to both hold themselves accountable and usher in long-needed changes.
14 There are people who are voiceless in society and nurses can be their voices.
15 Nurses who are active in unions are not professional.

been entrenched in protecting the comfort of nurses who have not been historically excluded. Most importantly, myths of diversity in nursing have allowed nurses to participate in all levels of racism (Jones, 2000). Naming and debunking myths are essential to hold white supremacists accountable for the harm and mistrust created over the decades. Without this process, nursing will not equitably thrive. Godsey et al. (2020) explain that nursing as a brand is inconsistent with the care delivered by the nursing profession. Godsey et al. (2020) examined the importance of nursing in healthcare but while doing so, they also created negative stereotypes. For example, the authors assume that Patients of Color seeking care may believe that they are unlikely to be mistreated, which is inaccurate. Table 11.1 *Myths That Serve as Vehicles of Oppression in Nursing* outlines additional misconceptions that serve as vehicles of oppression. These have scarred the integrity of nursing and there is much to be done to strengthen the backbone of the profession.

Bedrock of Empire Building, Colonialism, and White Supremacy

To examine nursing education in a manner that centers social justice is to situate nursing within a broader context of historical and ongoing colonial projects. Schools have been a vehicle for racist American empire building for decades. This includes Indian boarding schools, enacting genocide which continues to impact the physical, emotional, cultural, and spiritual health and safety of Indigenous peoples (Lajimodiere, 2014). The global diaspora of Filipino nurses, both in workforce demographics and COVID-19-related deaths among nurses, is due to American nurses' interventions to civilize Filipinos and build nursing programs after the Spanish American War in 1898. Their efforts set the stage for labor export policy, which is why Filipino nurses practice in more than 50 countries, with most working in acute care and long-term inpatient settings (Choy, 2003; Nazareno et al., 2021). The American system of education continues to invest in policies and practices that place Black/African American and Latine/x students into the school to containment pipeline (Morris, 2016; Nelson & Williams, 2019) while obfuscating mechanisms of exclusion (Au, 2016; Darder, 2005). The process of learning about and affirming the lived experiences, resistance, and contributions of historically excluded communities is aggressively silenced, entrenching false and harmful narratives (Goggins, 2021) that perpetuate the myth that white people are naturally the reference group in scientific endeavors (Bray & McLemore, 2021).

White supremacy culture reproduces harm, where workarounds influenced by fear and fragility are favored over bold systems change in academia, healthcare, and beyond. This stratifies nursing into practice, education, research, and policy while naturalizing the focus on disease process, specialization of organ systems, and hierarchy based on educational degree. Numerous scholars have examined the roots and ongoing manifestations of racism and cisheteropatriarchy in nursing and healthcare (Barbee, 1993; Bell, 2021; Carabez et al., 2015; Eaker, 2021; Essex et al., 2021; Hantke, 2021; Hassouneh, 2008; Iheduru-Anderson, 2021; Keeton, 2020; Koschmann et al., 2020; Puzan, 2003; Schroeder & DiAngelo, 2010; Smith, 2021; Threat, 2015; Truitt & Snyder, 2020; Valderama-Wallace & Apesoa-Varano, 2020). An enduring commitment to social justice requires systematic reckoning of what brought us to this point and investment in the imaginations and future-building efforts of historically excluded communities.

Another manifestation of white supremacy culture is the preoccupation with professionalism. Central to this is gatekeeping and the focus on autonomy, self-regulation, narrow conceptualizations of health, and prioritizing status above meeting the needs of society (Green, 2016; Valderama-Wallace, 2017; Nardi et al., 2020). These siloes worsen health inequities and prevent the normalization of humility, collaboration, ongoing learning, and systems-level changes to promote health equity. This climate favors superficial and ill-cited attempts to adopt the language of anti-racism, diversity, inclusion, and/or justice, protecting the status quo despite risks taken by students and faculty to create change. The power dynamics infused in the design, regulation, implementation, and evaluation of nursing education are such that racism, heteropatriarchy, ableism, transmisia, ageism, and classism endure, as does resistance.

Fear and Silencing in Nursing Education

Nursing education is influenced by white supremacy culture that firmly believes that past practices are the only way to develop successful future nurses. This ideology is generated through silencing throughout the educational path. Audre

Lorde (1984) noted that "… it is not difference which immobilizes us, but silence. And there are so many silences to be broken." (p. 39) Silencing occurs in schools where there are low-income, immigrants, vulnerable students, and historically forgotten who are accustomed to authoritarianism. Students who are suppressed are often not aware of or lack support from individuals who will support their vision. For example, imagine November 4, 1960 Ruby Bridges' first day at an all-white school and the significance of how that one day helped pave the way for Students of Color who attempted to pursue an equitable education. Systems of nursing education are in a continuous cycle of Ruby Bridges' November 4, 1960 experience, based on how many roadblocks Students of Color encounter along the way and the intense scrutiny that they receive while obtaining a nursing degree. The silencing of Students' of Color experiences is a continuation of white supremacy because of the harsh suppression of their lived reality.

Silencing in the classroom seeks to erase and destroy the past history of our ancestors fighting for freedom. Critical conversations are suppressed because faculty and staff lack the ability to discuss the role of racism and mistreatment of Students of Color. In recent years, policies have been created to prevent professors from discussing Critical Race Theory (CRT). Like many uncomfortable discussions, professors are pressured to participate in duties that do not reflect their values and there are still those who believe racism does not exist.

In the early 1900s, a large portion of the nursing profession was only white, and their non-inclusive practices have continued to control nursing education and healthcare organizations (D'Antonio & Whelan, 2009). As of now, we are starting to see more Nurses of Color entering the workforce, but it has not been enough to change the practices of the white instructors and the systems that regulate nursing education. Bennett et al. (2019) describe how the discomfort of discussing race leads to nursing faculty avoiding the topic all around. However, navigating difficult conversations in classrooms and clinical debriefings are vital in molding how future nurses perceive and interact with patients.

Unfortunately, if these topics are actively silenced, how can anyone in the nursing profession understand how to care for patients safely and effectively? If students do not feel comfortable speaking about these topics, then the environment must not be safe enough. Silencing also creates a disconnect amongst all students, controlling students' thoughts and downplaying their concerns, which does not foster an environment to learn how to navigate these topics safely and effectively (Bennett et al., 2019). Ultimately, institutionalized silencing impacts the future of nursing while uplifting colonialism.

Constructed and Gate Kept Siloes

Individual nurses who have satisfied the requirements put forth by colonial systems that protect the status quo are incentivized to perpetuate gatekeeping as they ascend to positions as deans, nurse executives, department chairs, journal editors, fellows, accreditation site visitors, authors of foundational nursing documents, and directors of professional nursing organizations. The pursuit of Magnet® status by hospitals also represents gatekeeping, building on bias against non-BSN nursing degrees. This structure of mobilizing Magnet® status comes with a criterion that only allows BSN nurses to practice in in-patient settings.

According to American Nurses Credentialing Center (ANCC), Magnet® recognition indicates nursing excellence that aligns with the safety of the patient and continuing the education of the healthcare provider (*Magnet Recognition Program®*| ANCC, 2020). The criteria reward those who follow the predetermined structures that favor those with Bachelor of Science in Nursing (BSN) degrees, while simultaneously limiting respect and inhibiting professional mobility to those with non-BSN degrees. For example, those with a Licensed Vocational Nurse (LVN) or Certified Nursing Assistant (CNA) certificate are not allowed to participate in the creation of the future of nursing as nurse leaders.

The ecosystem of nursing is rooted in the discretization of colonialism, which naturalizes and professionalizes siloes—narrowing the available paths in our minds and hearts while constricting the future of nursing and opportunities for more equitable health among future generations. These examples of constructed siloes include the false separations and misleading conflations of worth and promise based on degree programs, acute care and community health, social science and health science, critical thinking and liberatory imagination, nurse and patient, and health care and healing.

The Impact and Cost of Nursing Education Industries

Research has shown that standardized testing preparation companies attract more white students, making it less likely to create a diverse workforce (Au, 2016). The majority of historically excluded communities are from low-income families who lack the resources to support their child's education. It is irrational to believe that standardized test prep companies that cater to nursing such as Kaplan or Uworld are genuinely created to help nursing students succeed because they are both profit-based and convey that students will only be successful by utilizing their products. Furthermore, due to accreditation standards, faculty are also tied to teaching to the NCLEX (national licensing exam in the USA); prompting one to ask themselves, how do the historically forgotten overcome this challenge if they are not white? Will there be a change in testing companies to attract a larger population of people and not just one group? How can a Person of Color continue to succeed in the nursing profession if the education structures do not support them? These questions encourage one to think about the historical roots of nursing education and standardized testing.

The history of standardized testing, steeped in white supremacy, was developed to create an objective metric that measured students' academic knowledge on a particular topic. It is important to note that performance on tests do not accurately capture the intelligence and potential of learners. According to Walker (2021), Students of Color score lower on college admission tests, creating a substantial racial gap in enrollment. Likewise, the American Association of Colleges of Nursing (AACN), report that racial minority nursing students comprise only 34.2% of students in entry-level baccalaureate programs followed by 34.7% of master's students, and 33.0% of students in research-focused doctoral programs (AACN, 2019). These percentages are a reflection of the minorities who have successfully beat the odds of being accepted into a nursing program. Given the demographics mentioned above, we see harm throughout the college pipeline. Metrics and indicators upheld by nursing leaders, those overseeing nursing organizations, and regulatory bodies, serve as pillars that will continue to harm Brown and Black students.

In the 19th century, Henry Fischel invented exams to gauge students' overall performance on subjects in America (Lambert, 2022). History has shown that standardized tests marginalize Black and Brown communities, making it easier for the educational system to ignore students' ability to perform beyond the standardized test. The racial gap in education cannot be closed if organizations do not change their racist gatekeeping in nursing education. A nursing student should be evaluated on their ability to deliver patient-centered care. Nevertheless, nursing students in the United States are routinely required to take standardized tests to enter nursing school and to become licensed nurses, the latter being through a standardized national licensure exam (NCLEX). Successfully passing this test requires students to undergo extensive preparation through the use of commercialized testing companies mentioned above.

Ultimately the regulation of education leads to Students' of Color increased anxiety and fear of not being accepted and supported. Schools of nursing perpetuate this anxiety and fear through the use of educational testing surveillance which enslaves nursing students in a resemblance of slavery; in essence, students should control their education without the use of educational testing surveillance. Nursing educators operate from the dogma that not being proctored or monitored allows cheating- locking faculty into fear. The economy of technology capitalizes on faculty fears of cheating, linking to worries about program accreditation and intensifying student fears about success. Education surveillance controls students and incentivizes adherence to narrow approaches to knowledge, and the regurgitation of information without critical thinking. Effective nursing education should not be surveilled but instead work toward a supportive learning environment that enables students of all colors to receive an equitable education.

The Path Forward According to Existing Institutional Powers

The authors of the 2010 *Future of Nursing Report* (Institute of Medicine, 2010) put forth recommendations that focused on expanding nursing infrastructure, presence, and status. These recommendations held firm the status quo of the racist neoliberal health care industry. A number of updated foundational documents were released in 2021, including the *New Essentials of Nursing Education* from the American Association of Colleges of Nursing

(AACN, 2021) and the *Future of Nursing Report 2020–2030* (National Academies of Sciences, Engineering, and Medicine, 2021). Notably missing from these documents were critical and relational stances. The absence of critical and relational stances will not usher in the bold futures historically excluded communities have called for, are creating, and from which we would all benefit.

Future of Nursing 2030

In the *Future of Nursing 2020–2030* report by the National Academies of Sciences, Engineering, and Medicine (2021) an ongoing endorsement of the healthcare industry in all its myopia and profit-driven violence figures prominently. There is no mention of nursing's contributions to longstanding injustice, lack of diversity, and the ongoing resistance of historically excluded nurses and our accomplices. The authors' commitment to including health equity makes the lack of accountability for nursing's historical and ongoing investment in white supremacy culture and colonialism that much more glaring and unconscionable. This causes us to question; how will those not from historically excluded backgrounds be held accountable? How might spaces of nursing education become incubators where learners are fully in dialogue with and informing the world around them, beyond survival?

The New Essentials of Nursing Education

Similarly, the authors of the *New Essentials of Nursing Education* (American Association of Colleges of Nursing, 2021) frame the future as best imagined and brought forth by current oppressive structures, organizations, and leaders. The lack of reckoning in the *Future of Nursing Report* is also found here, endorsing ongoing erasure of the colonial and oppressive past. The authors of the *New Essentials* continue to tie the roots of nursing to Florence Nightingale, with a cursory mention of Mary Seacole. Further evidence of ongoing colonialism in this document includes competencies that are not indicative of "new thinking and new approaches," as they continue to focus on quantifiable measurements of behavioral objectives (Foth and Holmes, 2017; Schilling & Koetting, 2010). To facilitate learning under the auspices of the *New Essentials* document means cultivating a "work ready" workforce that accepts the current healthcare industry in its neoliberal machinery. The *New Essentials* authors' narrow conceptualizations limit the future of nursing and preclude genuine accountability to those whose health, self-determination, dreams, and futures we impact.

The Relevance of Accreditation

The Commission on Collegiate Nursing Education (CCNE), which regulates nursing education in the United States, released revised accreditation procedures in September 2021. The authors of these documents assert that they provide "an unbiased assessment of the quality of professional education programs" (CCNE, 2021). However, simultaneously every institution embodies particular epistemologies and stances, thus shaping nursing education in their image, which is never unbiased. An examination grounded in Critical Race Theory demands that we ask, "How is racism at work here?" In fact, asking how accreditation standards contribute to racism, colonialism, ableism, and various forms of overlapping systems of oppression would be a true next step in advancing health equity. Accreditation standards perpetuate a culture of fear, maintain the hidden curriculum (Giroux & Penna, 1979; Glicken & Merenstein, 2007), and veer away from centering communities as partners. Faculty decisions are shaped by the specter of attrition rates, adherence to the Essentials, NCLEX pass rates, and employment. These are benchmarks that buttress industries that profit from the health care industrial complex.

Calls to Action: Building a New Topography

Health inequities cannot be addressed without the interrogation of organizations and structures that benefit from the status quo, where pursuit of social justice is optional and silenced, and where the focus is on formal schooling rather than the whole of health care. Shedding the relentless pursuit for legitimacy and status will allow us to ask expansive questions and strategize possibilities. In order for the nursing profession to consider a radical imagination for the present-future, we pose the following series of questions, which can guide radical transformation. How might we transform the current healthcare industry into ecosystems of accountability, curiosity, and healing for generations to come? How might we learn from and build with peoples whose epistemologies and lifeways protect the health of populations and the planet- without voyeurism and appropriation? When the goal is internationalist justice for generations to come, how might the relevance of accrediting bodies, professional organizations, testing industries, and regulatory mechanisms shift? How might nursing and nursing care be reimagined in all settings if our study and practice were unmoored from the doctrine of profit over people and the purview of select educational institutions? How might deep study of the principles, practices, goals, and struggles of grassroots organizations and social movements transform nursing? How might we uplift and build on the health activism and liberatory work of the Black Panther Party, Zapatistas, ACT Up, the Young Lords, and the Combahee River Collective? How might nurses' conceptualizations of health be expanded by studying and acting in solidarity with Asian Pacific Islander Equality - Northern California, La Via Campesina, NDN Collective, the Poor People's Campaign, Red Canary Song, Sister Song, Mujeres Unidas y Activas, the International League of People's Struggle, International Migrants Alliance, and the Anti Police Terror Project? (Additional guiding questions are available in this chapter's online resources)

Diversity Is Not Enough

The above questions require that we contemplate and activate, beckoning us to consider; how can we address health inequities? Recently, nursing educational institutions began admitting more students from historically excluded backgrounds, resulting in a 2.2% increase in the admission rate of students into entry-level baccalaureate programs, from 66.7% in 2017-2018 to 68.9% in the 2018–2019 school year (Blash & Spetz, 2019). This minimal diversification of admissions was a response to the disparity in nursing in terms of ethnic representation, as identified by a 2017 survey, finding that 80.8% of active nurses in the workforce to be white/caucasian, a meager 0.3% increase from 2015 (AACN, 2021). Also factoring into this response was the growing need of cultural representation as the population of those from historically excluded backgrounds is projected to increase from 37% now to 57% by 2060 (D'Antonio & Whelan, 2009). Similar to the discussion in preceding sections, diversity is not enough to solve the problem if the same Euro-centric structures continue to uphold. There must be extensive rectification of the colonialist values within nursing. Initiatives designed around increasing racial diversity alone, in the absence of intersectionality and foundational changes, will circle around hiring practices and curricula to maintain status quo. Application of anti-racist strategies in nursing education would be the best path forward for a more equitable and anti-oppressive admissions process. These strategies include understanding frameworks such as Critical Race Theory, Decolonizing Theory, Race Equity Culture, Cultural Humility, or Strategic Empathy (Nardi et al., 2020, p. 700).

The admissions process controls the gateway into nursing and influences every aspect of the profession. In order for nursing to embody inclusion and diversity, admissions practices must be transformed. In 2016, the AACN made an agreement in which nursing programs that trained their staff to adopt a more holistic approach to admissions review, would receive more technical assistance through the Nursing Workforce Diversity Program. To increase diversity, many institutions utilize the Holistic Admissions Review (HAR) strategy, which is based on the EAM format that uses Experiences, Attributes, and Academic Metrics, to assess applications. However, the HAR does not prevent an admission committee member's personal biases from affecting the outcome of an applicant's acceptance/rejection into the program. It is also important to note that even though standardized testing is utilized in the admissions practices of nursing programs and is required for licensure in the United States, it is not a global phenomenon. Countries with healthy populations such as Norway, Finland, and the United Kingdom, do not have standardized testing for their nursing programs (Ensio et al., 2019; Sjetne et al., 2019). If these countries can maintain the health and well-being of their people without assessing the technical proficiency of their nursing students through standardized examinations, the United States can as well.

Systems of Accountability

Through the lens of justice and inclusion, there is no system in place that holds nursing faculty and leadership accountable. Sustained commitment to effective strategies that push beyond diversity will result from a lens focused on a robust understanding of systems of oppression being mutable, restrictive, hierarchical, and complex, (Adams & Bell, 2016). Given a more current review based on transformative justice, the four steps of accountability: self-reflect, apologize, repair, and change behavior would advance Justice, Equity, Diversity, and Inclusion (JEDI) (Mingus, 2019). To ensure these steps are being followed, we would need a uniformed, standardized system with a rigorous rubric aligned with non-oppressive values and practices, guided by socially just policies in genuine appreciation of each other.

A Call to Action for Nursing Leadership, (Nardi et al., 2020), was written by nurses for nurse leaders, aimed to dismantle racist structures within all levels of the nursing profession. They provided a set of recommendations, which we endeavor to build upon by critically analyzing and questioning them in regards to the educational setting. Based upon Nardi et al. (2020) suggestions, we recommend that nursing faculty engage in study, discussion, and collectively address institutional oppression in every space where faculty meet, work, strategize, assess, and teach. These steps and actions taken to address institutional oppression should be documented to show accountability. Nardi et al. (2020) further recommend incorporating opportunities for difficult racialized conversations to occur within senior guidance and support, but the authors do not outline who is considered "senior" and who has "qualified guidance." We question, who would be deciding these qualifications? And if nurses were averse to discussing racism, how would these conversations occur? Therefore, we recommend that faculty take note of the class environment, document the actions that were taken toward creating more open dialogue, and re-evaluate the effectiveness of those actions. Lastly, we advocate for nurse educators to undergo training on addressing conflict fairly, through self-reflection, apology, and repair in order to ensure they are qualified to facilitate this learning.

Conclusion

Uprooting contradictions and repairing harm that is entrenched throughout nursing education constitutes our work ahead. A multiplicity of epistemologies and liberatory approaches to learning and care continue to be silenced and siloed out of nursing curricula, learning materials, program policies, handbooks, committees, notions of success, lines of inquiry, and collective imagination. This does not mean, however, that there is an absence of guidance and solutions (Boyd et al., 2020; Garland & Batty, 2021; Garneau et al., 2021). That being said, the fact that the concerted pursuit of social justice through reckoning remains optional or the responsibility of Nurses of Color, demands disruption. Communities continue to suffer needlessly and resist in beautiful ways while much of nursing continues to invest in empires. We are committed to ecosystems where nursing students are not merely surviving an obstacle course of gatekeeping but are actively in critical internationalist dialogue and action, with health and liberation at the core.

References

AACN Fact Sheet - Enhancing Diversity in the Nursing Workforce. (2019). American Association of Colleges of Nursing. https://www.aacnnursing.org/news-information/fact-sheets/enhancing-diversity

Adams, M., & Bell, L. A. (2016). Theoretical foundations for social justice education. In *Teaching for diversity and social justice* (pp. 21–44). Routledge.

American Association of Colleges of Nursing. (October 20, 2008). The essentials of Baccalaureate education for professional nursing practice. Retrieved from http://www.aacn.nche.edu/education-resources/BaccEssentials08.pdf

American Nurses Association. (2015). Code of ethics for nurses with interpretive statements. https://www.nursingworld.org/practice-policy/nursing-excellence/ethics/code-of-ethics-for-nurses/coe-view-only/

American Association of Colleges of Nursing (2021). The Essentials: Core Competencies for Professional Nursing Education. https://www.aacnnursing.org/Portals/42/AcademicNursing/pdf/Essentials-2021.pdf

American Association of Colleges of Nursing. (2021). Procedures for accreditation of baccalaureate and graduate nursing programs.

Au, W. (2016). Meritocracy 2.0: High-stakes, standardized testing as a racial project of neoliberal multiculturalism. *Educational Policy*, 30(1), 39–62.

Barbee, E. L. (1993). Racism in US nursing. *Medical Anthropology Quarterly*, 7(4), 346–362.

Bell Jr, D. A. (1975). Serving two masters: Integration ideals and client interests in school desegregation litigation. *Yale. LJ*, 85, 470.

Bell, B. (2021). White dominance in nursing education: A target for anti-racist efforts. *Nursing Inquiry*, 28(1), e12379.

Bennett, C., Hamilton, E. K., & Rochani, H. (May 31, 2019) Exploring race in nursing: Teaching nursing students about racial inequality using the historical lens. *OJIN: The Online Journal of Issues in Nursing*, 24(2).

Blash, L., & Spetz, J. (2019). California Board of Registered Nursing 2017-2018 annual school report.

Boyd, R. W., Lindo, E. G., Weeks, L. D., & McLemore, M. R. (2020). On racism: a new standard for publishing on racial health inequities. *Health Affairs Blog*, 10(10.1377).

Bray, S. R., & McLemore, M. R. (2021). Demolishing the myth of the default human that is killing Black mothers. *Frontiers in Public Health*, 9, 630.

Breilh, J. (2021). *Critical epidemiology and the people's health.* USA: Oxford University Press.

Carabez, R., Pellegrini, M., Mankovitz, A., Eliason, M., Ciano, M., & Scott, M. (2015). "Never in all my years … ": Nurses' education about LGBT health. *Journal of Professional Nursing*, 31(4), 323–329.

CCNE: Commission on Collegiate Nursing Education. (2021). *Procedures for accreditation of baccalaureate and graduate nursing programs.* https://www.aacnnursing.org/Portals/42/CCNE/PDF/Procedures.pdf

Choy, C. C. (2003). Empire of care. *Nursing and Migration in Filipino American History.*

Darder, A. (2005). Schooling and the culture of dominion: Unmasking the ideology of standardized testing. *Critical Theories, Radical Pedagogies, and Global Conflicts Rowman & Littlefield,* 207–222.

D'Antonio, P., & Whelan, J. C. (2009). Counting nurses: The power of historical census data. *Journal of Clinical Nursing, 18*(19), 2717–2724. 10.1111/j.1365-2702.2009.02 892.x

Eaker, M. (2021). wâhkôtowin: A nehiyaw Ethical Analysis of Anti-Indigenous Racism in Canadian Nursing. *Witness: The Canadian Journal of Critical Nursing Discourse, 3*(1), 31–44.

Ensio A., Lammintakanen J., Härkönen M., et al. Finland. In A. M. Rafferty, R. Busse, B. Zander-Jentsch, et al., (Eds.), (2019). *Strengthening health systems through nursing: Evidence from 14 European countries [Internet].* European Observatory on Health Systems and Policies. (Health Policy Series, No. 52.).

Essex, R., Markowski, M., & Miller, D. (2021). Structural injustice and dismantling racism in health and healthcare. *Nursing Inquiry, 29*(1), e12441.

Foth, T., & Holmes, D. (2017). Neoliberalism and the government of nursing through competency-based education. *Nursing Inquiry, 24*(2), e12154.

Garland, R., & Batty, M. L. (2021). Moving beyond the rhetoric of social justice in nursing education: Practical guidance for nurse educators committed to anti-racist pedagogical practice. *Witness: The Canadian Journal of Critical Nursing Discourse, 3*(1), 17–30.

Garneau, A. B., Bélisle, M., Lavoie, P., & Sédillot, C. L. (2021). Integrating equity and social justice for indigenous peoples in undergraduate health professions education in Canada: A framework from a critical review of literature. *International Journal for Equity in Health, 20*(1), 1–9.

Giroux, H. A., & Penna, A. N. (1979). Social education in the classroom: The dynamics of the hidden curriculum. *Theory & Research in Social Education, 7*(1), 21–42.

Glicken, A. D., & Merenstein, G. B. (2007). Addressing the hidden curriculum: Understanding educator professionalism. *Medical teacher, 29*(1), 54–57.

Godsey, J. A., Houghton, D. M., & Hayes, T. (2020). Registered nurse perceptions of factors contributing to the inconsistent brand image of the nursing profession. *Nursing Outlook, 68*(6), 808–821. 10.1016/j.outlook.2020.06.005

Goggins, S. (2021). Reshaping public memory in the 1619 project: Rhetorical interventions against selective forgetting. *Museums & Social Issues, 14*(1–2), 60–73.

Green B. (2016). Decolonizing of the nursing academy. *The Canadian Journal of Native Studies, 36*(1), 131.

Hantke, S. (2021). *Still a Long Way to Go: Integrating Antiracist, Anti-oppressive Education in Nursing* (Doctoral dissertation, University of Saskatchewan).

Hassouneh, D. (2008). Reframing the diversity question: Challenging Eurocentric power hierarchies in nursing education. *Journal of Nursing Education, 47*(7), 291–292.

Iheduru-Anderson, K. C. (2021). The White/Black hierarchy institutionalizes White supremacy in nursing and nursing leadership in the United States. *Journal of Professional Nursing, 37*(2), 411–421.

Institute of Medicine. (2010). The future of nursing: Leading change, advancing health. https://books.nap.edu/openbook.php?record_id=12956&page=R1

Jones, C. P. (2000). Levels of racism: A theoretic framework and a gardener's tale. *American Journal of Public Health, 90*(8), 1212–1215. 10.2105/ajph.90.8.1212

Kaba, M. (2021). *We do this' til we free us: Abolitionist organizing and transforming justice.* Haymarket Books.

Keeton, V. F. (2020). What's race got to do with it? A close look at the misuse of race in case-based nursing education. *Nurse Educator, 45*(3), 122–124.

Knopf, A., Budhwani, H., Logie, C. H., Oruche, U., Wyatt, E., & Draucker, C. B. (2021). A review of nursing position statements on racism following the murder of George Floyd and other Black Americans. *Journal of the Association of Nurses in AIDS Care, 32*(4), 453–466. [available here]

Koschmann, K. S., Jeffers, N. K., & Heidari, O. (2020). "I can't breathe": A call for antiracist nursing practice. *Nursing Outlook, 68*(5), 539.

Ladson-Billings, G., & Tate, W. F. (2016). Toward a critical race theory of education. In *Critical race theory in education* (pp. 10–31). Routledge.

Lajimodiere, D. K. (2014). American Indian boarding schools in the United States: A brief history and legacy.

Lambert, T. (2022, January 16). Who invented exams? A history of examination. *Local Histories.* https://localhistories.org/who-invented-exams/

Lorde, A. (1984). *Sister outsider: Essays and speeches. Crossing Press feminist series.* Trumansburg, N.Y.: Crossing Press.

Magnet Recognition Program® | ANCC. (2020). ANA. https://www.nursingworld.org/organizational-programs/magnet/

McFarling, U. (Sept. 23, 2021). 'Health equity tourists': How white scholars are colonizing research on health disparities. *STAT.* https://www.statnews.com/2021/09/23/health-equity-tourists-white-scholars-colonizing-health-disparities-research/

Mingus, M. (2019, Dec 18). *The four parts of accountability: How to give a genuine apology part 1.* Leaving Evidence. Retrieved from https://leavingevidence.wordpress.com/2019/12/18/how-to-give-a-good-apology-part-1-the-four-parts-of-accountability/

Morris, M. (2016). *Pushout: The criminalization of Black girls in schools.* The New Press.

Nardi, D., Waite, R., Nowak, M., Hatcher, B., Hines-Martin, V., & Stacciarini, J. M. R. (2020). Achieving health equity through eradicating structural racism in the United States: A call to action for nursing leadership. *Journal of Nursing Scholarship, 52*(6), 696–704.

National Academies of Sciences, Engineering, and Medicine. (2021). *The future of nursing 2020–2030: Charting a path to achieve health equity.* Washington, DC: The National Academies Press. 10.17226/25982.

Nazareno, J., Yoshioka, E., Adia, A. C., Restar, A., Operario, D., & Choy, C. C. (2021). From imperialism to inpatient care: Work differences of Filipino and White registered nurses in the United States and implications for COVID-19 through an intersectional lens. *Gender, Work & Organization, 28*(4), 1426–1446.

Nelson, S. L., & Williams, R. O. (2019). From Slave Codes to Educational Racism: Urban Education Policy in the United States as the Dispossession, Containment, Dehumanization, and Disenfranchisement of Black Peoples. *JL Soc'y, 19,* 82.

Practicalnursing.org Staff Writers. (2021, November 9). *The importance of holistic nursing care: How to completely care for your patients.* PracticalNursing.Org. https://www.practicalnursing.org/importance-holistic-nursing-care-how-completely-care-patients

Puzan, E. (2003). The unbearable whiteness of being (in nursing). *Nursing Inquiry, 10*(3), 193–200.

Schilling, J. F., & Koetting, J. R. (2010). Underpinnings of competency-based education. *Athletic Training Education Journal, 5*(4), 165–169.

Schroeder, C. PhD, RN, DiAngelo, R. PhD (July/September 2010). Addressing whiteness in nursing education. *Advances in Nursing Science, 33*(3), 244–255. doi: 10.1097/ANS.0b013e3181eb41cf

Smith, K. 2021. Moving beyond florence: Why we need to decolonize nursing history. https://nursingclio.org/2020/12/17/black-before-florence-black-nurses-enslaved-labor-and-the-british-royal-navy-1790-1820/

Sjetne, I. S., Tvedt, C. R., Ringard, Å. (2019). Norway. In A. M. Rafferty, R. Busse, & B. Zander-Jentsch, et al. (Eds.) *Strengthening health systems through nursing: Evidence from 14 European countries [Internet].* Copenhagen (Denmark): European Observatory on Health Systems and Policies. (Health Policy Series, No. 52.)

Threat, C. J. (2015). *Nursing civil rights: Gender and race in the Army Nurse Corps.* University of Illinois Press.

Truitt, A. R., & Snyder, C. R. (2020). Racialized experiences of black nursing professionals and certified nursing assistants in long-term care settings. *Journal of Transcultural Nursing, 31*(3), 312–318.

Valderama-Wallace, C. P. (2017). Critical discourse analysis of social justice in nursing's foundational documents. *Public Health Nursing, 34*(4), 363–369.

Valderama-Wallace, C. P., & Apesoa-Varano, E. C. (2020). 'The Problem of the Color Line': Faculty approaches to teaching Social Justice in Baccalaureate Nursing Programs. *Nursing Inquiry, 27*(3), e12349.

Walker, J. R. A. T. (2021). *The Racist Beginnings of Standardized Testing | NEA.* National Education Association. https://www.nea.org/advocating-for-change/new-from-nea/racist-beginnings-standardized-testing

12 Open Nursing Science: Using Citizen Science to Make Nursing Knowledge Wide-Open

Patrick McMurray

I am a Black non-disabled cisgender-heterosexual man raised in the rural and southeastern United States. I identify as a Christian and am one of Jehovah's Witnesses. Like my mother before me, I am a registered nurse taking the community college pathway to enter into nursing. My nursing career has included clinical care in inpatient and outpatient settings and functioning as a nurse educator to Associate Degree Nursing (A.D.N.) and Practical Nursing (P.N.) students. I am an avid participant in various citizen science projects. I hold membership in several formal and informal groups and organizations: The Citizen Science Association (C.S.A.), The Disrupt and Reimagine Nursing (D.N.R.) Twitter group, and The Nursology Theory Collective (NTC).

Introduction

Citizen science first entered my awareness five years ago when I was desperately looking for ways to support causes I loved but did not plan to pursue as a career. As a nurse, I work most intimately with people in relation to the health sciences. My education was a curated mix of learning about and applying the social and natural sciences (as well as the arts), such as psychology, sociology, various biological sciences, and chemistry. Even though these things continue to fascinate me, I also love and am curious about marine science, astronomy, and ecology and what those disciplines could teach me about science as a practice and the world and society in which I practice nursing. Citizen science allowed me to expand my knowledge without shifting my career trajectory or having pre-established relationships in those science communities. In this essay, I hope to convey the wonder I feel when I consider the possibilities that citizen science could offer us in nursing as a research methodology and conceptual framework. Specifically, this essay addresses what we currently know about citizen science and nursing, and what we have yet to observe when the two intersect. This essay will discuss the possible implications of integrating citizen science into nursing from the standpoint of education, research/knowledge development, and practice.

DOI: 10.4324/9781003245957-18

Conceptual Framework

This essay draws heavily on the idea of open science. Open science concerns the assumptions and philosophies surrounding transparency in creating and disseminating knowledge (Fecher & Friesike, 2014). Beyond superficial transparency, the practice of open science challenges us to imagine a world where accessibility of knowledge is a starting point that leads to an open invitation to the creation, expansion, and dissemination of knowledge. Open science asks us to be hungry for futures where knowledge is not only consumable but also collaboratively defined and augmented by the global constituency. In many ways, open science positions us to confront the silos we have created in knowledge, pitting the physical sciences, social sciences, and humanities against one another (Sidler, 2014). Open science (or knowledge) offers a world where our historical ways of knowing and sharing knowledge can be challenged and where the future of knowledge can be marvelously wide-open to whatever wondrous imaginings that we can collectively weave into a tangible reality.

Honoring the legacy of knowledge within my community, this essay is also informed by the concept of "doing right by folks." This is a conceptual framework that likely has never been inscribed in a book or journal article. It is a theory or concept that has been passed along, both orally and experientially, in my family and community. It is a conglomeration of other concepts like Ubuntu (I am because we are), the golden rule (treat others as you wish to be treated), and countless other emotions and expressions for which the English language has no singular expression. The closest expression to this concept that I have read in literature are the words of the late Toni Morrison, who said, "Make a difference about something other than yourselves" (Morrison, 1998). Unlike the hero rhetoric we see being shared surrounding nurses and healthcare workers in the ongoing COVID-19 pandemic, these words do not ask one to martyr themselves to save the world but rather to be invested in something outside ourselves as we relate to our communities. Part of "doing right by folks" means ensuring they have a voice in the things that impact them, and this aptly aligns with the concept of citizen science.

Background

Nursing, as a profession, is at a precipice. COVID-19 has challenged our profession in ways that are both inspiring and devastating. However, unlike ever before, our profession is positioned to disrupt and reimagine how we take up space. Increasingly, we see a need for nurses to hold roles in the community and outside of traditional care settings like hospitals and clinics. One of the most fantastic things about nursing is the fact that it is dynamic. The profession of nursing is in a near-perpetual state of metamorphosis, both in ways that are exhilarating and others that are frustrating. Time and circumstance have validated that we need nurses to show up in new and creative ways to serve their communities as clinicians, innovators, entrepreneurs, and agents of change.

In many ways, nursing is like a root-bound plant in a pot, in desperate need of replanting into fertile soil to truly flourish and we share responsibility for our halting growth. Our profession has had its fair share of being complicit in historical and present atrocities and injustices, both actively and passively. However, COVID-19 and the exacerbation of numerous ongoing historical traumas in 2020 have made it increasingly clear that what we have always done and thought, as a profession and as an academic discipline, will be insufficient as we hurtle forward in time. As a practice and a body of knowledge, nursing needs to be liberated to stretch and imagine new ways of existing. Citizen science offers nursing an emancipatory approach to nursing practice and knowledge development.

What Do You Mean by Citizen Science?

Citizen Science is a form of participatory research where the public participates in the scientific process to address real-world issues including activities across the spectrum of scientific inquiry, from data collection and analyzation to formulating research priorities and questions (U.S. General Services Administration & Wilson Center, nd). It is often conducted in partnership with professional scientists and academic institutions, but not exclusively. The National Institute of Health (NIH) further describes citizen science as being driven by community concerns (Vohland et al., 2021). Citizen Science is sometimes referred to as crowd-sourced science, with citizen science being the most common term globally recognizable, and thus is the term used in this essay. However, **citizen science is for EVERYONE** and is **NOT dependent on an individual's or group's citizenship or immigration status to a country or region** (Audubon Center at Debs Park, 2018). The European Citizen Science Association (ECSA) presents citizen science as a flexible concept that can be applied to diverse situations and disciplines (Robinson et al., 2018). The ECSA also collaborated internationally to develop ten principles concerning the best practice of citizen science {See box 12.1: *The Ten Principles of Citizen Science*}.

Box 12.1   The Ten Principles of Citizen Science. Source: (ECSA 10 *Principles of Citizen Science, 2015*)

1   *Citizen science projects actively involve citizens in scientific endeavor that generates new knowledge or understanding. Citizens may act as contributors, collaborators, or as project leader and have a meaningful role in the project.*

2 Citizen science projects have a genuine science outcome. For example, answering a research question or informing conservation action, management decisions or environmental policy.

3 Both the professional scientists and the citizen scientists benefit from taking part. Benefits may include the publication of research outputs, learning opportunities, personal enjoyment, social benefits, satisfaction through contributing to scientific evidence e.g., to address local, national and international issues, and through that, the potential to influence policy.

4 Citizen scientists may, if they wish, participate in multiple stages of the scientific process. This may include developing the research question, designing the method, gathering and analysing data, and communicating the results.

5 Citizen scientists receive feedback from the project. For example, how their data are being used and what the research, policy or societal outcomes are.

6 Citizen science is considered a research approach like any other, with limitations and biases that should be considered and controlled for. However, unlike traditional research approaches, citizen science provides opportunity for greater public engagement and democratisation of science.

7 Citizen science project data and meta-data are made publicly available and where possible, results are published in an open-access format. Data sharing may occur during or after the project, unless there are security or privacy concerns that prevent this.

8 Citizen scientists are acknowledged in project results and publications.

9 Citizen science programmes are evaluated for their scientific output, data quality, participant experience and wider societal or policy impact.

10 The leaders of citizen science projects take into consideration legal and ethical issues surrounding copyright, intellectual property, data sharing agreements, confidentiality, attribution, and the environmental impact of any activities.

Activities that fit the description of citizen science are documented as far back as the 17th century (Mahr et al., 2018). In recent years, the concept of citizen science has seen a resurgence in attention, particularly in the environmental sciences and the impact of climate change at the local and continental levels (Hecker et al., 2018). Notably, citizen science also has a vibrant history with activities such as bird-watching (Vohland et al., 2021). It can be easy for folks to only legitimize science when done within the silo of academia to dismiss citizen science as little more than community projects; however, doing this would be a mistake. Citizen Science is a legitimate method of scientific inquiry that makes a real-world impact on both local and international levels (see Box 12.2 Examples of the real-world impact of citizen science).

Box 12.2   Examples of the Real-World Impact of Citizen Science

1   Citizen science has helped identify new worlds (exoplanets) and more in NASA-sponsored projects.
2   The Environmental Protection Agency (E.P.A.) relies on data collected from citizen science.
3   Citizen Scientists, using gaming focused on protein folding, contributed to discovering new and creative ways to design proteins.
4   A Study being completed by researchers at Columbia University allows those living with endometriosis to become citizen scientists and contribute to the research about their lived experiences using the Phendo App.
5   Patients like me is an ongoing medical information-sharing effort utilized by healthcare providers and the people they serve to improve patient experiences in healthcare and treatment.

(*Note*: Please visit the online resources that accompany this chapter to view these examples of the real-world impact of citizen science)

In an effort to utilize more inclusive language, there are sentiments to rebrand citizen science to community science (C. B. Cooper et al., 2021). However, it is important to note that community science and citizen science, while related in many ways, have distinct features. **Community science** (also called community-driven science) can be distinguished from citizen science in that in community science the ownership of the project is always in the hands of the community and may not include academic institutions and researchers at all, is also often driven by the need for social action relevant to the community (Lief, Louise, 2021). Furthermore, community science has a particular history of being linked to social action related to the protection and improvement of the community and human rights (C. B. Cooper et al., 2021). This is contrasted by citizen science, where final ownership of the project is most often in the hands of the institution or professional scientist leading the project and the project may not be sourced in social action but to other scientific causes or endeavors. Cooper et al. (2021) caution against co-opting the term community-driven science, so as not to detract from the specific goals of this approach. Community science includes and intersects with the ideas of community-based participatory research and similar participatory methods that are intended to produce social change for communities and special populations (C. B. Cooper et al., 2021).

What Does This Have to Do With Nursing, and Why Does It Matter?

A virtually unfilled gap exists in the peer-reviewed literature exploring the relationship nurses have with citizen science. This is not completely surprising, as citizen science being embraced in biomedical, public health, and health equity research is a relatively recent phenomenon (Wiggins & Wilbanks, 2019). However, citizen science is growing and becoming more ambitious in the types of questions it seeks to address (Irwin, 2018).

As a distinct role and practice, nursing can be traced in historical records noted as far back as the ancient Egyptian (Elhabashy & Abdelgawad, 2019), Babylonian, Indian, and Grecian (Hunt, 2017) empires. As an academic body of knowledge, nursing is relatively young when considering it from the perspective of what western academia has deemed academic or scientific. Nursing, as a science, has been described as the science of human caring and human response to care and illness (Manhart Barrett, 2002). Further noted by Manhart Barrett (2002) is the difficulty in creating a comprehensive definition of nursing, as the work and knowledge of nursing can be interpreted in numerous ways. However, one truth is evident to nursing scholars and practitioners who are paying attention: the development of nursing knowledge has been reserved for the privileged few (Brown et al., 2021).

One of the current dilemmas we face in nursing is those who are allowed to participate most intimately in the generation and manipulation of nursing knowledge come from a highly exclusive group within nursing. In a TEDx talk, citizen science advocate Dr. Caren Cooper noted that:

> There's some long standing stereotypes about science. That it's lofty. That it's separate from the rest of us ... Science typically takes place out of sight, behind closed doors. With science, you have to choose which side of the door you want to be on, and you're either all in or you are out ... What if we end the stereotype of scientists being special by changing science in a fundamental way? By eliminating the door (C. Cooper, 2017).

We see Dr. Cooper's words play out in the world of nursing science as well. The individuals who are allowed to most intimately interact with, define, and manipulate nursing science are mostly prepared with graduate degrees, most specifically the doctor of philosophy in nursing (Ph.D.). Some may view this as appropriate. However, this current system alienates the vast majority of nurses who do not hold such credentials or who hold advanced education in disciplines outside of nursing. Thus, we are left with the privileged few, almost exclusively white cisgender women, who hold the reins of power and influence over nursing knowledge (Salerno et al., 2017). Citizen science offers us the opportunity to create a portal that decentralizes power and influence in our science and knowledge (Vohland et al., 2021). Similar to the idea put forth by Dr. Cooper (2017), academic discussions about science (nursing science) often happen behind closed doors and to those with the inherent and (or) acquired privilege to have access to the world behind these doors.

As a Black man who entered nursing through the community college associate degree in nursing pathway, I have personal experience with being made to feel as if I was not worthy of being a nurse or scholar. To compound those violent feelings, when I regarded those presented as nursing scholars and theorists early in my career, I very rarely saw a face that reminded me of my own. Nursing remains disproportionately dominated by cisgender women, who identify as white (Smiley et al., 2018). Citizen science can act as a mechanism for changing our approach to developing and expanding nursing knowledge to validate that being a part of science, even nursing science, should not be limited to those with particular academic credentials or job titles. However, in nursing, the academy jealously guards who gets to be viewed as a scholar, scientist, theorist, leader, innovator, and change-maker.

Titles, such as scientists, are fiercely guarded, in part because of the social currency and authority the title holds (Pew Research Center, 2015). Nursing is no exception to this tendency. There are currently three primary doctoral paths in nursing, the practice-focused Doctor of Nursing Practice (D.N.P), the Doctor of Education with a focus in Nursing Education (Ed.D.), and the doctor of philosophy in nursing (Ph.D.) (Ketefian & Redman, 2015). We have many who attribute the title of nurse scientist to only that 1% population of nurses who have completed a Ph.D. in nursing (Broome & Corazzini, 2016). This tendency is limiting because this population is exceptionally small and slow-growing, with less than 1000 people being granted a Ph.D. in nursing each year in the last ten years, compared with an average of 4,900 D.N.P graduates in the United States (Campaign for Action, 2021). However, some nurses cast the net of the title or role of scientist to all nurses, including those working in direct care roles during the pandemic (Sullivan-Marx, 2021). This is an essential consideration because it expands the idea of what it means to generate nursing knowledge and who does this work.

Certainly, Ph.D.-prepared nurses, who are comprehensively trained in various research methodologies, are very qualified to advance nursing knowledge. However, the academe must investigate how it could ever rightly deny the artistic way nurses working in direct care roles embody the science of nursing in an applied and practical manner. It is time to ask, not how or if, we bring Diploma, ADN, and PN-prepared nurses into the so-called "fold" of nursing science, but rather why "the fold" excluded them in the first place? Can we truly say that nursing, as a discipline, is better for excluding nearly half of the nursing workforce because of their educational point of entry? Particularly given the fact that it is from this half (Diploma, ADN, and PN programs) that we find the primary source for what ethnic, gender, and socioeconomic diversity we currently have in nursing.

The science and practice of nursing are not separate concepts, despite how we discuss and implement them in nursing. Nursing science does not exist without practice and practice does not improve or change without science and knowledge.

Who are we to tell the nurse in a medical-surgical unit or long-term care facility that they are not scientists or part of nursing science? These are nurses who facilitate and regulate biochemical reactions via medication administration and pharmacology while also navigating individuals and communities' biophysical, sociopolitical, and human-environmental health experiences. Nurses in direct, indirect, and academic roles generate and expand on nursing knowledge utilizing varying mechanisms and mediums, not all of which are acknowledged as scholarly or valid by the academy. Consider that, every day, nurses working in non-academic roles collect data, not simply on the people they care for but also on their work environments and communities. Nurses utilize this data to alter staffing needs, assess for trends, maintain supplies for care, anticipate phenomena, and act on collected data, often in a narrow span of time.

What Does a Future With Nurses Embracing Citizen Science Look Like?

At the 2021 #CitSciVirtual Conference hosted by the Citizen Science Association (C.S.A.) I was able to view poster presentations that were the product of professional and non-professional citizen scientists with varying education levels, presenting their citizen science projects and posters alongside one another. In this conference, I caught a glimpse of a future where science belongs to everyone. It is a place where communities, and the individuals in them, are empowered to ask questions, seek answers, and disseminate knowledge in a way that is accessible and meaningful.

It's time for nurses (and others) to be a part of **doing science "out loud" and in the open.** As we forge new possibilities for the future, ones that will require us to work more meaningfully with communities, public and open science will be imperative. Communities want to be informed and involved. The future of nursing and citizen science is ours to design. We must seize the opportunity that citizen science gives us to reimagine nursing knowledge, practice, and education.

Research and Knowledge

For so long, not only in nursing, we have been guilty of what I call "researching **AT** people." Technology and social change demand that we start making the community **EQUAL PARTNERS** in the care processes we create and in scientific knowledge. It is time to do less "researching **AT** people and communities" and more "co-creating research **WITH** people and communities." Citizen science offers flexibility, on the part of researchers and the public, in ways that many may not have considered. It allows more people from all over the world to contribute to science/research. Citizen science and community science-driven studies can have varying levels of complexity and design, offering participants the chance to participate at varying levels (see Figure 12.1), from data collection to co-designing studies and establishing research priorities.

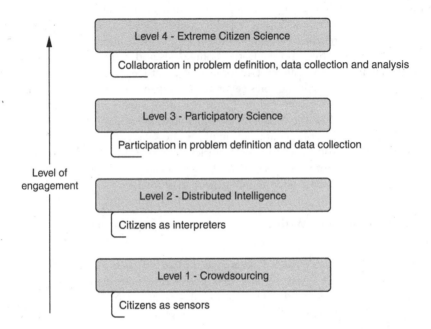

Figure 12.1 Levels of Citizen Science (Available via license: CC BY 4.0).

Citizen science, as well as its counterpart community science, offers a chance to help reconcile the gap between the academy and the community that occurred with the professionalization of science because it creates the circumstances where we can re-engage the public in science (Mahr et al., 2018). With the broader population of nurses engaging with nurse researchers, nursing is well-positioned to make an impact on making meaningful strides to be worthy of the trust of their communities. A Gallup poll has consistently demonstrated that a more significant portion of Americans rated nurses as the most honest and ethical professionals (Gallup Inc, 2020). However, we in nursing have not always made that trust meaningful nor have we always wielded and leveraged it responsibly. Citizen science allows us to restore the notion that science belongs to everyone and increases transparency, something that is foundational if we are to rebuild the public's trust in science (Boele-Woelki et al., 2018). It stands to reason that people are more likely to optimally understand and trust processes and projects in which they could participate and share ownership. However, we must be conscious that citizen science will be a starting point and will not easily cure some legitimate mistrust in the academy or research.

The mistrust of research and researchers in certain populations, such as the Black community, is rooted in a long history of the weaponization of science to justify racism and violence (Scharff et al., 2010). Beyond increasing participation and engagement in research, citizen science also positions communities to conduct their own citizen science projects and collect data in an enhanced way that external researchers could not. This lays the foundation for a future where science and knowledge development are no longer bound solely to academic institutions but are also within the realm of possibility for communities within their networks. Citizen science allows us to envision a future where people can come together to ask questions about phenomena that impact them, design a project, and collect data to illustrate their concerns and needs. In this future of decentralized and democratized science, professional scientists and researchers could be embedded in the community rather than behind the gates of universities and labs, to help facilitate and support the communities in their projects.

Practice

Citizen science offers flexibility in how nurses in clinical practice collect and utilize data. These nurses often do not have advanced training in research methodologies or the funds or time to complete "traditional" full-scale research studies. However, a citizen science approach permits these nurses to answer questions about their patient populations, their work environment, and more. Currently, in clinical practice, many nurses frequently collect data about phenomena that occur in their work environments, whether it is tracking the origin or rate of healthcare-acquired infections or tracking information about the occurrence of patient falls. Often, nurses in clinical practice approach data generation and responses to data via mechanisms like the Plan, Do Study, Act (PDSA) quality improvement (Q.I.) projects. However, the PDSA QI project approach is not without its limitations or drawbacks. Knudsen et al. (2019) advised caution in claiming that PDSA inherently leads to improvement; these projects typically lack enough data to make causal assumptions and often lack theoretical rationale and contain methodological limitations. We must consider that there exist many outcome-oriented PDSA and Evidence-Based Practice (E.B.P.) focused Q.I. projects that are often designed with the patient's experience in mind, but leave the interpretation of data and evidence solely to clinicians (Baumann, 2010). Further, we must confront that many outcome-oriented projects can be primarily fiscally driven, which could diminish claims of patient-centeredness.

Citizen science can empower nurses to collaborate with both patients and clinicians in varying types of care environments to develop projects that collect data on an ongoing basis, a limitation of many quality improvement project designs, and make the resulting actions meaningful for those engaged in this work. Websites such as "Patients Like Me" is an example of a citizen science-inspired effort that allows patients to collaborate in their health journey in a way that honors their lived experience (Patients Like Me, 2020). Epidemiologists created projects, such as "Flu Near You" (F.N.Y.) at Harvard, collect real-time data from citizen scientists, and visualize it so that community members and clinicians can understand local influenza trends (Flu Near You, nd). The Stanford University department of medicine has developed a citizen science-based intervention for health equity by allowing community members to document features in the community that impacts their ability to maintain their health (Stanford University Department of Medicine, nd). The Our Voice Citizen science program has resulted in the publication of several different peer-reviewed articles using citizen science to build healthier community environments (Hinckson et al., 2017).

Another aspect of citizen science is how it can help support policy changes at varying levels. An international group of researchers developed the Citizen Science Impact Storytelling Approach (CSISTA) to help citizen science practitioners communicate the impact of their citizen science project on policy (Wehn et al., 2021). Implementing citizen science as a tool and extension of nursing practice gives nurses at all levels of nursing practice the potential to directly impact how we practice nursing, deliver nursing care, and translate our knowledge into meaningful action for our communities.

Education

As we move forward, we increasingly see the importance of clinicians and the public having access to education that enhances their scientific literacy. In the classroom, citizen science holds immense potential as a pedagogical tool that has been shown to instill a sense of community awareness, promote critical thinking, and increase scientific literacy (Shah & Martinez, 2016). In higher education, citizen science can help students, even in non-STEM courses (Krieg & Kramer Theorodou, 2020), see science as relevant to their personal lives (Jenkins, 2011). Jenkins (2011) also discusses how implementing citizen science in the classroom offers a humanistic approach to science education, even when strict curriculum standards bind educators.

As an educator in a community college nursing education programs (for both associate degree and practical nursing students) the possibilities for citizen science to enhance the scientific literacy of students in these types of programs are not missed. Often in peer-reviewed literature, the role and training of registered nurses educated at the associate degree (A.D.N) and practical nursing diploma (P.N.) level have been mischaracterized as simple technical nurses with limited capabilities and critical thinking ability, most often in comparison to their baccalaureate-prepared RN counterparts. While there are differences between the scope of practice and role of Licensed Practical Nurses (L.P.N) and Registered Nurses, the difference is much less evident between registered nurses educated in A.D.N programs and Bachelor of Science in Nursing (B.S.N), who take the same licensure examination.

The divisive and segregational rhetoric plaguing nursing literature regarding diploma, A.D.N-prepared registered nurses, and practical nurses perpetuates harmful stereotypes and generalizations. We even see evidence of this thinking spilling over into the public, with a New Hampshire representative, Linda Tanner, denigrating community college-educated nurses in early 2021, later offering an "apology" (Graham, 2021). Dismissive rhetoric about nurses educated in community colleges or as practical nurses often particularly harms those from historically disadvantaged groups, who depend on these types of programs to enter the nursing profession (Mohammed et al., 2021; Orsolini-Hain & Waters, 2009). Licensed Practical Nurses make up the most ethnically diverse group of licensed nursing professionals (Livornese, 2012). In addition to perpetuating a hierarchical and classist view of nursing, these stereotypes and mischaracterizations of community college-educated nurses often lack a contextual understanding, and assumptions made about these programs have historically been based on minimal and outdated data or complete lack of data information (Mahaffey, 2002).

Implementing citizen science into the curriculum of all levels of undergraduate and graduate nursing education offers a new option for fortifying the scientific literacy and practical research skills of students of nursing. Particularly concerning A.D.N and P.N. diploma programs, citizen science offers these students to further demonstrate their ability to achieve scientific and research competency similar to that of their peers in baccalaureate programs and higher. It may be tempting for some to fall into the unimaginative and closed-minded view that nurses prepared at the diploma or associate degree level do not possess the skills and knowledge to meaningfully contribute to nursing knowledge. However, a shift in perspective is needed in this regard, for nursing knowledge is developed or has the potential to be developed in any of the ways which nurses practice. Beyond this, citizen science offers an opportunity to envision a world where nurse scientists co-create knowledge more intimately with the communities they serve and with nurses in a variety of direct and indirect care roles.

Respecting Indigenous, Traditional, and Local Knowledge

Citizen science, as well as community science, can also act as a conduit to uplift indigenous, traditional, and local knowledge (Tengö et al., 2021). These systems of knowledge and methodologies have always been legitimate to those communities that own the knowledge. However, both historical and present western ideologies about knowledge, knowledge development, and the dissemination of knowledge have attempted to diminish these ways of knowing. As highlighted by the ten principles of citizen science, an essential tenet of citizen science is to acknowledge the contributions of citizen scientists in the project (Robinson et al., 2018), which includes the contribution of indigenous and localized knowledge. Both nursing and the academy at large have historically and presently done a poor job of acknowledging traditional knowledge and understanding outside the historically white-centered western culture and status quo.

Thoughts to Carry Forward

Citizen science is not the be-all and end-all of research and knowledge development; it presents challenges and limitations, just as any other method of doing science. Despite the potential of citizen science to democratize and decentralize science and knowledge generation, it is still disproportionately inaccessible and underutilized by historically excluded groups in many places (Paleco et al., 2021). Questions and debates about how citizen science should intersect with institutional review boards (I.R.B.s) continue in the scientific community. There is a need to ensure that human subjects are protected and that citizen science projects are conducted ethically (Resnik, 2019). Simultaneously, we need meaningful conversations about I.R.B.s, who is included in them, and who goes unrepresented across all research realms. Beyond conversation, we desperately need a tangible reimagining of how to ethically facilitate public-driven research in a way that meaningfully centers and includes communities impacted by and engaged in the work of knowledge development. Citizen science presents us with a future where the ownership of science is open to anyone who wishes to be included. By making science within reach of EVERYONE who wishes to be included, we slowly begin to challenge the historical narrative of who gets to ask questions and how we find answers. There is an undeniable liberty in being able to ponder the world around us and yet even more freedom in being equipped to pursue and interpret truth for oneself. I impatiently await the future where communities and nurses are less dependent on inaccessible institutions to discover the answers to the age-old questions of how, if, who, what, when, where, and why.

References

Audubon Center at Debs Park. (2018, May 2). *Why We're Changing From "Citizen Science" to "Community Science."* Https://Debspark.Audubon.Org/. https://debspark.audubon.org/news/why-were-changing-citizen-science-community-science

Baumann, S. L. (2010). The limitations of evidenced-based practice. *Nursing Science Quarterly, 23*(3), 226–230. 10.1177/0894318410371833

Boele-Woelki, K., Francisco, J. S., Hahn, U., & Herz, J. (2018). How we can rebuild trust in science—and why we must. *Angewandte Chemie International Edition, 57*(42), 13696–13697. 10.1002/anie.201805342

Broome, M. E., & Corazzini, K. (2016). Nurse scientist or nursing scientist: Future considerations for the field. *Nursing Outlook, 64*(6), 523–524. 10.1016/j.outlook.2016.09.008

Brown, B. B., Dillard-Wright, J., Hopkins-Walsh, J., Littzen, C. O. R., & Vo, T. (2021). Patterns of knowing and being in the COVIDicene an Epistemological and Ontological reckoning for Posthumans. *Advances in Nursing Science.* 10.1097/ANS.0000000000000387

Campaign for Action. (2021). *Transforming Nursing Education: Number of people receiving nursing doctoral degrees annually.* https://campaignforaction.org/issue/transforming-nursing-education/

Cooper, C. (2017, May 15). *Citizen Science: Everybody Counts | Caren Cooper | TEDxGreensboro* [Youtube Video]. TEDx. https://youtu.be/G7cQHSqfSzI

Cooper, C. B., Hawn, C. L., Larson, L. R., Parrish, J. K., Bowser, G., Cavalier, D., Dunn, R. R., Haklay, M. (Muki), Gupta, K. K., Jelks, N. O., Johnson, V. A., Katti, M., Leggett, Z., Wilson, O. R., & Wilson, S. (2021). Inclusion in citizen science: The conundrum of rebranding. *Science, 372*(6549), 1386–1388. 10.1126/science.abi6487

Elhabashy, S., & Abdelgawad, E. M. (2019). The history of nursing profession in ancient Egyptian society. *International Journal of Africa Nursing Sciences, 11,* 100174. 10.1016/j.ijans.2019.100174

Fecher, B., & Friesike, S. (2014). Open science: One term, five schools of thought. In S. Bartling & S. Friesike (Eds.), *Opening Science* (pp. 17–47). Springer International Publishing. 10.1007/978-3-319-00026-8_2

Flu Near You. (nd). *Who We Are.* Flunearyou.Org. https://flunearyou.org/#!/who-we-are

Gallup Inc, G. (2020, January 6). *Nurses Continue to Rate Highest in Honesty, Ethics.* Gallup.Com. https://news.gallup.com/poll/274673/nurses-continue-rate-highest-honesty-ethics.aspx

Graham, M. (2021, February 4). Rep's "Elitist" slam of community college nurses inspires criticism, semi-apology [news]. *InsideSources.* https://insidesources.com/reps-elitist-slam-of-community-college-nurses-inspires-criticism-semi-apology/

Hecker, S., Haklay, M., Bowser, A., Makuch, Z., Vogel, J., & Bonn, A. (2018). Innovation in open science, society and policy – setting the agenda for citizen science. In S. Hecker, M. Haklay, A. Bowser, Z. Makuch, J. Vogel, & A. Bonn (Eds.), *Citizen Science* (pp. 1–24). UCL Press; JSTOR. http://www.jstor.org/stable/j.ctv550cf2.8

Hinckson, E., Schneider, M., Winter, S., Stone, E., Puhan, M., Stathi, A., Porter, M., Gardiner, P., Santos, D., Wolff, A., & King, A. (2017). Citizen science applied to building healthier community environments: Advancing the field through shared construct and measurement development. *International Journal of Behavioral Nutrition and Physical Activity, 14.* 10.1186/s12966-017-0588-6

Hunt, D.D. (2017). Chapter 2: Nursing and medicine in ancient times. In *Fast facts about the nursing profession: Historical perspectives in a nutshell. Chapter 2.* Springer Publishing. https://connect.springerpub.com/content/book/978-0-8261-3139-3/part/part01/chapter/ch02

Irwin, A (2018). No PhDs needed: How citizen science is transforming research. *Nature, 562,* 480–482. 10.1038/d41586-018-07106-5

Jenkins, L. (2011). Using citizen science beyond teaching science content: A strategy for making science relevant to students' lives. *Cultural Studies of Science Education, 6,* 501–508. 10.1007/s11422-010-9304-4

Ketefian, S., & Redman, R. W. (2015). A critical examination of developments in nursing doctoral education in the United States. *Revista Latino-Americana de Enfermagem, 23*(3), 363–371. 10.1590/0104-1169.0797.2566

Krieg, C., & Kramer Theorodou, R. (2020, June 15). *CSA Webinar: Using Citizen Science in Non-STEM Courses- Virtual Happy Hour* [Youtube Video]. https://youtu.be/OGsEKVL5Rx0

Knudsen, S. V., Laursen, H. V. B., Johnsen, S. P., Bartels, P. D., Ehlers, L. H., & Mainz, J. (2019). Can quality improvement improve the quality of care? A systematic review of reported effects and methodological rigor in plan-do-study-act projects. *BMC Health Services Research, 19*(1), 683. 10.1186/s12913-019-4482-6

Lief, L. (2021). *The Promise of Community-Driven Science.* 46–53.

Livornese, K. (2012). The advantages of utilizing LPNs. *Nursing Management, 43*(8), 19–21. 10.1097/01.NUMA.0000416409.60732.14

Mahaffey, E. H. (2002). The relevance of associate degree nursing education: Past, present, future. *Online Journal of Issues in Nursing, 7*(2), 3.

Mahr, D., Göbel, C., Irwin, A., & Vohland, K. (2018). Watching or being watched: Enhancing productive discussion between the citizen sciences, the social sciences and the humanities. In S. Hecker, M. Haklay, A. Bowser, Z. Makuch, J. Vogel, & A. Bonn (Eds.), *Citizen Science* (pp. 99–109). UCL Press. https://www.jstor.org/stable/j.ctv550cf2.14

Manhart Barrett, E. A. (2002). What is nursing science? *Nursing Science Quarterly*, 15(1), 51–60. 10.1177%2F089431840201500109

Mohammed, S. A., Guenther, G. A., Frogner, B. K., & Skillman, S. M. (2021). Examining the racial and ethnic diversity of associate degree in nursing programs by type of institution in the US, 2012–2018. *Nursing Outlook*, 69(4), 598–608. 10.1016/j.outlook.2021.01.009

Morrison, T. (1998, February 2). *The Salon Interview—Toni Morrison | Salon.com* [Live interview]. https://www.salon.com/1998/02/02/cov_si_02int/

Orsolini-Hain, L., & Waters, V. (2009). Education evolution: A historical perspective of associate degree nursing. *Journal of Nursing Education*, 48(5), 266–271. 10.9999/01484834-20090416-05

Paleco, C., García Peter, S., Salas Seoane, N., Kaufmann, J., & Argyri, P. (2021). *Inclusiveness and Diversity in Citizen Science*. 261–281. 10.1007/978-3-030-58278-4_14

Patients Like Me. (2020). *PatientsLikeMe | About us*. PatientsLikeMe. https://www.patientslikeme.com/about

Pew Research Center. (2015). *Public and Scientists' Views on Science and Society* (p. 111). American Association for the Advancement of Science (AAAS). https://www.pewresearch.org/science/2015/01/29/public-and-scientists-views-on-science-and-society/#about-this-report

Resnik, D. B. (2019). Institutional review board oversight of citizen science research Involving human subjects. *The American Journal of Bioethics*, 19(8), 21–23. 10.1080/15265161.2019.1619864

Robinson, L., Cawthray, J., West, S., Bonn, A., & Ansine, J. (2018). *Ten principles of citizen science: Innovation in Open Science, Society and Policy* (pp. 27–40). 10.2307/j.ctv550cf2.9

Salerno, J. P., Gonzalez-Guarda, R., & Hooshmand, M. (2017). Increasing the pipeline and diversity of doctorally prepared nurses: Description and preliminary evaluation of a health disparities summer research program. *Public Health Nursing (Boston, Mass.)*, 34(5), 493–499. 10.1111/phn.12341

Scharff, D. P., Mathews, K. J., Jackson, P., Hoffsuemmer, J., Martin, E., & Edwards, D. (2010). More than Tuskegee: Understanding mistrust about research participation. *Journal of Health Care for the Poor and Underserved*, 21(3), 879–897. 10.1353/hpu.0.0323

Shah, H. R., & Martinez, L. R. (2016). Current approaches in implementing citizen science in the classroom. *Journal of Microbiology & Biology Education*, 17(1), 17–22. 10.1128/jmbe.v17i1.1032

Sidler, M. (2014). Open science and the three cultures: Expanding open science to all domains of knowledge creation. In S. Bartling & S. Friesike (Eds.), *Opening science: The evolving guide on how the internet is changing research, collaboration and scholarly publishing* (pp. 81–85). Springer International Publishing. 10.1007/978-3-319-00026-8_5

Smiley, R. A., Lauer, P., Bienemy, C., Berg, J. G., Shireman, E., Reneau, K. A., & Alexander, M. (2018). The 2017 national nursing workforce survey. *Journal of Nursing Regulation*, 9(3), S1–S88. 10.1016/S2155-8256(18)30131-5

Stanford University Department of Medicine. (nd). *The Our Voice Approach*. https://med.stanford.edu/ourvoice/the-our-voice-model-page-2.html

Sullivan-Marx, E. (2021, April 27). *Nurses are also scientists*. Scientific American. https://www.scientificamerican.com/article/nurses-are-also-scientists/

Tengö, M., Austin, B. J., Danielsen, F., & Fernández-Llamazares, Á. (2021). Creating synergies between citizen science and indigenous and local knowledge. *BioScience*, *71*(5), 503–518. 10.1093/biosci/biab023

U.S. General Services Administration, & Wilson Center. (nd). *About CitizenScience.gov* [Government Website]. CitizenScience.Gov. https://www.citizenscience.gov/about/#

Vohland, K., Land-Zandstra, A., Ceccaroni, L., Lemmens, R., Perello, J., Ponti, M., Samson, R., & Wagenknecht, K. (2021). *The science of Citizen Science*. Springer Nature. https://library.oapen.org/handle/20.500.12657/46119

Wehn, U., Ajates, R., Fraisl, D., Gharesifard, M., Gold, M., Hager, G., Oliver, J. L., See, L., Shanley, L. A., Ferri, M., Howitt, C., Monego, M., Pfeiffer, E., & Wood, C. (2021). Capturing and communicating impact of citizen science for policy: A storytelling approach. *Journal of Environmental Management*, *295*, 113082. 10.1016/j.jenvman.2021.113082

Wiggins, A., & Wilbanks, J. (2019). The rise of citizen science in health and biomedical research. *The American Journal of Bioethics*, *19*(8), 3–14. 10.1080/15265161.2019.1619859

13 Posthuman Pedagogy: Metamorphosing Nursing Education for a Dying Planet

Brandon Blaine Brown (He/Him/His)

Author Positionality—Situating Myself Amongst and Within the Extinctive Process

I write this essay as a white man thinking behind a comfortable desk within the academy about the history and present context of nursing, higher education, climate change, and environmental activism while imaging a radical alternative future for the discipline. As part of this process, I believe it is essential to claim my salient identities and privileges as an integral part of my movement toward unlearning and relearning to employ an ecologically-centered praxis and pedagogy. I identify as a white, cisgender man, who is non-disabled, queer, a nurse, a settler-colonizer, and a clinical assistant professor. I benefit from white-male privilege, white supremacy, capitalism, and dispossessed Indigenous lands. This has led me to have biases around gender, ableism, oppression, colonization, racism, and racial trauma, and I am on the path of critical self-reflection. I also embody the following assumptions: I am skeptical of the underpinnings of nursing education, and I believe that equity and justice are ongoing foundational components of nursing and educational work. I aspire to and believe in a radical future where nursing education has the potential to be liberatory and freeing in nature. I also firmly believe nursing has the potential to expand the environs of care to include: nonhumans, plants, animals, and Earth itself (Zoë) (Figure 13.1).

The Burning of Our Sublunary Planet

Nursing is built upon the principle foundation of caring. While initially, it seems that this simple value is centered upon caring for human beings, digging further reveals that there is much more to be discovered. Upon a more in-depth inspection, other hegemonic forces are at play within a broader global and societal context. These powers often manifest as vehicles of violence and oppression, including the profound and often contemptuous relationship that humans have with the environment. Currently, the primary foundation

DOI: 10.4324/9781003245957-19

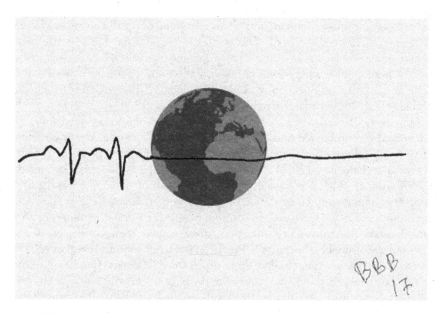

Figure 13.1 Caring for a Postmortem Planet.
Source: Image Created by Brandon Blaine Brown (2017).

of our human-centered relationship with Earth is under threat. We are living in a time of unprecedented change in which the planet we rest our feet upon continues to unravel, threatening the existence of life. Kolbert (2014) describes that we are currently living and dying in the 6th great extinction—a geological epoch that is filled with an abundant ongoing threat to human and non-human life. Colloquially geologists refer to our present time as the Anthropocene, an era that is defined by the unfettered reign of the Anthropos (the Greek root for human) upon Earth by shaping and reforming all corners of the planet while extinguishing life through the neoliberal interests of a capitalist society (Yusoff, 2018). The causes of the Anthropocene are not ambiguous, having burst forth from the depths of anthropocentrism (human exceptionalism), technological advancement, capitalism, and ongoing ecological extraction, including forced human labor and dispossessed Indigenous lands (Braidotti, 2019a; Yusoff, 2018).

Undeterred by the perils of the Anthropocene, paradoxically, we are also living in a time that economists refer to as the fourth great industrial revolution—a time of human progress, prosperity, great wealth, rising quality of life, and the infiltration of digital technology into all corners and crevices of our interwoven material reality (Braidotti, 2019a; Schwab, 2016). As part of this economic revolution, the lines between the physical, the digital, the biotic (living), and abiotic (nonliving) spheres of the world have become intertwined (Haraway, 2016; Schwab, 2016). However, the fourth industrial revolution does not come without pain—pain inflicted upon Earth, upon humans who have never been considered human, and all the denizens who call this planet home (Haraway, 2016; Yusoff, 2018). The economic panacea put forth by the neoliberal empire is plagued by rising rates of income inequality, health disparities, racism, homophobia, transmisia, police brutality, and ongoing environmental colonial projects resulting in ecocide (Braidotti, 2019a; Dillard-Wright & Shields-Haas, 2021; Dillard-Wright et al., 2020; LeClair et al., 2021).

Moreover, Chakrabarty (2021) describes that our human-centered foray of unchecked growth has led us down a path of undeniable damage to our environment that results in climate change and its associated threats to planetary health. Nicholas and Breakey (2017) describe climate change as an unfolding urgent health crisis in which nursing will be at the forefront of alleviating the harmful effects of environmental degradation on people worldwide and locally. These adverse impacts include increased deaths from heatwaves, respiratory illnesses, natural disasters, life-threatening infectious diseases, and their consequences on food and water supplies (Nicholas & Breakey, 2017). Nicholas and Breakey (2017) specify that those who must endure these effects will be those who are already most at risk. Furthermore, those who contribute the most to climate change at the population, community, and nation-state levels are the least likely to bear the effects (Stoddard et al., 2021). Environmental racism is hard at work, with disproportionate impacts documented in historically underserved communities (LeClair et al., 2021; Salas, 2021). Thus, addressing these hazards of the Anthropocene is of utmost importance for nursing education and practice. However, Leffers et al. (2017) note that while nursing education has the potential to advocate for change in many areas of society, it lags in productivity, thinking, and resources. This is due to multiple societal and global forces, including the construction of nursing knowledge and practice based upon colonialism, eurocentrism, and capitalism (McGibbon et al., 2014). These basic constructs permeate nursing education and the broader healthcare system of the United States, preventing ecological justice from taking root in nursing classrooms and practice areas.

In 2015, in the U.S., President Obama "convened a White House Summit on climate change and health, inviting deans from nursing, public health, and medical schools" to foster a commitment to the development of curricula and research to tackle climate change and ultimately lessen the impacts on human health (Sullivan-Marx & McCauley, 2017, p. 593). Despite this push from the federal government, nursing education in the U.S. has failed to attend to the effects of climate change on planetary health. Sullivan-Marx and McCauley (2017) further note that nurses who are experts on climate change are currently lacking due to an already overcrowded curriculum in nursing and a lack of funding for health-based climate research.

Humans are not the only beings-bodies that are at risk in the Anthropocene. Ecofeminist scholar Donna Haraway (2016) describes the profound entanglement that humans share with more than human worlds, including nonhuman entities such as plants, water, fish, land animals, and bacteria on which humans depend for survival and flourishing. As Haraway (2016) puts it, "we are at stake to each other" sharing an enduring common ground in an intertwined space of shared living and dying (p. 55). Similarly, feminist scholar Rosi Braidotti (2013) describes that we are living in posthuman times with an imminent and embodied connection "between the self and other, including the non-human or 'Earth' others" (p. 48). Given the deep relationality that humans share with other worlds and the ongoing threat to planetary health in the Anthropocene causes one to question: how will nursing education honor these bonds, cultivate a kinship with Earth, and engage in bidirectional eco-centered epistemological practices with students? It is clear that answering that question and addressing these more than human problems will require reconceptualizing the way in which we educate the nurses of the present and future. Becoming and being nurses during this time of entanglement will require nursing education to press forward with a reimagined ontological and epistemological foundation of discipline that promotes not only human but terrestrial flourishing. Located among this imperative is the need to transform nursing education with a turn toward our current posthuman reality, expanding the environs of care to a planetary level (LeClair & Potter, 2022). It is clear that our posthuman time is in urgent need of a posthuman education.

Therefore, given our posthuman condition, I wonder: How do faculty educate nurses to become caregivers of Earth—of all biotic and abiotic lifeforms in the Anthropocene? How does the professoriate educate nurses to care for the relational embeddedness of our lifeworld? This chapter will visit these particular questions by beginning with a brief overview of the conceptual framework and philosophical underpinnings that guide my thinking. From there, the chapter moves forward by unpacking the humanistic onto-epistemological underpinnings of the discipline and then situating them within the commodified territories of nursing and higher education that enshrine the extractive modes of capitalism while perpetuating the reign of the Anthropos. Stemming from these origins, I then propose a speculative vision for reimagining the ontological foundation for the discipline to propel nursing education toward rhizomatic (non-linear) learning and relational educational practices in hopes of these radiating out into a planetary caring praxis. The ultimate goal of which is to flatten hierarchies, abolish the dichotomy that separates humans from nature, and embrace multiple ways of knowing and educating that will allow us to better attend to the complexities of the Anthropocene.

Conceptual Framework—Blazing Through a Posthuman Tunnel Without Lights

Navigating the Anthropocene and moving forward during entangled times will require nursing to develop new modes of thinking that reframe the ontological premise of the discipline and redesign the foundational assumptions from which nurses are educated. Accomplishing these goals will require nursing to shift its current conceptual frame that centers upon humanism toward the philosophy of critical posthumanism that is grounded in new materialist perspectives. Critical posthumanism emphasizes a post-anthropocentric approach to thinking that de-centers the "the human in relation to the nonhuman," removing the onto-epistemological privilege of the human (Ferrando, 2019, p. 54). This allows one to think beyond the dualisms that have been constructed in western thought such as nature/culture, man/woman, human/animal, and alive/dead (Ferrando, 2019).

New materialism is an ontological feminist approach emanating from post-humanism that is grounded in quantum physics that allows us to recognize the material agency of non-human things, bodies, and beings—the agency of matter itself (Ferrando, 2019). In new materialism, the subject (the human) is no longer the center of thought or discourse, and there is no center, the focus is on all matter—the material substances that compose everything in the Universe (Bennett, 2010). Bennett (2010) explores this idea further by postulating that "matter is not the raw material for the creative activity of humans and Gods" (p. xiii), but it is rather our bodies, your body, my body, but also the bodies of whales, maple trees, ants, airplanes, feeding tubes, ventilators, and COVID-19. In new materialism, there is no separation or duality in these entities. Instead, they are all mixing and churning together—becoming compost (Haraway, 2016).

Utilizing a new materialist framework for nursing education requires educators and students to think through rhizomatic networks, and the assemblage of the subject (you, me, us, and others) and how it is formed, and to think in terms of matter beyond the anthropocentric frame (Bennett, 2010). Applying a new materialist lens in educational practices results in students and educators seeing living and nonliving matter—human and nonhuman—as radically active with po-tentiality and meaning. Ultimately, removing the human from the central position of thinking allows students and faculty to understand the possibilities in devel-oping nursing care from a planetary perspective that is "geo-centered, mediated, and has a non-anthropocentric frame of reference" (Braidotti, 2019b, p. xiv).

Despite the possibilities in thinking with new materialism, it is important to be critical of the way in which new materialist and posthuman philosophy participates in the co-optation of Indigenous knowledge systems. The threads and linkages to Indigenous epistemologies run deep, but these connections are often co-opted and appropriated without credit, reference, or citations (Bignall & Rigney, 2019). Furthermore, Bignall and Rigney (2019) note that new ma-terialism is not new philosophical thought, beckoning those who use it to in-terrogate this with critical reflection. I recognize the messiness of posthumanism and wonder how to navigate this as a white settler-colonizer. Understanding that moves such as these may be described as settler-moves to innocence and must be countered with action supporting Indigenous leadership, sovereignty, and land reparations (Tuck & Yang, 2012).

The Ethos of "Humanism"—The Ontological and Epistemological Foundation of Nursing Education

Nursing is built upon the fundamentals of humanism and human-centered caring practices (McCaffrey, 2019). Bennett (2010) describes that when a discipline operates from a humanistic frame, it prevents folks from seeing the capability of agency in more than human matter. Explaining the ways in which nursing came to develop a humanistic foundation first requires an examination of the eurocentric heritage of the discipline and how it infiltrates the present. McGibbon et al. (2014) describe that the guiding theoretical knowledge of nursing's metaparadigm and grand theories was developed by white women of privilege during the 1970s-1980s as a way for nursing to differentiate itself from medicine. Furthermore, McGibbon et al. (2014) state that these theories offer us "ethically inadequate modes" of thinking and doing within the context of globalization and capitalism, which promote environmental destruction (McGibbon et al., 2014, p. 184). Jakubec and Bearskin (2020) further note that "nursing knowledge and practice do not fully address the dimensions of power or sufficiently work to challenge such deep, and often taken for granted, structures of oppression" (p. 244). It is from these underpinnings drenched in eurocentrism and whiteness that nursing has and continues to theorize its disciplinary perspective, seen notably in the metaparadigm.

The primacy of the human rings forth from all corners of the theoretical groundwork of the discipline through the conceptualization of its various grand theories and the metaparadigm advanced by Fawcett and Desanto-Madeya (2013). Historically nursing knowledge has been constructed under the purview of its metaparadigm—providing structure, anchors, boundaries, and borders to disciplinary knowledge development (Fawcett & Desanto-Madeya, 2013). In the 1980s, Fawcett (2013) advanced the metaparadigm concepts of human beings, environment, health, and nursing. According to the hegemony of the academy, it is from these four concepts in which all nursing knowledge, research, care, and practice should emanate. The metaparadigm concepts within nursing describe the essence, meaning, and nature of nursing practice. Although there are contemporary moves away from these defining domains of the discipline, the metaparadigm still serves as a historical force of influence for the organization of knowledge development—foreclosing open networks of knowledge generation, diverse perspectives, and multiple ways of knowing (Kalogirou et al., 2020). For example, in 2022, Fawcett described the metaparadigm concept of the environment as needing "decolonization" (p. 263). However, Fawcett's (2022) vision for the future still centers an anthropocentric framing that is based in humanism, lacking attention to the posthuman planet and the material agency of matter. Ultimately, historical and contemporary conceptualizations of the environmental domain of the metaparadigm leave the discipline's understanding of the environment in a state of stasis.

Environment as Static—Nature/Culture Divide in Nursing Science

In 1986, nurse scholar Chopoorian critiqued the metaparadigm concept of the *environment*, suggesting that the "environment is rigidly conceptualized within nursing as a static entity that does not inform the nursing paradigm in a substantive manner, nor does it foster comprehensive images and relationships" (p. 41). Likewise, Kleffel using an ecofeminist framework (1991), stated that "the image of the environment as the immediate surroundings or circumstances of an individual or family has kept nurses from addressing the larger social, political, economic, and global structures that affect health" (p. 6). Therefore, nursing practice has traditionally occurred in the immediate surroundings of patients or directly on the human body focusing solely on the individual and their responses to the environment around them (Chopoorian, 1986; Kalogirou et al., 2020; Kleffel, 1991). Kalogirou et al. (2020) take this analysis further by postulating nursing's lack of engagement in planetary health results from the discipline's limited conceptualization of the environment in its metaparadigm and foundational grand theories—translating into shortcomings in addressing climate change and environmental degradation.

From these critiques, it is clear that the way in which the theoretical concept of the *environment* is constructed within the discipline has limited the purview of nursing work to individuals with persistent humanist and anthropocentric framings. Operating from this narrow assumption eclipses transformative action in the sociopolitical and environmental systems in which folks are caught up in. Furthermore, the discipline's limited view of the environment forecloses nursing's engagement with issues surrounding planetary health such as climate mitigation strategies to reduce its causative factors, and instead focuses on the individual downstream effects (Dillard-Wright et al., 2020; Kalogirou et al., 2020). Many nurse educators have been socialized into this paradigm of thought, imparting a human-centered onto-epistemological understanding of the environment to students where it infiltrates classrooms in conscious and unconscious ways—limiting possibility.

Given the historical disciplinary footing of nursing and the perils of the Anthropocene, the time has come for nursing to reconceptualize its environmental domain that honors our thick posthuman present. Reimagining the environment from a new materialist perspective promulgates the understanding that the environment ultimately is shaped by complex relationships beyond the human, with the environment not only affecting humans but vice versa—impacting the health and wellbeing of all matter. To accomplish this, the professoriate needs to educate from a relational new materialist conceptualization of the environment that focuses on the health of the planetary system. However, this reimagining will not be possible until the academy reckons with the ways in which nursing and higher education are constrained within the neoliberal market, which will be discussed next.

Industrializing Care: The Commodified Territory of Nursing Education in the United States

For nursing education to address the hazards of the Anthropocene, it must consider its present location in the commodified territories of higher education and the neoliberal healthcare system. We are currently living components and actors in what Braidotti (2019a) describes as the corporatization of the university impacting knowledge production practices and leading to the industrialization of the academy. Stoddard et al. (2021) explain that operating within this commodified setting privileges the knowledge-making practices associated with industrial modernity, making it difficult for students and faculty to construct a new social imaginary for the future that addresses climate change. Furthermore, agreeing with Bradiotti (2019a), Stoddard et al. (2021) explicate that the neoliberal educational agenda stifles creativity and critical analyses of the present, perpetuating neoliberal futures.

Nursing education is fettered to the neoliberal academic movement. This manifests with a monetized world bursting forth, bringing a penchant love for evidence-based practice, high-stakes testing, marginalizing admissions practices, competency-based education, and standardized licensure examinations (Fontenot & McMurray, 2020; Foth & Holmes, 2017; Holmes et al., 2006). These material forces coalesce and hold nursing curricula hostage to the market constraints of capitalism while upholding neoliberal walls around discipline. Educating from the logic of capitalism limits the possibilities of nursing education to address climate change and educate for a posthuman planet. Moreover, the corporatized structure of the academy perpetuates a grounding of nursing education that is based in eurocentrism and post-positivism, focusing on individuality and espousing anthropocentric ideas, while eliding kinship with Earth (Brown et al., 2022).

Preparing Workforce Ready Graduates and Licensure Examinations

The way in which nursing arrived into the commodified territory of higher education presents a complex cartography. The historical threads that have contributed to this moment are vast, but a significant factor includes the mandate by healthcare employers that nursing education prepares work-ready graduates who are fit for the marketplace and ready to become actors in the commercialized industrial healthcare complex. As evidence, The American Association of Colleges of Nursing (AACN), which guides the curricular development activities of baccalaureate, masters, and doctoral programs in the United States, put forth their new guidelines entitled the *Essentials: Core Competencies for Professional Nursing Education* in 2021. The most recent version of the AACN *Essentials* focuses on maintaining the ongoing industrialization of education/care through prescriptive curricular guidance to prepare graduates for the workplace (American Association of Colleges of Nursing, 2021). The *Essentials* includes a provision to educate entry-level registered nurses to "understand the impact of climate change on environmental and population health" (American Association of Colleges of Nursing, 2021, p. 36). However, humanism still figures prominently, with an absence of mitigation strategies at the entry to practice level. The entire *Essentials* document lacks awareness of multispecies responsibilities in a posthuman world. Planetary health is given a cursory mention as an essential component of a liberal education that is integrated within nursing, but the document does not explain how it should be integrated or how planetary health is framed (American Association of Colleges of Nursing, 2021).

The National Council Licensure Examination (NCLEX in the US) is another pillar of corporatization within the academy and perpetuates the monetization of knowledge—forestalling engagement with multispecies planetary health. The NCLEX exam forces faculty into pre-curated curricula based on the testing plan put forth by institutions and governing bodies such as the National Council of States Boards of Nursing (NCSBN)—obligating nursing education to privilege the biomedical model. This model is steeped in the ethos of humanism that focuses on quantitative empirical measures while averting an upstream focus on climate change (Dillard-Wright & Shields-Haas, 2021). The NCLEX prepares students for situations of certainty, but students undoubtedly encounter un-certain situations on a daily basis. The posthuman world requires us to think in terms of species and planetary systems (Chakrabarty, 2021), which are fore-closed upon by standardized testing. Standardized testing is incompatible with the deep thought that nursing requires to address the perils of the Anthropocene (Dillard-Wright & Shields-Haas, 2021). Furthermore, the NCLEX acts as a mode of policing and suppressing nursing curricula on the basis of pass rates and accreditation by state boards of nursing, requiring faculty to teach to the test with little room for deviation.

Sullivan-Marx and McCauley (2017) note that nursing has an overburdened curriculum preventing the inclusion of climate-related content. Sullivan-Marx and McCauley (2017) fail to note that perhaps the reason the curriculum is so overburdened is due to the way in which the neoliberal market infiltrates nursing education, serving the capitalist healthcare enterprise. In neoliberal modes of education, what counts as knowledge is authorized by the institutions steeped in white supremacy and privileges ways of knowing based on the western ideals (Whyte, 2016), not how to care in a posthuman world.

Toward a Posthuman Pedagogy—Cultivating a Sense of Multispecies Responsibility

Addressing planetary degradation, reckoning with the humanistic under-pinnings of the discipline, and disentangling nursing education from the neo-liberal economy will require new pedagogical practices beyond the virtues of what Braidotti (2013) calls the Vitruvian man. Nursing education must im-plement teaching practices that decenter the discipline's white, eurocentric, humanistic foundations. Posthuman pedagogical practices grounded in new materialist perspectives are potential tools to move beyond these historical cornerstones—illuminating a multispecies responsibility for students and fa-culty. Braidotti (2019a) describes that the benefits of a posthuman approach to education "targets both Humanism and anthropocentrism" (p. 141) while simultaneously working toward resisting the commodified models of higher education and life. A posthuman approach to education gives nurse educators the tools that they need to foreground planetary health in their classrooms and clinical spaces. Utilizing such an approach has the potential to center planetary justice. Ulmer (2017) describes that justice certainly affects humans, but justice is also found outside the realm of human relations. Ulmer (2017) explained that "justice can also be material, ecological, geographical, geological, geopolitical, and geo-philosophical. Justice is a more than human endeavor" (Ulmer, 2017, p. 833). Educating students toward Ulmer's (2017) vision of justice will require the enactment of pedagogies that decenters the human and embraces multiple ways of knowing.

Rhizomatic Knowing—Educating With bios and Zoë

Envisioning rhizomatic (non-linear) ways of knowing and pedagogical practices begin by resisting the impulses of western science and humanism and moving beyond the dualistic binaries that it imposes. When educators operate within a humanistic frame, it perpetuates what Chandra Pescord Weinstein refers to as white empiricism, preserving colonialism and anthropocentrism (Prescod-Weinstein, 2020). Instead, the academy needs to educate nurses to think in terms of species, moving beyond the canon of empirical knowledge and its biomedical undercurrents. This means shifting from educating for *bios* which refers to the "life humans have organized in society" to educating for Zoë which refers "to the life of all living beings" (Braidotti, 2019a, p. 10). Adopting this new materialist orientation within nursing education urges students and faculty to care for our entangled world, beckoning us as humans to consider the critical point that we are "not in the world but of the world" (Haraway, 2016, p. 14). Orienting pedagogical practices in this manner opens the door to co-creating knowledge alongside non-human entities and shifts the focus of education beyond the individual to the planetary system. Educating from a planetary perspective invites students and faculty to attend to the complexities of the Anthropocene, including the ways in which humans have contributed to the degradation of Earth and the more than human world (LeClair & Potter, 2022).

Ultimately, in this pedagogical reconceptualization, a more expansive view of the environment takes hold and the planetary community becomes the central focus of the discipline—moving beyond the human/nature opposition. Teaching from this perspective invites students and educators to reimagine how they conceive the center of the discipline as no longer human, but instead the environment intermingling and in cohabitation with matter, health, and healing in which there are no boundaries, borders, or lines of demarcation.

Relational Learning

How might posthuman pedagogy be enacted in the classroom? Well, it begins with relational modes of learning and knowledge production that are embodied and collaborative in nature with Zoë (Braidotti, 2019a). Furthermore, Braidotti (2019a) notes that centering Zoë is crucial in posthuman pedagogical practices and in turn, abolishes the epistemological hierarchy that privileges the human. Here I will try to illustrate a brief example of how nurse educators may implement this philosophy in their classrooms.

In pharmacology, student learning can be linked to more than human connections. Rainforests are integral to the planet's survival and mitigating the effects of climate change, but are under immense threat from the consequences of anthropogenic-driven climate change (Harris et al., 2021). Rainforests also provide humans with medications to treat various ailments, 25% of all medicines used today are extracted from the rainforest (Holland, 2021), and two-thirds of all chemotherapeutic medications come from rainforest plants (Earth Talk, 2019). Environmental biologist Kimmerer (2013) notes "that even a wounded world is feeding us" (p. 327). However, highlighting the connection that rainforests are beneficial to humans is not enough—a more apt approach would be to consider what humans do to benefit the rainforest.

Moreover, human forays for medications have stretched beyond the plants to include animals. The common drug exenatide used to treat diabetes was derived from the saliva of the Gila monster, a venomous lizard that is native to the Southwestern portions of North America (Furman, 2012). Here again, we see benefits to the human, but what is the benefit for the Gila monster? The Gila Monitor's survival is under threat from climate change due to decreasing water and humidity patterns in the desert (Howard, 2016). How will nurse educators impart these connections with a turn toward ecological justice for species, rainforests, humans—for all matter? These few examples highlight the exchange of meaning and knowledge-making practices that are occurring with more than human worlds in the classroom. Haraway (2016) describes this practice as tentacular thinking—the threading together of experiences—"the patterning of possible worlds and possible times, material-semiotic worlds, gone, here, and yet to come" (p. 31). Just maybe, educating in this way will propel students and faculty to "stay with the trouble" of the Anthropocene (Haraway, 2016, p. 1). I do not pretend to have the answers and maybe I am too naive, but I wonder if small steps like this with action, might prompt students and faculty to think deeply about relationality, giving them pause to consider not just the health of humans but the planet.

Conclusion

Nursing education holds great potential in the present-future to advance planetary health and multispecies kinship. Fostering a posthuman education within nursing allows students and faculty to recognize their relational and rhizomatic lifeways in an entangled world of shared living. Adopting a post-human frame also provides us with opportunities to deconstruct the past and interrogate the present—presenting us with the potential to reimagine nursing education and create a planetary-informed praxis that pursues justice. However, initiating a turn toward a posthuman pedagogy requires us first to examine ourselves as members of a planetary species and to recognize our accountability for the disastrous planetary destruction that is taking place as a consequence of anthropocentrism.

I would also be remiss not to mention that the struggles of the Anthropocene have become code for universalism and white supremacy, sweeping away pasts (from which I benefit) and turning climate change into a white man's lament (Braidotti, 2019c). Larocque et al. (2021) stated, "No More Settler Tears, No More Humanitarian Consternation" when describing white-settler "discoveries" (p.7). Linking to the discussion of planetary justice in this chapter, it is essential to state that I am building on the labor of centuries of people who have been working for planetary health, including Indigenous land and water protectors, risking their lives and leading protest movements. As Braidotti (2019a) elucidates, "we are all in this together, but we are not one and the same" (p. 52). **There is no ecological justice without social justice.** Larocque et al. (2021) explain that "racism is the driver of necropower" (p. 8), forcing us to acknowledge the structural oppressions and white supremacy that undergird nursing and society at large. This must be seen as part of planetary justice. Likewise, Braidotti (2013) describes, "If humanism has a future at all it has to come from outside the western world and bypass the limitations of eurocentrism" (p.25). It is clear that a posthuman world already impacts nursing education. Therefore, my hope is that this chapter will serve to unravel our posthuman context and invite others to consider posthuman pedagogies—opening the door, causing rupture, and nursing for the planet.

References

American Association of Colleges of Nursing. (2021). *The essentials: Core competencies for professional nursing education.* https://www.aacnnursing.org/Portals/42/AcademicNursing/pdf/Essentials-2021.pdf

Bennett, J. (2010). *Vibrant matter: A political ecology of things.* Duke University Press.

Bignall, S., & Rigney, D. (2019). Indigeneity, posthumanism, and nomad thought: Transforming colonial ecologies. In R. Braidotti & S. Bignall (Eds.), *Posthuman ecologies: Complexity and process after Deleuze* (pp. 159–181). Rowman & Littlefield International.

Braidotti, R. (2013). *The posthuman.* Polity Press.

Braidotti, R. (2019a). *Posthuman knowledge.* Polity.

Braidotti, R. (2019b). Preface: The posthuman as exuberant excess. In F. Ferrando, *Philosophical posthumanism* (pp. xi–xvi). Bloomsbury Academic.

Braidotti, R. (2019c, August 3). *Necropolitics and ways of dying.* https://youtu.be/UnFbKv_WFN0Brandon

Brown, B.B. (2017). *Caring for a Postmortem World*, [Digital Image].

Brown, B. B., Dillard-Wright, J., Hopkins-Walsh, J., Littzen, C. O. R., & Vo, T. (2022). Patterns of knowing and being in the COVIDicene: An epistemological and ontological reckoning for Posthumans. *Advances in Nursing Science, 45*(1), 3.

Chakrabarty, D. (2021). *The climate of history in a planetary age.* The University of Chicago Press.

Chopoorian, T. J. (1986). Reconceptualizing the environment. In P. Moccia (Ed.), *New approaches to theory development* (pp. 39–54). National League for Nursing.

Dillard-Wright, J., & Shields-Haas, V. (2021). Nursing with the people: Reimagining futures for nursing. *Advances in Nursing Science, 44*(3), 195–209. 10.1097/ANS. 0000000000000361

Dillard-Wright, J., Walsh, J. H., & Brown, B. B. (2020). We have never been nurses: Nursing in the Anthropocene, undoing the Capitalocene. *Advances in Nursing Science, 43*(2), 132–146. 10.1097/ANS.0000000000000313

Earth Talk. (2019). Tropical rainforests are nature's medicine cabinet. *Thought Co.* https://www.thoughtco.com/tropical-rainforests-natures-medicine-cabinet-1204030# :~:text=Rainforest%20Plants%20Produce%20Life%2DSaving,properties%20come %20from%20rainforest%20plants

Fawcett, J. (2022). Thoughts about environment. *Nursing Science Quarterly, 35*(2), 267–269. 10.1177/08943184211070578

Fawcett, J., & Desanto-Madeya, S. (2013). *Contemporary nursing knowledge: Analysis and evaluation of nursing models and theories* (3rd ed). F. A. Davis Co.

Ferrando, F. (2019). *Philosophical posthumanism.*

Fontenot, J., & McMurray, P. (2020). Decolonizing entry to practice: Reconceptualizing methods to facilitate diversity in nursing programs. *Teaching and Learning in Nursing, 15*(4), 272–279. 10.1016/j.teln.2020.07.002

Foth, T., & Holmes, D. (2017). Neoliberalism and the government of nursing through competency-based education. *Nursing Inquiry, 24*(2), e12154. 10.1111/nin. 12154

Furman, B. L. (2012). The development of Byetta (exenatide) from the venom of the Gila monster as an anti-diabetic agent. *Toxicon, 59*(4), 464–471. 10.1016/j.toxicon. 2010.12.016

Haraway, D. J. (2016). *Staying with the trouble: Making kin in the Chthulucene.* Duke University Press.

Harris, N. L., Gibbs, D. A., Baccini, A., Birdsey, R. A., de Bruin, S., Farina, M., Fatoyinbo, L., Hansen, M. C., Herold, M., Houghton, R. A., Potapov, P. V., Suarez, D. R., Roman-Cuesta, R. M., Saatchi, S. S., Slay, C. M., Turubanova, S. A., & Tyukavina, A. (2021). Global maps of twenty-first century forest carbon fluxes. *Nature Climate Change, 11*(3), 234–240. 10.1038/s41558-020-00976-6

Holland, J. (2021). Nature's pharmacy: The remarkable plants of the Amazon rainforest—and what they might cure. *The Telegraph.* https://www.telegraph.co.uk/ travel/cruises/articles/how-to-be-a-botanical-buff/

Holmes, D., Murray, S. J., Perron, A., & Rail, G. (2006). Deconstructing the evidence-based discourse in health sciences: Truth, power and fascism. *International Journal of Evidence-Based Healthcare, 4*(3), 180–186. 10.1111/j.1479-6988.2006.00041.x

Howard, B. C. (2016). Colorful, venomous lizard is declining due to climate change. *National Geographic.* https://www.nationalgeographic.com/animals/article/gila-monsters-threatened-climate-change#:~:text=The%20name%20Gila%20monster%20comes, climate%20in%20their%20natural%20habitat

Jakubec, S. L., & Bearskin, R. L. B. (2020). Decolonizing and anti-oppressive nursing practice: Awareness, allyship, and action. In *Ross-Kerr and Wood's Canadian Nursing Issues & Perspective-E-Book: Issues and Perspectives* (pp. 243–268). Elsevier Health Sciences.

Kalogirou, M. R., Olson, J., & Davidson, S. (2020). Nursing's metaparadigm, climate change and planetary health. *Nursing Inquiry, 27*(3). 10.1111/nin.12356

Kimmerer, R. (2013). *Braiding sweetgrass: Indigenous wisdom, scientific knowledge and the teachings of plants.* Milkweed Editions.

Kleffel, D. (1991). An ecofeminist analysis of nursing knowledge. *Nursing Forum, 26*(4), 5–18.

Kolbert, E. (2014). *The sixth extinction: An unnatural history* (First edition). Henry Holt and Company.

Larocque, C., Foth, T., & Gifford, W. (2021). No more settler tears, no more humanitarian consternation: Recognizing our racist history and present now! *Witness: The Canadian Journal of Critical Nursing Discourse, 3*(1), 7–10. 10.25071/2291-5 796.107

LeClair, J., Luebke, J., & Oakley, L. D. (2021). Critical environmental justice nursing for planetary health: A guiding framework. *Advances in Nursing Science, Publish Ahead of Print.* 10.1097/ANS.0000000000000398

LeClair, J., & Potter, T. (2022). Planetary health nursing. *AJN, American Journal of Nursing, 122*(4), 47–52. 10.1097/01.NAJ.0000827336.29891.9b

Leffers, J., Levy, R. M., Nicholas, P. K., & Sweeney, C. F. (2017). Mandate for the nursing Profession to address climate change through nursing education: Climate change nursing education. *Journal of Nursing Scholarship, 49*(6), 679–687. 10.1111/jnu.12331

McCaffrey, G. (2019). A humanism for nursing? *Nursing Inquiry, 26*(2), e12281. 10.1111/nin.12281

McGibbon, E., Mulaudzi, F. M., Didham, P., Barton, S., & Sochan, A. (2014). Toward decolonizing nursing: The colonization of nursing and strategies for increasing the counter-narrative. *Nursing Inquiry, 21*(3), 179–191. 10.1111/nin.12042

Nicholas, P. K., & Breakey, S. (2017). Climate change, climate justice, and environmental health: Implications for the nursing Profession: Climate change and environmental health. *Journal of Nursing Scholarship, 49*(6), 606–616. 10.1111/jnu.12326

Prescod-Weinstein, C. (2020). Making black women scientists under white empiricism: The Racialization of Epistemology in physics. *Signs: Journal of Women in Culture and Society, 45*(2), 421–447. 10.1086/704991

Salas, R. N. (2021). Environmental racism and climate change—Missed diagnoses. *New England Journal of Medicine, 385*(11), 967–969. 10.1056/NEJMp2109160

Schwab, K. (2016). The fourth industrial revolution: What it means, how to respond. *World Economic Forum.* https://www.weforum.org/agenda/2016/01/the-fourth-industrial-revolution-what-it-means-and-how-to-respond/

Stoddard, I., Anderson, K., Capstick, S., Carton, W., Depledge, J., Facer, K., Gough, C., Hache, F., Hoolohan, C., Hultman, M., Hällström, N., Kartha, S., Klinsky, S., Kuchler, M., Lövbrand, E., Nasiritousi, N., Newell, P., Peters, G. P., Sokona, Y., … Williams, M. (2021). Three decades of climate mitigation: Why haven't we bent the global emissions curve? *Annual Review of Environment and Resources, 46*(1), 653–689. 10.1146/annurev-environ-012220-011104

Sullivan-Marx, E., & McCauley, L. (2017). Climate change, global health, and nursing scholarship: Climate change, global health, and nursing scholarship. *Journal of Nursing Scholarship, 49*(6), 593–595. 10.1111/jnu.12342

Tuck, E., & Yang, K. W. (2012). Decolonization is not a metaphor. *Decolonization: Indigeneity, Education & Society, 1*(1). https://jps.library.utoronto.ca/index.php/des/article/view/18630

Ulmer, J. B. (2017). Posthumanism as research methodology: Inquiry in the Anthropocene. *International Journal of Qualitative Studies in Education, 30*(9), 832–848. 10.1080/09518398.2017.1336806

Whyte, K. (2016). Indigenous experience, environmental justice and settler colonialism. *Environmental Justice and Settler Colonialism.* 10.2139/ssrn.2770058

Yusoff, K. (2018). *A Billion Black Anthropocenes or none.* University of Minnesota Press.

14 #AbolishNursing: An Ethics for Creating Safer Realities

Em Rabelais (fae/femme/faer)

On #AbolishNursing

#AbolishNursing is an ethics and a response to how nursing engages in its practices, policies, ethics, narrativizations (the stories that nursing tells about itself), engagements, and other formations with each other, our students, our patients, our students' future patients, and the communities that we keep saying that we care about. This chapter has two sections: the first discusses what whiteness is and the ways in which whiteness manifests in nursing (briefly, *whiteness* names what is (ab)normal about and are (in)appropriate uses of the body); the second offers the ways in which we can bring about liberatory futures in whatever nursing is to become.

I'm writing not only as an abolitionist health ethicist and nurse but also as one of the many who desperately needs safer realities in nursing. I am white, disabled, queer, and non-binary/agender. Note the verb "am"; my identities *are*. I do not "identify as" any more than a white cisgender heterosexual non-disabled person would state that they "identify as" any of their descriptors. As noted by Eb (2017), Devon Price (2021), and many others, communities led by disabled people consistently use disability-first language. Person-first language requires that we disabled people erase ourselves in order to meet the comfort of non-disabled people. We are "not a personal tragedy" (Eb, 2017). Importantly, I am a trans feminine person, and it is this identification of mine that elicits tremendous violence from nursing and nurses, in addition to the wealth of violence from society and government. I write from this positionality, just as nurses who are white, cisgender/cissexual, heterosexual, abled/non-disabled women are writing from their own positionalities within the violences of normative whiteness. Just as any nurse, who is inculcated into nursing's demands for normative whiteness and feminist-appropriations through whiteness praxis, acts from these violent positionalities. Importantly, one need not be a white, cisgender, heterosexual, abled/non-disabled woman to enact nursing's violence precisely because the exercise of nursing itself is an exercise of white supremacy. Whiteness doesn't just consume everyone, but covertly demands that everyone adhere to its requirements.

DOI: 10.4324/9781003245957-20

Educators of nurses teach students how to be nurses, and they do this through the formal and informal requirements of nursing education, its accreditation, educators' interpretations, and the oppression, repression, other violence, and whatever community and interpersonal care that is or is not structurally built in. As with medical education (Burgess et al., 2010; Good, 1994; Spatoula et al., 2019), nursing education changes the nursing student's understandings of bodies, other people, and communication with and onto other people, no matter how much a student works to resist this transformation. For example, a medical student described learning medical interviewing as:

"I felt that it was a great privilege for me to hear some intimate details of their lives," and she would spend time listening to what patients wanted to talk about. By the fourth year, however, she said "you start to develop this sense of 'well, I have a job to do here and I'm doing something for you, so I'm going to just do it as efficiently as I can'".

(Good, 1994, p. 78)

The learning objective for section one (Nursing's White Supremacy: Reviewed) of this chapter is simple, and unfortunately it's something that needs to be named: believe students when they tell us that we are oppressive and violent. Our students have expertise. We need to listen to them, believe them, and act only when we can act from that belief. It's not just our students that we need to believe but our patients as well. Simply stated, *when we do not believe our students, we are actively teaching them to not believe their patients.* For example, recall the many TikTok videos made in 2019 and later by healthcare clinicians that claimed patients were lying about pain and other symptoms and see #PatientsAreNotFaking on Twitter (Barbarin, 2019). Your clinical education taught you to not believe your patients. If you, as a nurse or other healthcare professional, do believe your patients at their literal word, then you must have done reflective work on your interpersonal communication skills at some point to unlearn what nursing education enforces (for more on this, see Chapter 3 in this volume).

The learning objective for section two (Abolish Nursing) is also simple: act from our belief in students and patients. Acting from belief requires that we fully give up control of the process and it demands reflection. Students and patients name the violence of our methods and content. Because they are most hurt by our violence, students and patients are the only ones who can name and create alternative and less or non-violent processes. We must also reflect upon the violence we participate in as educators of nurses and as nurses for patients. We can start with our language and the ways that we name, discuss, frame, deny, support, dismiss, and misconstrue; how we reinforce structuralized violence; and how we gatekeep and gaslight (Murray & Holmes, 2013).

I don't doubt that some readers will be taken aback, and that's okay. For those of you who are, I suggest reading about transformative justice, which was de-veloped as a collective response to violence and harm without creating further violence and harm (Mingus, 2019c; Project Nia & Barnard Center for Research on Women, 2020). Resources include texts by Mia Mingus, especially those on her website (https://leavingevidence.wordpress.com/), including the two-part discussion of accountability and how to give a good apology (2019a, 2019b), as well as those by Mariame Kaba (Kaba, 2021; Kaba & Hassan, 2019) and Creative Interventions (2012). Transformative justice generally involves support for the survivors around healing and safety, working with the person(s) who caused harm to take accountability of that harm, building community members' capacities such that they can facilitate transformation and/or take accountability for the harm they cause, and to build skills to prevent or interrupt violence from happening. Calls for abolition must include these components of transformative justice, as the two frameworks are tightly bound together (see Kaba, 2021). Abolitionist activist and organizer Mariame Kaba famously teaches us that "nothing that we do that is worthwhile is done alone." An Aboriginal rights activist group from Queensland, Australia, though often attributed to group member Lila Watson, stated that "If you have come to help me you are wasting your time. But if you have come because your liberation is bound up with mine, then let us work together." Abolition is a community event.

Nursing's White Supremacy: Reviewed

This first section is a brief review of white supremacy in nursing. For in-depth discussion and analysis, please see other chapters in this text as well as the cited references. This review includes explanations of how nursing and nursing education are oppressive and violent. In nursing, we hold close and teach many concepts and enactments including a strict adherence to whiteness, which comprises the mandates of white supremacy culture (McGibbon et al., 2014; Okum, 2001, 2021; Waite & Nardi, 2017). Whiteness sets about the requirements of what is normal or abnormal about and appropriate or inappropriate uses of the body; foremost here, of course, is race, but whiteness goes far, far beyond skin color (Rabelais & Figueroa, unpublished data, as cited in Rabelais & Walker, 2021).

Whiteness makes requirements about biological essentialisms. Most important here is biological racism, in which science has included "race science" as a formative element of the biological basis of existence. Importantly, race is not biological, genetic, nor biogeographic (Tishkoff & Kidd, 2004). Race is a sociopolitical invention used for white supremacy. Race is not a variable nor risk factor that should ever be used to understand the human condition in any form: biological, genetic, psychological, social, etc. (Chadha et al., 2020; Rabelais & Figueroa, unpublished data, as cited in Rabelais & Walker, 2021). More appropriately, if even possible to measure, the correct predictive variable is racism or white supremacy.

Biological racism has contributed to what Harriet Washington calls medical apartheid (Washington, 2006), which is a condition of systematized racism within the healthcare establishment, just as it is in white supremacy culture within medicine, that sees Black people as merely bodies upon which to experiment and to subjugate. This idea is endemic in all of healthcare, including nursing, because white supremacy culture was part of the sociopolitical milieu at the origins of medicine, nursing, and other health professions.

Systematized racism continues in healthcare today. Manifestations of this include discussion of implicit or unconscious bias—as if they are different than explicit/conscious biases, which they are not—rather than simply naming racism, ableism, sex, fat-phobia, transmisia and transmisogyny, homophobia, xenophobia, and other enactments of white supremacy. In 2003 the text *Unequal Treatment* called for an end to disparities research and instead to begin health equity work, which requires investigators to look far, far upstream to the source inequities which are the actual causes of systematized and structuralized racism and other oppressions (Institute of Medicine, 2003). However, we have a seemingly unending interest in disparities, which are outcomes, rather than addressing structural causes that create inequity and what are sometimes called social and other determinants of health (Rabelais & Walker, 2021). By continuing to investigate disparities we are only furthering the mission of white supremacy by delaying any chance to disrupt and dismantle white supremacy culture. It is already abundantly clear what the structures and systems are that created and uphold white supremacy in what is called the United States. These include the very basis of white people navigating to this land and then killing and/or wresting control of the land from those who had been living here before the late 15th century (Koch et al., 2019). White supremacy culture exists within the founding documents of the United States. These include public works, police forces, and all the social, legal, political, medical, and other structures that are generally understood as integral to this country, despite them being established to take and destroy land and humans while insisting upon ruling ideologies that include colonialism, capitalism, and Christianity. While this may seem a broad and perhaps unsubstantiatable claim, colonialism, capitalism, and Christianity have been the driving forces of white people and our white supremacy for the past 530 years. *Note:* I am white, as are the vast majority of nurses, and thus am a part of settler colonialism and will always be (initially) seen as a representative of white supremacy culture.

Ableism is another oppression upheld by nursing that manifests by indicating that disabled people, like me and so many of my students, cannot be nurses or educators of nurses. A common response I hear goes something like, "people with disabilities [sic] cannot be nurses because nurses take care of people with disabilities [sic]." Notably, ableism was inherently entwined with racism since at least the mid-15th century when the Portuguese began an enslavement trade between sub-Saharan West Africa and Europe, as well as within Europe (Lewis, 2019). Ableism continues to be enmeshed within legal and carceral systems in what we now call the United States (Lewis, 2018). Beyond gatekeeping, excluding disabled people in nursing is ableist because of nursing's own definition of what might be allowed to be disability. The American Nurses Association's document outlining the scope and standards of practice for nursing indicates that disabled people face "inherent suffering" (p. 22) and that competence requires "ability," which is "the capacity to act effectively. It requires listening, integrity, knowledge of one's strengths and weaknesses, positive self-regard, emotional intelligence, and openness to feedback" (p. 52) disability can be "prevented or resolved" (American Nurses Association, 2021). An early draft of this document stated that disability can be "prevented or resolved" and contained no acknowledgment that disability generally is a chronic condition that is lifelong (Valderama-Wallace et al., 2020). My and my students' disabilities will be resolved when we're dead. If disability is something that requires an accommodation in order for the disabled person to find access, then you should note that shoes, glasses, nitrile gloves, medical masks, potholders, personal vehicles, public transportation, and elevators are all accommodations.

The second biological essentialism held by nursing and the rest of healthcare is gender essentialism. Quite often gender is also confused with sex, and both are understood within a binary. Neither sex (Fausto-Sterling, October 25, 2018) nor gender are binary. Because gender is fluid, there are innumerable genders, and gender is not defined by body parts nor what someone wears. Gender is not female or male (both are sex terms). Biological essentialism fuel transmisia (hatred of transgender people) and transmisogyny, violence coming from the idea that masculinity dominates femininity such that trans feminine people are subverting the power of men while simultaneously violating the purity, virtuosity, etc. of what it means to be a woman (Harsis, 2020b; Serano, 2016). While trans masculine people are included in the violence of transmisia and can experience misogyny, along with cisgender women and trans feminine people, it is generally only trans feminine people who are subjected to physical violence and death within the trans community (for analysis on power between transmisogyny-exempt and transmisogyny-affected people, see: Harsis, 2021). Notably, gender and sex assignments at birth are entirely unimportant in healthcare settings. This naming provides no benefit to any healthcare task, nor does it offer any clues about what an individual's upbringing was like, including the fallacy of socialization (Price, 2 August 2021). Transmedicalists, also called truscum, are those who demand that transgender people adhere to cisheteropatriarchal notions of gender safety (Harsis, 2020a), including having "gender dysphoria," and are confused in their need for gender/sex designations rather than a person's pronouns, organ inventory, and medical and surgical histories.

Cisheteropatriarchy, the notion that cisgender and heterosexual people are to be seen as "normal" and to exist within a sex and gender hierarchy in which men are more important and dominant, is another violent form of white supremacy that invades nursing. Patriarchy, especially, is well integrated into nursing's feminist-appropriations through whiteness. White women and so-called "white feminism" control the white supremacy culture of nursing (along with education and social work), and white women in nursing use the dominating ideas from patriarchy to enact their power and gatekeeping over the profession. Gatekeeping is ensured through measures such as racist restrictions on how hair looks and is worn, transmisic and especially transmisogynistic definitions of who is/can be a woman, preventing disabled people from entering or succeeding in nursing training programs, and in general holding up whiteness through demands about how bodies are deemed (ab)normal or are used (in)appropriately. White women learned patriarchy from white men and use it to continue to hold their power over others. Only those who inculcate themselves into white woman supremacy culture—no matter their race, gender, sexuality, disability status, etc.—are acceptable for moving "up the ladder" and into leadership positions. These include, for example, Black women faculty leaders who are "Onlys," pay a personal price for their authenticity, and understand that they are the illusion of diversity and inclusion while trying to survive academia, all while having to balance change versus appeasing the white majority (Iheduru-Anderson et al., 2022). Nursing's white women continue the tradition of dominating Black women and taking credit for their contributions, only supporting Black women when helps white women themselves (hooks, 1994) and always demanding emotional attention and care (to "white women's tears") when Black women protest white women's injustices (Hamad, 2020).

Patriarchy plays out in nursing in all of its relationships: instructors over students, nurses over patients, senior nurses over junior nurses (see: "nurses eat their young"), and nurses over others in the healthcare team (nursing/medical assistants, desk and custodial staff, and others). Cisheteropatriarchy appears through reinforcing gendered roles and gender stereotypes with assumptions that cisgender and heterosexual is normal and that a person is heterosexual and cisgender, based upon the false notion of "binary biological sex" through sex and gender essentialism (Fausto-Sterling, October 25, 2018). Nursing education textbooks discuss and display families containing a man and woman, who are married, with children, and repeat patriarchy's demands of men being the dominant actor in the family. Nursing's cisheteropatriarchy excludes trans people, especially transmisogyny-affected people, because of the threat that cisgender white women imagine is placed against white womanhood.

Nursing's patriarchy upholds Christianity as foundational to nursing. This is because many Catholic nuns were and are nurses, and the narrow history of nursing as seen through people like Florence Nightingale prioritizes a harmful Protestant ethic in the breadth of nursing. Related to our misplaced praise of Florence Nightingale, who was racist (Stake-Doucet, 5 November 2020), so many Christianity-inspired imperatives mandate that students/nurses speak and act white, reinforced through a Christian appropriation of Aristotle's virtue ethics to reinforce purity and propriety demands for the good woman/nurse. This links directly to so-called "white feminism" and white normativity, both explicit and implicit, in nursing. Nurses are taught sacrifice as a value, whereby nurses are to work hard and long to ensure that all the work is complete no matter the staffing situation. Nurses prove themselves through sacrifice within our capitalist system, even to their detriment, including volunteering for covid safety relief (triage, screening, vaccine administration, and more) despite funds being made available to pay for the increase healthcare need *and* travel nurses being paid up to four times more than staff nurses on the same unit during the ongoing COVID-19 global pandemic. At the same time, and related to sacrifice, nursing's "white feminist" requirements hold saviorism on a pedestal. White savior feminist professors push "Western-centered narratives, not least the right of white and Western women to pass judgement on the rest of the world's" people (Zakaria, 2021, p. 177).

An example of this, that is directly relevant to nursing, is in spoken word artist FreeQuency's (2018) discussion of Christianity's whiteness and saviorist roles in colonialism: from portraits of a white-skinned, blue-eyed Jesus to missionaries spreading Christianity "like a biblical plague" where rivers "flowed red" and "how they used their god to justify the taking of what ours had blessed us with for centuries, how they claim to introduce god to our lands and our lands birthed even their humanity." It is incredibly common for nurses and other healthcare professionals to frame voluntourism and medical mission trips (where *mission* refers to Christian mission and can require attendance at a religious meeting to receive care) to formerly-colonized countries as global healthcare (Cole, 2012; No White Saviors).

For nursing and medicine, global healthcare is the delivery of healthcare or another project from whiteness-dominated United States to an, generally, overseas country whose population consists of Black or Brown people. Nursing's global health is new "charity care." In doing so nursing, through Christianity and whiteness, is naming which Black and Brown people are deserving of care. Ebony Stewart (2017, 2022), a Black woman, reinforces this point in her poem *Compassion Fatigue*, a phrase used in nursing, where she addresses the white women tired of hearing about race:

> I'm not sure if compassion fatigue happens
> because no one taught you how not to be oppressed
> or because no one taught you how not to be the oppressor,
> but your comment reminds us that *no one cares about us but us* (49).

The Black and Brown people living alongside urban academic medical centers are not seen as deserving until their existence is reframed into an opportunity for a "*domestic* global health experience" for health professions students (Rabelais & Rosales, 2020). Global saviorism manipulates the narrative around colonialism and capitalism—a "we have resources to help those unfortunates" rather than the hoarding of wealth and preventing peoples and whole nations from which colonization has stolen natural and human resources—in order to appease white people's guilt, shame, and especially the knowing ignorance of white women around the abuses of capitalism, colonialism, and Christianity. This indoctrination into/reinforcement of whiteness also places demands upon the kinds of information that are considered valid in a scholarly work. And while my inclusion of spoken word poetry in the classroom and during talks has been tremendously effective, that discussion is outside the scope of this chapter.

Christianities, cisheteropatriarchy, white saviorism, and the rest of white supremacy culture all demand adherence to respectability and civility. Respectability politics, civility rhetoric, and all professionalisms are mandates of white supremacy that are used to control bodies by making and enforcing rules such as how we dress, speak, behave, form and hold relationships, hold power, and otherwise express ourselves. Power is never held by the patient or student, neither of which are allowed to express knowledge/expertise about bodies, their own or otherwise, without correction. Nurses, especially when teaching, are to have a coldness or at least a distance from students and patients. Love must not show up in the classroom nor the bedside because doing so would supposedly lose objectivity, authority/domination, and the fear of our students. And yet, those seen as objective both aren't and are also poor communicators, and when students do not fear faculty or competitively chase grades, "when we teach with love we are better able to respond to the unique concerns of individual students while simultaneously integrating those of the classroom community" (hooks, 2003, p. 133). Professionalisms demand knowing ignorance of one's own emotional self as well as weaponization of that same emotional self. For example, see Hamad's (2020) discussion of the weaponization of white women's emotions, especially their tears, to dominate Black women while benefiting from and taking credit for the labor of Black women and only supporting them when it helps white women themselves (hooks, 1994).

Nursing demands that nurses and patients adhere to white supremacy culture. Nurses must speak and act white, even when they aren't. Nurses are to maintain respectability politics, civility rhetoric, the white supremacy of professionalisms, and overall propriety. Nurses must be nondisabled and cisgender; those who are disabled and/or transgender are safe so long as they hide their disabilities and gender. Importantly, no nurse need to look the part of white supremacy to enact white supremacy culture. We are inculcated into this culture and must do the work to disrupt its influences on us.

Abolish Nursing

Just like Mariame Kaba (12 June 2020), by abolition I do literally mean that we should abolish nursing. This second section outlines how we get to our liberatory futures. Abolition involves destroying what is oppressive, creating something else that is not oppressive, and this creation can only be done by those who have been hurt the most. It is not likely that those of us who are authors or have access to this published text are the people who should lead creation of something new.

We already have answers for how to move forward and attain our liberatory futures: we have been told for centuries what it is we need to do (Rabelais, 2020). Obviously, we have not been listening or, more importantly, believing and acting from that belief. After the news in September 2020 that nurse whistleblower Dawn Wooten revealed that US Immigration and Customs Enforcement, unsurprisingly though still absolutely devastatingly understood, was committing genocidal acts, Monica McLemore wrote, "Action and Changed Behavior is all I want to see. I'm done with the meetings, done with the discussions, done with lip service. DONE" (15 September 2020).

Moving forward from Dr. McLemore's demand, the very first step toward our liberatory futures is to follow these steps:

- Those in leadership must step down.
- Those of us who are white must stop talking. We should get out of the way.
- Create ease in the transition of control by:

  - Those of us who are white must make it easy for our Black and Brown colleagues to both take over and tell us what to do.
  - Those of us who are cisgender must make it easy for our transgender colleagues to both take over and tell us what to do.
  - Those of us who are non-disabled must make it easy for our disabled colleagues to both take over and tell us what to do.
  - Those of us who are Christian must make it easy for our atheist and other religious practicing colleagues to both take over and tell us what to do.
  - "Colleagues" here includes our students, patients, and junior or former faculty members and nurses who were excluded from nursing spaces, promotion, or leadership.
  - "Colleagues" includes the communities that we live in and serve.

- Most importantly, for those of us who must cede power:

  - Don't question.
  - Do.

We have been reforming for centuries. We're even reforming yet again with the American Nurses Association and American Association of Colleges of Nursing's misguided approaches to policy change. The World Professional Association for Transgender Health is preparing for policy changes that will make life even harder for transgender children. We, nurses and other healthcare professionals, are still doing terrible things—even when or if we say we don't want to be. This has to stop. Abolition is the only sure thing. Reform has consistently failed.

We don't, though, have abolition yet. We don't yet have leaders who will embrace abolition—not even in an appropriative way, such as how "diversity" efforts are handled. We don't yet have white people who will cede power to Black and Brown people. We don't yet have non-disabled people who will cede power to disabled people. We don't yet have cisgender people who will cede power to transgender people; we do not even have transmisogyny-exempt people who will cede power to trans women and other trans feminine people, who are all transmisogyny-affected. What until then?

Until then: Believe people, believe us, when we tell you something. Listen, reflect—until you can believe. Once you believe us, then you can ask us how you can support us; you can ask us how to support what we are already doing. Believing does not mean that you know the answers, nor even fully understand. Believing does not mean that you continue to hold your power.

Until then: Participate in community care, allowing those who need the care to lead.

There is no other path forward.

Believe your students. Believe your patients. None of them/us are lying.

Once again, abolition is a community event.

References

American Nurses Association. (2021). *Nursing: Scope and standards of practice* (4th ed.). American Nurses Association.

Barbarin, I. (2019). *#PatientsAreNotFaking*. Retrieved March 18 from https://twitter.com/Imani_Barbarin/status/1197960305512534016

Burgess, D. J., Warren, J., Phelan, S., Dovidio, J., & van Ryn, M. (2010, May). Stereotype threat and health disparities: What medical educators and future physicians need to know. *Journal of General Internal Medicine, 25 Suppl 2*, S169–S177. 10.1007/s11606-009-1221-4

Chadha, N., Lim, B., Kane, M., & Rowland, B. (2020). *Toward the abolition of biological race in medicine: Transforming clinical education, research, and practice.* https://belonging.berkeley.edu/race-medicine

Cole, T. (2012). *The white-savior industrial complex*. The Atlantic. Retrieved March 18 from https://www.theatlantic.com/international/archive/2012/03/the-white-savior-industrial-complex/254843/

Creative Interventions. (2012, 2018). *Creative interventions workbook: Practical tools to stop interpersonal violence*. Retrieved March 18 from https://www.creative-interventions.org/toolkit/

Eb. (2017). *Disability 101: Where does the person go?* Retrieved March 15 from https://twitter.com/EbThen/status/916056864273682433

Fausto-Sterling, A. (October 25, 2018). *Why sex is not binary*. The New York Times. Retrieved April 20 from https://www.nytimes.com/2018/10/25/opinion/sex-biology-binary.html

FreeQuency. (2018, May 3). *The gospel of colonization* [Video]. YouTube. https://youtu.be/3C6mKP7_dc0

Good, B. J. (1994). *Medicine, rationality, and experience: An anthropological perspective*. Cambridge University Press.

Hamad, R. (2020). *White tears/brown scars: How white feminism betrays women of color*. Catapult.

Harsis, C. (2020a). *Transmedicalism and the validity trap*. Retrieved March 18 from https://purecatharsis.medium.com/transmedicalism-and-the-validity-trap-ed44bafd80e2

Harsis, C. (2020b). *We need to talk about transmisogyny*. Retrieved March 18 from https://purecatharsis.medium.com/we-need-to-talk-about-transmisogyny-6bdf0e79d29c

Harsis, C. (2021). *On transmisogyny exempt privilege dynamics*. Retrieved March 18 from https://purecatharsis.medium.com/on-transmisogyny-exempt-privilege-dynamics-874f3969ae1d

hooks, b. (1994). *Teaching to transgress: Education as the practice of freedom*. Routledge.

hooks, b. (2003). *Teaching community: A pedagogy of hope*. Routledge.

Iheduru-Anderson, K., Okoro, F. O., & Moore, S. S. (2022). Diversity and inclusion or tokens? qualitative study of Black women academic nurse leaders in the United States. *Global Qualitative Nursing Research*, 9, 23333936211073116. 10.1177/23333936211 073116

Institute of Medicine. (2003). *Unequal treatment: Confronting racial and ethnic disparities in health care*. National Academies Press. 10.17226/12875

Kaba, M. (12 June 2020). *Yes, we mean literally abolish the police*. The New York Times. Retrieved June 30 from https://www.nytimes.com/2020/06/12/opinion/sunday/floyd-abolish-defund-police.html

Kaba, M. (2021). *We Do This Til We Free Us: Abolitionist organizing and transforming justice*. Haymarket Books.

Kaba, M., & Hassan, S. (2019). *Fumbling toward repair: A workbook for community accountability facilitators*. Project Nia and Just Practice.

Koch, A., Brierley, C., Maslin, M. M., & Lewis, S. L. (2019). Earth system impacts of the European arrival and Great Dying in the Americas after 1492. *Quaternary Science Reviews*, 207, 13–36. 10.1016/j.quascirev.2018.12.004

Lewis, T. A. (2018). the birth of resistance: Courageous dreams, powerful nobodies & revolutionary madness. In A. Wong (Ed.), *Resistance and hope: Essays by disabled people: Crip wisdom for the people* (pp. 80–94). Alice Wong.

Lewis, T. A. (2019, 18 November). *Longmore lecture: Context, clarity & grounding*. https://www.talilalewis.com/blog/longmore-lecture-context-clarity-grounding

McGibbon, E., Mulaudzi, F. M., Didham, P., Barton, S., & Sochan, A. (2014, Sep). Toward decolonizing nursing: The colonization of nursing and strategies for increasing the counter-narrative. *Nursing Inquiry*, 21(3), 179–191. 10.1111/nin.12042

McLemore, M. (15 September 2020). *Action and changed behavior ...* Retrieved November 1 from https://twitter.com/mclemoremr/status/1305938626774102016

Mingus, M. (2019a). *The four parts of accountability: How to give a genuine apology, Part 1*. Retrieved March 18 from https://leavingevidence.wordpress.com/2019/12/18/how-to-give-a-good-apology-part-1-the-four-parts-of-accountability/

Mingus, M. (2019b). *How to give a genuine apology, Part 2: The apology – the what and the how*. Retrieved March 18 from https://leavingevidence.wordpress.com/2019/12/18/how-to-give-a-good-apology-part-2-the-apology-the-what-and-the-how/

Mingus, M. (2019c). *Transformative justice: A brief description*. Retrieved March 18 from https://leavingevidence.wordpress.com/2019/01/09/transformative-justice-a-brief-description/

Murray, S. J., & Holmes, D. (2013, Jul). Toward a critical ethical reflexivity: Phenomenology and language in Maurice Merleau-Ponty. *Bioethics*, 27(6), 341–347. 10.1111/bioe.12031

No White Saviors. *No white saviors: Decolonizing missions and development work*. Retrieved March 18 from https://nowhitesaviors.org

Okum, T. (2001). *White supremacy culture*. dRworks. https://www.dismantlingracism.org/uploads/4/3/5/7/43579015/okun_-_white_sup_culture.pdf

Okum, T. (2021). *White supremacy culture*. Retrieved March 18 from https://www.whitesupremacyculture.info/

Price, D. (2 August 2021). *"Female socialization" is a transphobic myth*. Retrieved November 1 from https://devonprice.medium.com/female-socialization-is-a-transphobic-myth-97747 d1c7fb2

Price, D. (2021). *Such HUGE red flags*. Retrieved March 15 from https://twitter.com/drdevonprice/status/1454561571787747330

Project Nia, & Barnard Center for Research on Women. (2020, March 11). *What is transformative justice?* https://youtu.be/U-_BOFz5TXo

Rabelais, E. (2020, 16 October). *"This whole country is full of lies / you're all gonna die, and die like flies / I don't trust you anymore": Normative and bio- ethics produce racist violence* American Society for Bioethics and Humanities 2020 Annual Meeting, Virtual Event. https://youtu.be/Gh6ODFgX34w

Rabelais, E., & Rosales, E. (2020). Response to "How Should Academic Medical Centers Administer Students' 'Domestic Global Health' Experiences?" Ethics and Linguistics of "Domestic Global Health". *AMA Journal of Ethics, 22*(5), E458–E461. 10.1001/amajethics.2020.458

Rabelais, E., & Walker, R. (2021). Ethics, health disparities, and discourses in oncology nursing's research: If we know the problems, why are we asking the wrong questions? *Journal of Clinical Nursing, 30*(5–6), 892–899. 10.1111/jocn.15569

Serano, J. (2016). *Whipping girl: A transsexual woman on sexism and the scapegoating of femininity* (2nd ed.). Seal Press.

Spatoula, V., Panagopoulou, E., & Montgomery, A. (2019, 2019/08/03). Does empathy change during undergraduate medical education? – A meta-analysis*. *Medical Teacher, 41*(8), 895–904. 10.1080/0142159X.2019.1584275

Stake-Doucet, N. (5 November 2020). *The racist lady with the lamp*. Retrieved November 1 from https://nursingclio.org/2020/11/05/the-racist-lady-with-the-lamp/

Stewart, E. (2017, May 3). *Compassion fatigue* [Video]. YouTube. https://youtu.be/Z5Z3gc9p6DY

Stewart, E. (2022). *Home. Girl. Hood.* Button Publishing, Inc.

Tishkoff, S. A., & Kidd, K. K. (2004, Nov). Implications of biogeography of human populations for 'race' and medicine. *Nature Genetics, 36*(11 Suppl), S21–S27. 10.1038/ng1438

Valderama-Wallace, C., Nouredini, S., Engelman, A., Valdez, A. M., Rabelais, E., Walker, R., & Alliance for Disability in Health Care Education. (2020). *On ableism in nursing: AACN Essentials National Faculty Meeting Feedback*. Retrieved March 18 from https://drive.google.com/file/d/19zkCN90tbLY0N1hseX4jnSgVHsAmZMhs/view?usp=sharing

Waite, R., & Nardi, D. (2017). Nursing colonialism in America: Implications for nursing leadership. *Journal of Professional Nursing, 35*(1), 18–25. 10.1016/j.profnurs.2017.12.013

Washington, H. A. (2006). *Medical apartheid: The dark history of medical experimentation on Black Americans from colonial times to the present*. Doubleday.

Zakaria, R. (2021). *Against white feminism: Notes on disruption*. W.W. Norton & Company.

Epilogue Is Prologue

In naming this concluding section "Epilogue is Prologue," we wish to simultaneously acknowledge that this is just a starting place for activating a radical imagination for nursing and invite folks in who may wish to engage further. The work of imagining the world as it might otherwise be is not and cannot ever be done (Haiven & Khasnabish, 2014). This is a relentless, continuous praxis, in part because the moment we stop imagining, those radical possibilities evaporate and in part, because this praxis is a kernel of hope (Benjamin, 2020; Sonenstein & Wilson, n.d.). So, while this volume has outlined thoughts about nursing's history, cataloged the present, imagined radically, and strategized to bring radical visions to life, we are just getting started. We invite you to join us—in whatever might come next, in radical imagination, in collective solidarity. Scan the QR code shown in Figure 15.1 to navigate to nursingfuturities.org and then click on **BOOK: NURSING A RADICAL IMAGINATION** tag to access additional resources that accompany this work, including discussion guides and further reading. You can share your thoughts, dreams, visions, ideas, comments, and feedback on a Padlet board located in this resource repository. We conclude with parting thoughts from the collaborators who contributed to this text. May these visions stoke your radical imagination, fuel your actions, rally your solidarity, and contribute to a more just, equitable present/future for us all.

Figure 15.1 QR Code Link to Additional Resources.

MY PRIMARY HOPE, AND IT HAS BEEN THE SAME FOR YEARS, IS THAT NURSING (AND NURSES) WILL BECOME MORE PHILOSOPHICAL AND ULTIMATELY MORE POLITICAL.

Dave Holmes

ONLY IN AN INORDINATELY UNFAIR WORLD WOULD THESE CHANGES TO EDUCATION, NURSING, AND SOCIETY THAT ARE FUNDAMENTAL TO THE HEALTH AND SAFETY OF SO MANY PEOPLE BE DEEMED 'RADICAL'. IN A WORLD THAT HELD EVERY PERSON IN THE SAME REGARD, CHANGES TOWARDS JUSTICE WOULD BE COMMON SENSE.

Blythe Victoria Bell

CAN OUR COMMUNITIES AND FUTURE GENERATIONS TRULY BE HEALTHY IN THE ABSENCE OF JUSTICE, HEALING, AND LIBERATION?

Claire Valderama-Wallace

BY DENATURALIZING THE STRUCTURES WHICH
UNDERGIRD OUR PROFESSION AND OUR
DISCIPLINE, WE CAN SEE HOW EVERYTHING WAS
BUILT. ONCE WE UNDERSTAND THAT, WE CAN
DISMANTLE AND REBUILD, THIS TIME WITH
JUSTICE AS OUR FOUNDATION.

Cory Ellen Gattrall

OUR COMMITMENT TO A RADICAL IMAGINATION FOR NURSING IS
SYNONYMOUS WITH OUR COMMITMENT TO THE SURVIVAL OF OUR
PROFESSION. OUR ABILITY TO CARE FOR OUR PATIENTS,
COMMUNITIES AND SELVES RESTS UPON OUR WILLINGNESS TO
BE BE SPECULATIVE AND CRITICAL ABOUT WHO WE HAVE BEEN,
WHO WE ARE, AND WHO WE DARE TO DREAM BECOMING.

Danisha Jenkins

NO PARTICULAR VERSION OF NURSING, NO TECHNOLOGY, AND
INDEED NO IMAGINED FUTURE IS INEVITABLE. THE STORIES WE
TELL, THE WORLDS THOSE STORIES CONSTRUCT, AND THE
POSSIBILITIES CREATED OR EXCLUDED BY THOSE WORLDS
REPRESENT HUMAN CHOICES IN THE CONTEXT OF VARIOUS
ARRANGEMENTS OF POWER. CREATING NEW AND MORE
LIBERATORY FUTURES - FOR NURSES, COMMUNITIES WE
ACCOMPANY IN CARE, AND ALL LIFE ON OUR SHARED PLANET
DOESN'T JUST MEAN USING NEW WORDS OR METAPHORS. IT ALSO
MEANS REDISTRIBUTING POWER: OVER DATA, OVER NARRATIVES,
AND OVER DESIGN AND USE OF RESOURCES. PERSONS WHOSE
LIVED REALITIES HAVE BEEN MARGINALIZED, STIGMATIZED OR
ERASED UNDER CURRENT REGIMES MUST BE CENTERED IN THE
DECISION-MAKING, AND THOSE OF US USED TO WIELDING
UNEARNED POWER NEED TO CEDE IT.

Rae Walker

WHAT EVER SPECULATIVE FUTURE WE IMAGINE TOGETHER IT CAN NOT BE LED OR BUILT ONLY BY CISHET WHITE NURSES BUT MUST BE FORGED BY AND ALONGSIDE TOGETHER WITH PEOPLE WHO REFLECT THE FULL SPECTRUM OF HUMAN EXPERIENCES. THE RADICAL FUTURE MUST ALSO BE FORGED WITH ACCOMPANIMENT AND SOLIDARITY, AND ALIGNMENT OF VALUES AND ACTIONS FOR LIBERATION FOR OPPRESSED PEOPLE AND COMMUNITIES AND CARE FOR OUR PLANET AND NON HUMAN AND MORE THAN HUMAN MATTER.

Jane Hopkins Walsh

TO IMAGINE A RADICAL FUTURE FOR NURSING IS PERHAPS MOTIVATION TO DELVE INTO THE PAST, AND TO BEGIN THE CHALLENGING WORK OF DISASSEMBLING THE INEQUITABLE AND NON-INCLUSIVE FOUNDATIONS THAT HAVE SHAPED THE PROFESSION OVER ITS ENTIRE EXISTENCE. PERHAPS IN DOING SO, WE MAY FINALLY DISCOVER WHAT IS INDEED UNIQUE, SENTINEL, AND DEFINITIVE OF NURSING AT ITS MOST ACTUALIZED—AND INDEED, ERADICATE THE INFLUENCES THAT HINDER ITS SCIENTIFIC, PEDAGOGICAL, AND PRACTICAL GROWTH AND DEVELOPMENT.

Candace Burton

IN 2019, WE BELIEVED WE UNDERSTOOD THE EXTENT OF THE PHYSICAL, PSYCHIC AND MORAL WOUNDS OUR PROFESSION COULD INFLICT. WE THOUGHT WE KNEW THE TERMS OF OUR RELATIONSHIPS WITH OUR INSTITUTIONS AND COMMUNITIES. BUT PRE-PANDEMIC EXPECTATIONS OF SUPPORT AND MUTUAL INTEREST IF NOT HUMANITY OR COMPASSION SEEM EMBARASSINGLY NAIVE IN THE FACE OF THE GROTESQUERIES OF THE SUBSEQUENT YEARS. NURSING WAS RADICALLY UNDERMINED IN MYRIAD WAYS, ITS FOUNDATIONS EXPOSED AS INADEQUATE AND UNTENABLE. ITS FUTURE DEPENDS ON ITS RADICAL REIMAGINATION AND RECONSTRUCTION.

Jon McIntyre

[...] AS WE MOVE FORWARD IN TIME AND CIVILIZATION, WE WILL INCREASINGLY FIND THAT OUR IMAGINATION — AND OUR AUDACITY TO TRANSLATE THE IMAGINED INTO REALITY — WILL BE THE KEY TO OUR COLLECTIVE LIBERATION.

Patrick McMurray

Index